aromatherapy

aromatherapy

A COMPLETE GUIDE TO THE HEALING ART

second edition

Kathi Keville

and Mindy Green

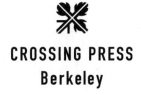

CROSSING PRESS
Berkeley

Library of Congress Cataloging-in-Publication Data
Keville, Kathi.
   Aromatherapy : a complete guide to the healing art / Kathi Keville and Mindy Green. — 2nd ed.
      p. cm.
   Includes bibliographical references and index.
   Summary: "A comprehensive guide to the art and science of creating therapeutic essential oils and herbal preparations, and using them in health, beauty, body care, massage, and more"—Provided by publisher.
   1. Aromatherapy. I. Green, Mindy. II. Title.
   RM666.A68K48 2009
   615'.3219—dc22

                                                    2008022226

ISBN-13: 978-1-58091-189-4

Printed in the United States of America on recycled paper (30% PCW)

Cover design by *the*BookDesigners
Front cover photograph by George Doyle/Stockbyte/Getty Images
Text design by Katy Brown

3 4 5 6 7 8 9 10----13 12 11

Second Edition

Contents

Preface

The word *aromatherapy* conjures up images of people magically alleviating their depression or insecurities with wonderful scents. But aromatherapy is much more than that. Incorporating aromatherapy into your life enhances your overall health, beauty, and psychological well-being. Aromatherapy can reduce stress, improve sleep, and give you more energy. It can improve your complexion, treat annoying itchy skin, and eliminate a stomachache.

Since writing our first edition of this book, aromatherapy has entered the mainstream. We see it everywhere—being used in clinics and hospitals to relax patients, as well as their families, to sell products, and to enhance everyday life.

Perhaps the best thing about aromatherapy is that engaging in it is so easy and pleasurable. Few people will complain about receiving a prescription to bathe with scented oils or apply fragrant body oil—two of the most popular aromatherapy techniques.

Essential oils give plants their characteristic odors, enabling us to take deep drafts of a fragrant rose bloom or drink in the perfume of lilacs and lavender. Because essential oils are by their very nature aromatic, the therapy involving their use has been christened *aromatherapy.*

We can use fragrance in healing in two main ways: One is through inhalation alone, which has its most significant impact on mood and emotions but also produces physical reactions, such as lowered blood pressure. The other route is the physical application of essential oils to the body—by massage, for example, or by applying antiseptic oil to stop infection. Of course, anytime you use

aromatherapy oil medicinally, the fragrance can't help but do double duty as it is inhaled.

Exactly how aromatherapy works is still unclear. Some researchers speculate that odors influence feelings because the nasal passage opens directly to the part of the brain that controls emotion and memory. Others believe that fragrance compounds interact with receptor sites in the central nervous system. Psychic healers believe that fragrances work on subtle, still-undiscovered energies in the body.

What we do know is that merely smelling a fragrance can influence us physically and emotionally not only by affecting thoughts and emotions, but also by altering hormone production, brain chemistry, stress levels, and general metabolism.

The many books on herbs and aromatherapy do not address their joint application. Encouraged by our combined seventy-five years' experience studying and teaching the healing uses of plants, we decided to join efforts and write about aromatherapy from the herbalists' perspective. We hope that this book conveys our enthusiasm, love, and appreciation of plants in all their varieties and that it inspires you to connect more deeply with the green world. May aromatherapy be as much of a healing journey for you as it has been for us!

It is an inspiration for us to see people get excited about the aromas and healing power of plants. If you wish to become more familiar with plants, we recommend that you observe them in nature, grow them, taste them (cautiously), pick and dry them, and use them to make your own medicine. Most of all, give thanks for them.

Acknowledgments

We would like to acknowledge the efforts of all those in the field of aromatherapy and herbal education who work to promote personal and planetary healing through the use of plant medicines.

Sincere thanks to all those who helped make this book possible: Evelyn Leigh, Ron Stringer, Julia Fischer, and Mary Greer, for their editing suggestions; Marianne Griffeth, for her samples and technical information; Kurt Schnaubelt, for his contributions, generosity, and patience with endless questions; John Steele, for his inspiration and teachings; Galina Lisin, for her technical editing; Jean-Claude Lapraz, Daniel Penoel, and Pierre Franchomme, for their contributions to aromatherapy research and education (many of their teachings are reflected in this book); Robert Tisserand, for technical information; and to our students, who are always an inspiration to both of us.

— Kathi Keville and Mindy Green

My heartfelt appreciation to Ron Bertolucci for his support and assistance in making this book a reality, for his skill in blending fragrances, and for sharing with me his passion for aromatherapy.

—Kathi

I give my heartfelt love and gratitude to my grandmother Alice Solem, for her encouragement, support, and faith in my abilities. I'd especially like to honor Rosemary Gladstar, for her inspiration and guidance in my lifelong work with plants, and James Green, for his encouragement in writing about my work.

—Mindy

As a child, I was drawn to the wonderful smells around me, and some of my most distinct memories are associated with those smells: my grandmother Irene's Chinese potpourri jar filled with rose petals, my grandmother Janna's cookie jar, the pine-scented woods where we went camping, and the great variety of fragrant plants that abound in southern California, including the pungent sages of the desert. But my real exposure to olfactory delight began with my first herb garden. Every visitor who came by was dragged outside, usually without much protest, to sniff pineapple sage, coconut, geranium, lemon verbena, and cinnamon basil. The potpourri of scents never failed to evoke plenty of smiles and dreamy, faraway gazes!

—Kathi

I'll never forget the first time I smelled the fruity fragrance of essential oil of carrot seed. I was instantly, dramatically, and emotionally transported to my youth in the tropics. I saw myself as a child on a seesaw, surrounded by hundreds of mango trees. I could feel the humid tropical heat. I remembered the safe, carefree feeling of that moment. I felt again, and strongly, the love I had had for that place and for our housemaid, who served me that delicious fruit. All of this happened in an instant! In that brief moment, years of memories floated effortlessly back into consciousness—for me, a clear example of the unconscious power of scent association, memory, and emotional programming.

—Mindy

PART I

theory

The rose distils a healing balm
The beating pulse of pain to calm.

—*Thomas Moore*

CHAPTER 1

A History of Fragrance

MUCH OF THE ancient history of fragrance is shrouded in mystery. Anthropologists speculate that primitive perfumery began with the burning of gums and resins for incense. Eventually, richly scented plants were incorporated into animal and vegetable oils to anoint the body for ceremony and pleasure. From 7000 to 4000 BC, the fatty oils of olive and sesame are thought to have been combined with fragrant plants to create the original Neolithic ointments. Perhaps fragrant leaves or flowers accidentally dropped into fat as meat cooked over a fire. Somehow, early peoples discovered that aromatic plants preserved and added flavor to food. When mixed into animal fats, these same plants became unguents that healed wounds and smoothed dry skin.

Eventually, fragrant fats—the forerunners of our modern massage and body lotions—were used to scent the wearer, protect skin and hair from weather and insects, and relax sore muscles. And they altered emotions. As civilizations became more advanced, incense and body oils were made into blends to heal body, mind, and spirit. Thus, throughout the world, aroma became an integral part of healing and laid the foundation for our use of

aromatherapy today. The earliest items of commerce were most likely spices, gums, and other fragrant plants reserved for religious purposes. Fortunately, gums, seeds, and herbs could be dried, and fragrant plants could be infused into oil or solid perfumes that retained, and even improved, their properties while making them extremely portable.

Early Beginnings: Egypt and the Middle East

In 2800 BC, when the Egyptians were learning to write and make bricks, they already had a word for "incense," *ntyw,* and were importing large quantities of myrrh. King Isesi sent an expedition to obtain myrrh and other gums from Punt on the African coast (Pwenet, or modern Eritrea). The great Queen Hatshepsut knew a business opportunity when she saw one. As one of her greatest accomplishments, she sent ships to bring thirty-one myrrh trees back to Egypt. They were planted to line the walkway leading to her massive temple of Deir al-Bahari near Thebes. On the temple walls, you can still see the images of the myrrh trees carved in bas-relief.

Other queens also made their mark on aromatic history. When the Queen of Sheba paid her famous visit to the courts of Israel's King Solomon, it was to discuss the fragrance trade. Some sources say she was from southwestern Arabia, the land of frankincense and myrrh, but it is more likely that she was a queen of a north Arabian tribe that traded the fragrant terebinth resin from pistachio trees.

On a 1974 archaeological expedition to the Indus Valley (which runs the length of modern Pakistan), Paolo Rovesti, PhD, found an unusual terra-cotta apparatus, displayed along with terra-cotta perfume containers, in a Taxila museum. It looked like a primitive still, although the 3000 BC dating would place it four thousand years earlier than most sources date the invention of distillation. Then a vessel of similar design, from around 2000 BC, was discovered in Afghanistan. Mesopotamian cuneiform tablets from the thirteenth to the twelfth centuries BC describe elaborate egg-shaped vessels containing coils; again, their function is unknown, but they are quite similar to Arab *itriz* used for distillation much later in the history of the region.

Even if essential oils were available at such an early date, most man-made fragrances were still in the form of incense and ointments. During the reign of the Egyptian pharaoh Khufu, builder of the Great Pyramid (c. 2700 BC), papyrus manuscripts recorded the use of fragrant herbs, choice oils, perfumes, and temple incense, and told of healing salves made of fragrant resins. Throughout the African continent, people coated their skin with fragrant oils to protect themselves from the hot, dry sun. This practice extended to the Mediterranean, where athletes were anointed with scented unguents before competing.

From this same era, the *Epic of Gilgamesh* tells of the legendary king of Ur in Mesopotamia (modern Iraq) burning *ntyw,* incense of cedarwood and myrrh, to put the gods and goddesses into pleasant moods. A tablet from neighboring Babylonia contains an import order for scented ointments; a third suggests medicinal uses for cypress. Still farther east, the *Chinese Yellow Emperor Book of Internal Medicine,* written in 2697 BC, explains various uses of aromatic herbs.

Trade routes to obtain fragrant goods were established throughout the Middle East well before 1700 BC and were well traveled for the next thirty centuries. The Old Testament describes one group of early traders as "a company of Ishmaelites [Arabs] from Gilead, bearing spicery, balm and myrrh, going to carry it down to Egypt." Overland trade meant grueling months, or even years, crossing arid deserts and negotiating difficult mountain passes while being threatened by bandits. But it was the only way to move the precious spice cargo. Then, possibly as early as 1500 BC, monsoon winds began carrying double-outrigger canoes along the cinnamon route. Egyptian and eventually Roman traders took advantage of these same winds to take them to India in the summer and home again in the winter.

Egypt's penchant for producing unguents and incense was to become legendary. A statue of King Thothraes IV, carved into the base of the Sphinx at Giza, has offered devotional incense and oil libations since 1425 BC. There is little doubt that Egyptian aromas were potent: calcite pots filled with spices, such as frankincense preserved in fat, still gave off a faint odor when opened in King Tutankhamen's tomb three thousand years later. Egyptians were particularly creative with scent and did not restrict it to religious rites. As depicted in wall paintings, solid ointments of spikenard and other aromatics, called "bit cones," were worn on the heads of dancers and musicians, where they were allowed to gradually—and dramatically—melt down over hair and body. An individual's special odor, or *khaibt,* was represented with a hieroglyphic of a fan and was considered capable of influencing the emotions of others.

The most famous Egyptian fragrance, *kyphi* (the name means "welcome to the gods"), was said to induce hypnotic states. The City of the Sun, Heliopolis, burned resins in the morning, myrrh at noon, and *kyphi* at sunset to the sun god Ra. *Kyphi* had more than religious uses, however. It could lull one to sleep, alleviate anxieties, increase dreaming, eliminate sorrow, treat asthma, and act as a general antidote for toxins. Several recipes are recorded, one of the oldest being a heady blend of calamus, henna, spikenard, frankincense, myrrh, cinnamon, cypress, and terebinth (pistachio resin), among other ingredients. Cubes of incense were prepared by mixing ground gums and plants with honey similar to a technique used by the Babylonians and later adapted by both Romans and Greeks.

The Hebrews employed fragrance to consecrate their temples, altars, candles, and priests. The book of Exodus (c. 1200 BC) provides the recipe for the holy anointing oil given to Moses for the initiation of priests: myrrh, cinnamon, and calamus, mixed with olive oil. Although Moses decreed severe punishment for anyone who obtained holy oils and incense for secular use, not all aromatics were restricted to religious use. We learn in the bible's book of Proverbs that "ointment and perfume rejoice in the heart" (27:9), while in the Song of Solomon (1:13–14) we read:

> *A bundle of myrrh is my beloved unto me;*
> *He shall lie all night between my breasts;*
> *My beloved is unto me as a cluster of camphire (henna)*
> *In the vineyards of En-gedi.*

The Classical Ancient World: Greece and Rome

Today cities prosper and fail with the fluctuating price of oil. So, too, did they in ancient times. However, it was fragrant herbs and spices that sparked growth of key cities along the avenues of commerce. With the introduction of camels as pack animals, the city of Alexandria developed into an active trading hub linking several trade routes including one to Arabia that was two thousand miles away. As trade routes expanded, Africa, South Arabia, and India began to supply spikenard, cymbopogons, and ginger to Middle Eastern and Mediterranean civilizations; Phoenician merchants traded in Chinese camphor and Indian cinnamon, pepper, and sandalwood; Syrians brought fragrant goods to Arabia. True myrrh and frankincense from distant Yemen finally reached the Mediterranean by 300 BC, by way of Persian traders. Traffic on the trade routes continued to swell as demand increased for roses, calamus, orris root, narcissus, saffron, mastic, oak moss, cinnamon, cardamom, pepper, nutmeg, ginger, costus, spikenard, aloeswood, grasses, and gum resins.

A thriving market developed in Babylon for the solid perfume trade, extensively offering cedar of Lebanon, cypress, pine, fir resin, myrtle, calamus, and juniper. When the Jews returned from captivity in Babylon, they brought back a heightened appreciation of fragrance, especially in the form of incense. In the seventh century BC, Athens was a mercantile center famous for the hundreds of perfumers that set up shop there. Trade was heavy in fragrant herbs such as marjoram, lily, thyme, sage, anise, rose, and iris, infused into olive, almond, castor, and linseed oils to make thick unguents and solid incense/perfumes. These were sold in small, elaborately decorated ceramic pots, similar to the smaller jars still sold in Athens today. Phoenician merchants brought Chinese camphor, cinnamon, black pepper, and sandalwood from India. Africa, South Arabia, and India supplied lemongrass, ginger, and spikenard. Astute traders knew which locales produced the best products.

The ancient Greek world was also rich in fragrance. Just one Greek word, *arómata,* describes incense, perfume, spices, and aromatic medicines. One such concoction, manufactured by a perfumer named Megallus, was the legendary *megaleion,* which contained burnt resin, cassia, cinnamon, and myrrh, and was used in the treatment of wounds and inflammation. At Delphi, the oracle priestesses sat over smoldering fumes of bay leaves to inspire an intoxicating trance; holes in the floor allowed the smoke to "magically" surround them.

While Socrates heartily disapproved of perfume, worrying that it might blur distinctions between slaves (who smelled of sweat) and free men (who apparently did not), it was not so with Alexander the Great. When he entered the tent of the defeated King Darius after the battle of Issos, Alexander contemptuously threw out the king's box of priceless ointments and perfumes, but later, after a few years of travel in Asia, he learned to love aromatics. And in his wake, he left the lands he conquered desiring more aromatics. In the fourth century BC, he sent deputies to Yemen and Oman to find the source of the Arabian incense with which he anointed his body and that burned constantly by his throne. To his Athenian classmate Theophrastus of Eresus, he sent plant cuttings obtained during his extensive travels, thus establishing a botanical garden in Athens. Theophrastus's treatise *On Odors* covered all the basics: blending perfumes, shelf life, using wine with aromatics, properties that carry scent, and the effect of odor on the mind and body. Alexander's teacher, Aristotle, organized odors into the classifications of pungent, harsh, astringent, and rich. This was also the time of the Alexandria school of medicine, which drew scholars from Europe and the Middle East. Hippocrates, called the "Father of Medicine," was a great Greek healer with a school on the Isle of Cos. His Hippocratic oath

is still repeated by doctors today, and he is credited with freeing Athenians from the plague by burning aromatic plants in the city. In happier times, he recommended the healthful use of aromatic oils in the bath.

By the first century AD, Rome was going through about 2,800 tons of imported frankincense and 550 tons of myrrh per year. Both men and women literally bathed in perfume while attended by slaves called *cosmetae.* Three types of perfume were applied to the body: solid unguents, scented oil, and perfumed powders, all purchased from the shops of *unguentarii,* who were regarded every bit as highly as doctors. The Romans even referred to their sweethearts as "my myrrh" and "my cinnamon," much as we use the gustatory endearments "honey" and "sweetie pie." Since ancient times, the wealthy and powerful have been able to drown themselves in fragrance. In fact, one unfortunate Roman literally did die. He was asphyxiated when the carved ivory ceilings in his dining rooms, which had been fitted with concealed pipes, sprayed down mists of fragrant waters on guests below, while panels slid aside to shower guests with fresh rose petals. This was in 54 AD, and Nero had spent the equivalent of $100,000 to scent the party.

The Roman historian Pliny, author of the impressive first-century AD *Natural History,* mentions thirty-two remedies prepared from rose, twenty-one from lily, seventeen from violet, and twenty-five from pennyroyal. Famous Roman blends of the era include *susinon,* which served not only as a perfume but also as a diuretic and women's anti-inflammatory tonic, and *amarakinon,* used to treat indigestion and hemorrhoids and to encourage menstruation. A similar spikenard ointment was suggested for coughs and laryngitis.

Mention of fragrance occurs, at least symbolically, throughout the New Testament records. The frankincense and myrrh brought to the Christ child were more valuable than the gift of gold (if indeed it was gold; some New Testament scholars speculate that the three wise men (magi) may have been carrying gold-colored, fragrant ambergris).

One of the most famous gospel scenes involves Judas Iscariot complaining about Mary Magdalene anointing Christ's feet with costly spikenard. Even the Greek word for "Christ," *Christos,* means "anointed" from the Greek *chriein,* "to anoint."

Indeed, the first century AD was a time of accelerated development of aromatherapy's source sciences. Aromatic plants were one of the five sections covered in the Greek physician Dioscorides' famous *Herbal,* which remained a popular medical reference for the next thousand years. In the third century, BC, he had the entire city of Athens fumigated with the smoke of aromatic plants to successfully eradicate the plague, a practice that would later be adopted in medieval Europe. The first written description of a distiller in the Western world is of one invented by Maria Prophetissima and described in *The Gold-Making of Cleopatra,* an Alexandrian text from around the first century. (Her design was used initially to distill essential oils, but it also proved useful for alcoholic beverages.) Gnostic Christians from the first to the fourth century AD, whose beliefs were deeply rooted in Egyptian philosophy, held fragrance in high regard. Seeking release from the limitations of the material world, they embraced the symbology of essential oils, which represented the soul of the plant.

Orientalia

Distillation of essential oils and use of aromatics also progressed in the Far East. Like the Gnostic Christians, Chinese Taoists believed that extraction of a plant's fragrance represented the liberation of its soul. Like the Greeks, the Chinese had just one word, *heang,* for perfume, incense, and fragrance. Moreover, *heang* was classified into six basic types according to the mood induced: tranquil, reclusive, luxurious, beautiful, refined, or noble.

The Chinese upper classes made lavish use of fragrance during the Tang dynasty, which began in the seventh century AD, and continued to do so until the end of the Ming dynasty in the seventeenth century. Their bodies, baths, clothes, homes, and temples were all richly scented, as were ink, paper, sachets tucked into their garments, and cosmetics. The ribs of fans were carved from fragrant sandalwood. Huge, fragrant statues of the Buddha were carved from camphor wood. Spectators at dances and other ceremonies could expect to be pelted with perfumed sachets.

To facilitate trade, the Chinese adopted the Indian system of counting. By the eleventh century, Arabs were navigating spice-laden ships from India to China with the Chinese compass and balanced stern rudders on their ships. During the next century, the Chinese navy grew from three thousand to fifty thousand sailors to accommodate large vessels that each hauled as much as six thousand baskets filled with fragrant herbs and spices. Jasmine-scented sesame oil arrived from India, Persian rosewater was brought via the Silk Route, and eventually, Indonesian aromatics—cloves, gum benzoin, ginger, nutmeg, and patchouli—came through India.

Numerous texts related to aromatherapy were published in China. The *Hsian Pu* treatise by Hung Chu, written about 1100 AD, and devoted to making incense, was followed by several similar works. The sixteenth century saw publication of the famous Chinese materia medica *Pen Ts'ao,* which discusses almost two thousand herbs, including a separate section on twenty essential oils. Jasmine was used as a general tonic; rose improved digestion, liver, and blood; chamomile reduced headaches, dizziness, and colds; ginger treated coughs and malaria.

It was the Japanese, however, who turned the use of incense into a fine art, even though incense didn't arrive in Japan until very late, around 500 AD. By then, the Japanese had also perfected a distillation process. By the fourth to the sixth centuries, incense pastes of powdered herbs mixed with plum pulp, seaweed, charcoal, and salt were pressed into cones, spirals, or letters, then burned on beds of ashes. Special schools taught (and still teach) *kodo,* the art of perfumery. Students learned how to burn incense ceremonially and performed story dances for incense-burning rituals. According to this tradition, the scent of incense keeps one both alert and peaceful.

From the Nara through the Kamakura periods (710–1333), small lacquer cases containing perfumes hung from a clasp on the kimono (the container for today's Opium brand perfume was inspired by one of these). An incense-stick clock changed its scent as time passed, but also dropped a brass ball in case no one was paying attention. A more sophisticated clock announced the time according to the chimney from which the fragrant smoke issued. A special headrest called a *koh-makura* imparted perfumed smoke to a lady's hair as her attendant was combing it. Geisha girls calculated the cost of their services according to how many sticks of incense had been consumed.

Clothing was scented by hanging it over a rack that contained sticks of incense inside. The world's first novel, *Prince Genji*, written by Lady Murasaki Shikibu in eleventh century Japan, describes the practice of scenting the sleeves of one's kimonos. Small incense burners were "held for a moment inside each sleeve" so that scent floated about whenever a motion was made with the hand. Japan's earliest anthology of poems, the *Kokinshu* from 905 AD, refers to this practice, saying, "Whose scented sleeves have brushed the blossoms in my garden?"

The Middle Ages

The spread of Islam helped to expand appreciation and knowledge of fragrance. Muhammad himself, whose life spanned the sixth and seventh centuries, is said to have loved children, women, and fragrance above all else. His favorite scent was probably camphire (henna), but the rose came to permeate the Muslim culture. Rosewater purified the mosque, scented gloves, flavored sherbet, and Turkish delight, and was sprinkled on guests from a flask called a *gulabdan*. Prayer beads made from gum arabic and rose petals released their scent when handled.

Following the translation of the Western classics into Arabic in the seventh century, Arab alchemists in search of the "quintessence" of plants found it represented in essential oils. The *Book of Perfume Chemistry and Distillation* by Yakub al-Kindi (803–870) describes many essential oils, including imported Chinese camphor. Gerber (Jabir ibn Hayyan) of Arabia, in his *Summa Perfectionis,* wrote several chapters on distillation. Credit for improving (and sometimes, erroneously, for discovering) distillation goes to Ibn-Sina, known in the West as Avicenna (980–1037), the Arab alchemist, astronomer, philosopher, mathematician, physician, and poet. His primary work, *Al-Qanun fi'l Tibb,* or the *Canon of Medicine,* became one of the most influential treatises in the Middle East on Tibb medicine and eventually influenced Western medicine, where it was translated at the end of the twelfth century. Essential oils and aromatic herbs were used extensively in his practice, and one of his hundred books was devoted entirely to roses.

A thirteenth-century text written by the Arab physician Al-Samarqandi was also filled with aromatherapeutic lore, with a chapter on aromatic baths and another on aromatic salves and powders. Steams and incenses of marjoram, thyme, wormwood, chamomile, fennel, mint, hyssop, and dill were suggested for sinus or ear infection. Herbs were burned in gourds, breathed as vapors, or sprinkled on hot stones or bricks.

The Muslim ruler Barbur, one of India's Mogul kings, declared, "One may prefer the fragrance of India to those of the flowers of the whole world." The twelfth-century East Indian text, the *Someshvara,* described a daily bath ritual in which fragrant oils of jasmine, coriander, cardamom, basil, costus, pandanus, agarwood, pine, saffron, champac, and clove-scented sesame oil were applied. Participants in Tantric ceremonies were also anointed with oils, the men with sandalwood, the women with the bouquet of jasmine on their hands, patchouli on their necks and cheeks, amber on their breasts, spikenard on their hair, musk on their abdomens, sandalwood on their thighs, and saffron on their feet. In other rituals, women called *dainyals* held cloths over their heads to capture Tibetan cedar smoke, which would send them into prophetic chanting. Special finger rings held small compartments filled with musk or amber. Indian temple doors carved from sandalwood invited worshipers to enter (and conveniently deterred termites).

In Europe, a shining light of the Middle Ages was the abbess Saint Hildegard of Bingen (1098–1179), an herbalist whose four treatises on medicinal herbs included *Causae et Curae (Causes and Cures of Illness)*, in which she spoke highly of fragrant herbs—especially of her favorite, lavender (some sources credit her with the invention of lavender water). European nuns and monks closely guarded the formulas for "Carmelite water," which contained melissa, angelica, and other herbs, and for *aqua mirabilis*, a "miracle water" used to improve memory and vision, and to reduce rheumatic pain, fever, melancholy, and congestion.

From the ninth to the fifteenth centuries, the Medical School of Salernum (Salerno) in Italy drew scholars from both the West and the East and crowned its graduates with bay-laurel wreaths. Here much Western knowledge, preserved and refined by the Muslims after the fall of Alexandria, was reestablished in the West. The school's *Regimen Sanitatis Salernitanum* was a kind of medical bible for many centuries.

Influence of the Spice Trade

In the thirteenth and fourteenth centuries AD, Italy monopolized the Eastern trade that had been established during the Crusades. Although certainly not the intention, the Crusades that spanned the eleventh through the twelfth centuries acquainted the European population with Arabian ideas and fostered an appreciation of Eastern aromatics. This was despite repeated warnings by the medieval Catholic priesthood that fragrance was associated with Satan (a stance that later changed as incense became an important feature of Catholic Mass). Crusaders returned bearing gifts of perfumes and fragrant oils and waters. Soon the European elite demanded rosewater, and Italians could not live without the addition of orange water to their sweet confections.

The guilds—grocers, spicers, apothecaries, perfumers, and glovers—controlled the import of enormous quantities of spices used to disinfect cities against the plague and other maladies. Spices were burned in public squares to fight infection. The purpose of Marco Polo's late-thirteenth-century journey to Kublai Khan's court in China was to establish direct trade. His merchant family in Italy dreamed of bypassing Muslim middlemen and their 300 percent markup in price by convincing the Orient to trade directly with Genoa. The plan proved so successful that throughout the thirteenth and fourteenth centuries, Italy monopolized Eastern trade with Europe. Spain was not to be outdone. When Christopher Columbus stumbled on the New World in 1492, he intended to finally make Spain a bigger player in the spice trade by beating out the competition. His route to the East was shorter. Tobacco, coca leaves, vanilla, potatoes, and chilies of the Americas were of great interest to the rest of the world. Columbus kept looking for cloves and cinnamon but never did find these spices.

It was the good fortune of the Portuguese to establish a route around the tip of Africa, or "Cape of Storms," which was later renamed "Cape of Good Hope." They had managed to circumvent Alexandria and Constantinople. In 1498, Vasco da Gama's sailors cheered, *"Christos e espiciarias!"* ("For Christ and spices!") as they neared India and her wealth of cloves, ginger, benzoin, and pepper. They returned with so much spice, the streets of London were said to be rolling in nutmeg! (Jealous, Venice persuaded the Muslim traders to fight the Portuguese, who now controlled the spice trade, but they were not successful.) The trade thus shifted from the Mediterranean to the Atlantic.

India—always prominent in the spice trade, although more as a pawn than a player—offered a rich variety of scents that included seventeen types of jasmine alone. The amazing number of aromatic and medicinal plants there was eventually described when the British published an extensive set of volumes on medicinal and fragrant botanicals titled *The Wealth of India*. It was the British, following the lead of the Portuguese, who finally attained a share of the action in the seventeenth century. After building forts and exploiting the friction between the Muslims and Hindus, the Dutch then forcibly took control of India and established the Dutch East India Company. Their range also extended into parts of Indonesia. In areas where they couldn't take control, they simply uprooted spice trees, such as cloves and nutmeg. However, the French did manage to slip some plants out from under Dutch noses. These were planted in the French West Indies and especially on the island of Bourbon, now called Réunion. Essential oils bearing the names of Bourbon or Réunion still come from there.

The Americas

Columbus's assumptions were correct in one respect at least. The Americas indeed held fragrant treasures: balsam of Peru and tolu, juniper, American cedar, sassafras, and tropical flowers such as vanilla, heady with perfume. Like other indigenous peoples around the world, the Native Americans had a long history of burning incense and using scented ointments. Throughout the Americas, massage with fragrant oils was a common form of therapy.

The Aztecs were as extravagant with incense as the Egyptians, and they too manufactured ornate vessels in which to burn it. Injured Aztecs were massaged with scented salves in sweat lodges, or *temazcalli*. The Incas made massage ointments of valerian and other herbs thickened with seaweed. In Central America, the Mayans steamed their patients one at a time in cramped clay structures.

Throughout the continent, North Americans "smudged" sick people with tight bundles of fragrant herbs or braided "sweet grass" (*Hierochloe odorata),* which smells like vanilla. Congestion, rheumatism, headaches, fainting, and other ills were treated with smoke from burning plants, or with a strong herb infusion thrown over hot rocks to produce scented steam. The people of the Great Plains used echinacea as a smoke treatment for headaches; many tribes used pungent plants such as goldenrod, fleabane, and pearly everlasting for therapeutic purposes.

Scents and "Sophistication"

Even after losing control over the spice trade, Italy remained the European leader for cosmetics and perfumes. As Venice became more cosmopolitan, it began to produce scented pastes, gloves, stockings, shoes, shirts, and even fragrant coins. Our word *pomander* comes from the French words *pomme d'ambre,* a scented ball made of ambergris, spices, wine, and honey, carried in a perforated container on the belt or on a string around the neck. Dried medicinals were stored in beautiful porcelain pots, and botanical waters were kept in Venetian glass.

The Italian influence swept through France, helped along by Caterina de Medici's marriage to France's Prince Henri II. Making the journey with her were her alchemist (who probably made her poisons too, but that's another story) and her perfumer, who set up shop in Paris. The towns of Montpellier and Grasse, already strongly influenced by neighboring Genoa, had long produced the perfumed gloves that were in high style among the elite.

The gloves were most often perfumed with neroli or with animal scents such as ambergris and civet. Apparently, this wasn't always appreciated. A seventeenth-century dramatist, Philip Massinger, complained, "Lady, I would descend to kiss thy hand/but that 'tis gloved, and civet makes me sick." These towns took the lead, as France's growing fragrance trade began to predominate over Italy's.

England was also influenced by the Italian love of scent. A pair of scented gloves so captured the attention of Queen Elizabeth I, she had a perfumed leather cape and shoes made to match. Sixteenth-century Elizabethans powdered their skin, hair, and clothes with fragrant powders and toned their skin with scented vinegars and fragrant waters. Like the Roman blends, these waters doubled as internal medicines.

The number of plants distilled expanded in the sixteenth century, and many books appeared on alchemy and the art of distillation. In 1732, when the Italian Giovanni Maria Farina took over his uncle's business in Cologne, he produced *aqua admirabilis,* a lively blend of neroli, bergamot, lavender, and rosemary in rectified grape spirit. This was splashed on the skin and used for treating sore gums and indigestion. French soldiers stationed there dubbed it *eau de Cologne,* and Napoleon is said to have gone through several bottles a day—an endorsement that made it so popular that thirty-nine competitors and half a century of lawsuits resulted. Other fashionable fragrances included rose, violet, and patchouli, which were used on the imported Indian shawls made popular by Napoleon's famous consort, Josephine.

The Modern World

In the nineteenth century, two important changes occurred in the Western world of fragrance. The 1867 Paris International Exhibition exhibited perfumes and soaps apart from the pharmacy section, thus establishing an independent commercial arena for "cosmetics." Even more significant was the product of the first synthetic fragrance, *coumarin* (which smells of newly mown hay) in 1868, followed twenty years later by musk, vanilla, and violet. Eventually this list expanded to many hundreds, even thousands, of synthetic fragrances—the first perfumes unsuitable for medicinal use.

France became the leader in reestablishing the therapeutic uses of fragrance. The perfume industry had been divorced from medicinal remedies for fifty years, but slowly began to reclaim its medicinal heritage. The term *aromatherapy* was coined in 1928 by French chemist René-Maurice Gattefossé. His interest in therapeutically using essential oils was stimulated by a laboratory explosion in his family's perfumery business in which his hand was severely burned. He plunged the injured hand into a container of lavender oil and was amazed at how quickly it healed.

By the 1960s, a few people, including the French doctor Jean Valnet, MD, and the Austrian-born biochemist Madame Marguerite Maury, were inspired by Gattefossé's work. As an army surgeon in World War II, Dr. Valnet used essential oils such as thyme, clove, lemon, and chamomile on wounds and burns and later found fragrances successful in treating psychiatric problems. But while Valnet helped inspire a modern aromatherapy movement when his book *Aromatherapie* was translated into English as *The Practice of Aromatherapy,* the 1977 appearance of masseur Robert Tisserand's book *The Art of Aromatherapy,* strongly influenced by the work of Valnet and Gattefossé, successfully captured American interest. At present, there are many books available on aromatherapy.

Most important, the efforts of pioneers such as Valnet, Maury, Tisserand, and others have turned aromatherapy into a disciplined healing art, rediscovering the uses of fragrance from ancient times and sparking a revival of aromatherapy that has swept throughout the world.

CHAPTER 2

The Sense of Smell

FEW THINGS can move us so deeply or have so profound an impact on our psyches as the memories evoked by specific smells. A smell can take us back to childhood or conjure up a lost love or sadness as real as the day we first experienced it. Smells invoke long-term memory and make the past present as none of the other senses can. The most direct of all of our senses, smell has an immediate impact, uninfluenced by language and unimpaired by the passage of time.

Sensitivity to fragrance is—to a large extent—culturally determined, and there is no doubt that the culture in which we live influences our perceptions of which scents are "acceptable," "normal," or "pleasant." Individual emotions that are associated with scent can change our perception of what we experience. That's why different people can have very different emotional responses to the same odor. The reaction to vanilla, for instance, seems to vary among cultures: it is comforting to Americans, but has little effect on most Japanese people, probably because the unfamiliar scent has no link to their childhood memories. At one time, a strong body odor could disqualify men from the Japanese military service. Since Asians have fewer hair follicles, and therefore fewer apocrine glands

than Westerners, they are culturally less accustomed to body odor. In a 1991 address to Summit 2000: Preparing for the First Global Civilization, Susan Schiffman, MD, a psychology professor at Duke University in North Carolina, speculated that exposing people to the smells from clothing, foods, and other items of different cultures engenders tolerance for others and promotes world peace. She suggests that children purposely be exposed to multicultural scents so they grow into tolerant adults. We do know that unidentified odors tend to make a person anxious.

Because our reactions to different scents are influenced by our personal experiences, a culture's general attitude toward certain scents can change over time. For example, the clean scent of lemon, and especially lemon eucalyptus, reminds many people of furniture polish, cleaning products, or bug repellents. Monell Chemical Senses Center's Susan Knasko says that everything is scented, which affects her research since people are learning to recognize scents out of context and not from their true origin. She found that subjects who are eighteen to forty-five years old often think the woodsy scent of pine is a cleaning product or mistake it for lemon since the two are so commonly used in these products. Young people are more accustomed to synthetic, chemical smells that are replacing natural ones.

Whatever your personal perceptions and preferences, there is no denying that the impact of odor is profound, if subtle. In her book *Scent*, Annick LeGuerer wrote the following:

> *Humans produce a characteristic odor in the air around them that reflects their diet and/or health, their age, their sex, occupation, and race. It can be argued that because of the physiology of the olfactory apparatus, the most direct and profound impression we can have of another person is his (or her) smell. Indeed, smell bypasses the thalamus in the brain and penetrates directly to that organ's oldest part, the rhinencephalon, known to the Greeks as the "olfactory brain," where it produces, willy-nilly, pleasure or repugnance.*

Smell is our most direct means of communication with nature. We smell with every breath we take, constantly monitoring the world around us, although we are not always conscious that we are doing so. (Just eight molecules of a substance can trigger an electrical impulse in a nerve ending, whereas roughly forty nerve endings must be stimulated before we become conscious of any smell.) In the words of twentieth-century writer, philosopher, explorer, and anthropologist Laurens Van Der Post, "Scent . . . is not only biologically the oldest but also the most evocative of all our senses. It goes deeper than conscious thought or organized memory and has a will of its own which human imagination is compelled to obey."

To fully understand aromatherapy and the effects of essential oils, we must arrive at a basic understanding of two physiological processes: how the olfactory apparatus works and how essential oils are absorbed into the body.

How the Brain Processes Odor

Odors are the effects of volatile molecules that float through the air, rushing through our nostrils as we inhale. There are three stages in the process of smelling: Fragrance begins with the *reception* of odor molecules, which, as they are inhaled, travel inside the nose to dissolve in the mucous within a membrane called the olfactory epithelium (receptor cells that contain, in all, some twenty million nerve endings). Odor *transmission* occurs when a message is fired to the right and left olfactory bulbs, located above and behind the nose at the base of the brain, each about the size and shape of a small lima bean. At this point, a variety of cells and neurons interpret, amplify, and transmit the message to the limbic system. This system contains the hypothalamus, Proust's hippocampus, olfactory cortex, and amygdala. *Perception* takes place when the message is received by the hypothalamus. Acting as a relay station, the hypothalamus sends information to other parts of the brain, such as the pituitary gland, which sends chemical messages into:

- the bloodstream
- the olfactory cortex, which helps distinguish odors
- the thalamus, which helps connect odor messages with higher thought functions
- the neocortex, which finely analyzes odor messages, relating them to the other senses, as well as to the higher brain functions that stimulate conscious thought

All this happens in less than a second. Columbia University researchers isolated, for the first time in medical history, what they believe to be odor receptors. This large family of genes—perhaps numbering as many as one thousand—is much more complex than the three types of receptors the eye uses to distinguish a few thousand colors. The average adult can process about ten thousand different odors in an area of the brain about one square inch.

The ability to detect so many different odors is also crucial to our sense of taste. While the tongue's receptors distinguish only a few tastes, all other sensations perceived as taste are in fact odors. Taste is usually described as only the basic four: sweet, sour, salty, and bitter. However, in his book *Sensory Neurophysiology,* former University of Texas taste physiologist James C. Boudreau, PhD, said he believes that there may be more than twenty distinct human taste sensations. Some that he adds to the basic four are two types of sweet, insipid, metallic, pungent, burning, warm and cool (as in menthol), astringent-dry, and astringent-tangy. Even so, it is estimated that about 80 percent of taste sensations rely on our sense of smell. Just about everyone has experienced a cold that deadens the sense of smell, resulting in a loss of taste.

Smell is the only sense with receptor nerve endings in direct contact with the outside world, providing a direct channel, as it were, to the brain. The "blood-brain barrier" is a lipid-rich (that is, oil-rich) membrane that sheathes and protects the brain. Oxygen and some nutrients can pass through this membrane, but large molecules, such as those of most therapeutic drugs, cannot. Because the olfactory nerves evolved before the brain, they are not protected by this sheath.

No one actually knows how the olfactory receptors react. Their response could be related to the scent molecule's shape, size, or electrical charge, or a combination of all of these. For many years, biophysicist Luca Turin, PhD, former University College London lecturer and author of *The Secret of Scent: Adventures in Perfume and the Science of Smell,* has worked on the theory that smell receptors act like switches tuned to different frequencies. This would mean that when a molecule of odor with the correct vibration binds to a smell receptor, it throws the switch and allows electrons to flow. This signal is then amplified and sent to the brain for interpretation. Since each molecule has a distinctive vibration pattern, it would relate only its own unique smell to the brain. Turin has no doubt that this is why scent has such a strong impact on emotions. He explains, "We don't smell with our noses, we smell with our brains so we shouldn't be surprised that fragrance has a direct effect on our moods."

The idea that something as noninvasive as natural odors can directly affect the mind is quite exciting. Medical researchers hope someday to be able to use this pathway to access specific areas of the brain with fragrance to treat various disorders, including Alzheimer's disease. For now, studies suggest that essential oils directly affect the central nervous system, modifying the brain's reactions. In 2006, Richard Axel and Linda Buck won the Nobel Prize for Science for their research on the popular lock and key theory that each odor has its own shape that fits into specific receptors.

The brain's response to a change in odor may be influenced by our thought patterns. Certain brain waves, called "contingent negative variation" (CNV), are very sensitive to emotional changes and are activated by particular fragrances. Aromatherapist Robert Tisserand, author of several books including *Aromatherapy: To Heal and Tend the Body,* thinks that "euphoric" odors such as clary sage and grapefruit stimulate the thalamus to secrete neurochemicals called enkephalins, natural painkillers that also produce a general feeling of well-being. Odors that stimulate the endorphin-secreting pituitary gland include the aphrodisiac scents jasmine and ylang-ylang. The pituitary also releases chemical messengers into the bloodstream to regulate other glands, such as the thyroid and the adrenals. Sedative odors such as marjoram stimulate the area of the brain called *raphe nucleus,* triggering the secretion of the neurochemical serotonin, which helps us sleep.

Essential Oil Absorption through the Skin

As with their journey into the brain and central nervous system, the absorption of essential oils through the skin is quick and easy due to their lipid-solubility, their extremely small molecular size, and to the natural oiliness of the skin itself. Essential oils also enter the bloodstream through the lungs and small capillaries; they affect the nervous and lymphatic systems when they contact with these vessels in the dermal layer of the skin.

Studies show that after a full body massage with a 2 percent dilution of lavender essential oil in vegetable oil (about 10 to 12 drops of essential oil per ounce of carrier oil), detectable amounts of linalol and linalyl acetate, the main chemical constituents of lavender, are found in the blood. Concentrations are highest after twenty minutes and diminished to undetectable levels within ninety minutes. The study concluded that not only are essential oils lipophilic (oil soluble) by nature, but also that massage with a vegetable oil accelerates absorption of essential oils by the skin. You can experiment with this theory at home: garlic rubbed on the feet can later be smelled on the breath.

Fragrance and Health

During the Black Plague in seventeenth-century Europe, stench was linked, quite naturally, to disease, decay, and death. (In France, the term *peste* described both the disease and the odor associated with it.) People sniffed pomander balls and boxes containing cedarwood and used hollow-topped walking sticks containing aromatic substances to warn off the plague. Nosegays were used for the same purpose; they were so popular that a London Bill of Mortality for 1635 gave precise instructions for their preparation (the recipe included vinegar, rice, wormwood, and rosewater). "Strewing herbs" were spread upon the floor, their fragrance rising when crushed underfoot.

Many perfumers—and glove makers who perfumed their products—escaped the plague. We now know that their secret was antibacterial properties of the essential oils to which they were exposed in their daily work. It is said that Bucklersbury, England, was spared from the plague because it was the center of the lavender trade, and even today the French city of Grasse, where so much perfume is produced, is known for having very low rates of respiratory illness.

Still, negative symptoms traceable to synthetic colognes and perfumes are increasing. These range from sinus pain to anaphylactic shock and seizures. The problem is a result of the increased strength of fragrances today, coupled with a rise in the use of synthetic chemicals. The U.S. Food and Drug Administration estimates that four thousand different chemicals are currently used in fragrances, with a rise in the use of single perfumes that often contain several hundred chemicals. There is particular concern about synthetic musklike fragrances that have been associated with damage to the central and peripheral nervous systems.

The sense of smell has a time-honored role in the diagnosis of disease. Typhoid fever is said to smell like freshly baked bread, diabetes like sugar, the plague like apples, yellow fever like a butcher shop, and nephritis like ammonia. Chemist John N. Labows, PhD, well known for his work on pheromones, has cataloged odor profiles to help identify numerous types of infections at the Monell Chemical Senses Center in Philadelphia. The Center has been working on multidisciplinary research on taste and smell since 1968.

Finally, specific odors provide a pathway through the central nervous system that activates the immune system's protector cells. The way the immune system and the central nervous system operate is only vaguely understood, but researchers know that they do communicate with one another. Current research suggests that it may be possible to teach the body to jump-start its own immune response through aromatherapy, although exactly which odors should be used is not yet clear. However, new evidence indicates that we may exercise direct control over health and disease through the hypothalamus.

Olfactory Deprivation

It is estimated that two million Americans have *anosmia,* the inability to smell or taste, a condition traceable to a number of factors. Still more people experience a partial loss of their sense of smell, or *hyposmia,* and a few people are born without a sense of smell. Curiously, the inability to smell is often associated with depression and decreased sexual drive. Another smell disorder is *parosmia,* when a scent is perceived although none exists or a familiar odor smells different. Researchers believe that most adults are "odor blind" to at least one group of chemical compounds.

Hormonal changes, such as menopause, diet, exposure to radiation, and the natural process of aging, may also damage the sense of smell, as can head injury, some surgeries, pharmaceutical antidepressants and anti-anxiety drugs, and exposure to toxic chemicals. The University Medical Center in Durham, North Carolina, found the ability to detect odors, distinguish between different smells, determine the strength of a scent, and even to identify it begins to decline around age sixty. The sense of smell also decreases after menopause. Gradual reduction of the ability to smell, as well as taste, is associated with several illnesses, including viral infection, neurological disorders, brain tumors, multiple sclerosis, Bell's palsy, Alzheimer's disease, high blood pressure, diabetes, and liver and kidney diseases. Probably everyone has experienced the temporary loss or distortion of smell that results from having a cold, sinus infection, or other type of upper respiratory infection; infected teeth or gums can likewise cause a loss of taste and smell.

In some instances, a deficiency of the mineral zinc has been implicated in smell disorders—as well as in some cases of infertility. Zinc sulfate supplements sometimes help bring back the sense of smell, even when no deficiency is apparent. However, nutrients are most effective in restoring an impaired sense of smell—as well as taste—when there is an existing deficiency. Taking supplements of vitamins A (as beta-carotene) and the B complex, especially B$_3$ (niacin), may also be helpful. Eliminating infection or inflammation, when this is the source of smell loss, also helps restore the sense of smell. The most drastic measure is intranasal cryosurgery, a procedure used to surgically restructure the inside of the nose when smell is inhibited by structural problems.

Several research centers have received funding from the National Institutes of Health to explore how the sense of smell works. The University of Pennsylvania Smell and Taste Center tested 638 people for their smell acuity. Not surprisingly, those who smoked had a decreased perception of smell that directly corresponded to how many cigarettes they smoked a day. On the other hand, the construction company Shimizu Corporation claims that the scented air they pump into their workplace reduces workers' urge to smoke. To prove their point, they did a study in which habitual smokers were deprived of cigarettes. Sniffing various scents reduced their cravings to light up. Curiously, the odors that the smokers rated as unpleasant decreased their cravings the most.

The largest database of clinical chemosensory information in the United States is at the Connecticut Chemosensory Clinical Research Center, which is exploring how the sense of smell relates to smoking, as well as aging and diseases such as diabetes. Their researchers also evaluate patients with smell and taste problems to discover how to use fragrance to reduce side effects from chemotherapy, kidney dialysis, and radiation therapy. At Children's Hospital in Minneapolis, the Integrative Medicine and Cultural Care Clinic uses essential oils in palliative care for kids undergoing stressful medical procedures. They have conducted two clinical studies showing that gender and ethnicity preferences do exist in children.

It is possible to increase your ability to smell through "scent exercising." In doing research for Johns Hopkins, Robert Anholt, PhD, professor of zoology genetics at North Carolina University, found that most people have the potential to detect subtle differences in smell, but that it takes practice. Test subjects exposed themselves to as many natural odors as possible, thereby training their noses to recognize more scents.

Dieting, Aromatherapy Style

People who lose their ability to smell often gain weight. Alan Hirsch, MD, head of Chicago's Smell and Taste Treatment and Research Foundation, wondered if the opposite was true, that scents could help weight loss. They gave over three thousand overweight individuals aromas to inhale. These longtime dieters had tried just about everything since they were in their twenties; a total of sixty-six different diet programs were represented. They were instructed to simply take six sniffs of an aromatic blend whenever they felt hungry. In six months, those sniffing sweet smells lost almost five pounds a month. It is thought that aromatherapy tricks the satiety center in the brain's hypothalamus into thinking the body has eaten enough. There's probably a lot of truth to this. We have noticed that we often overcome the cravings of a certain food by being satisfied simply by the odor or even by sniffing another pleasant aroma.

CHAPTER 3

Odor and Eros

IN HER BOOK *A Natural History of the Senses,* Diane Ackerman wrote, "Because females have often been responsible for initiating mating, smell has been their weapon." To the unconscious mind, perfumes reveal an aspect of sex appeal often hidden from consciousness. A kiss—the word means "smell" in many languages—is a prolonged sniffing of a loved one, an expression of the desire to linger where the beloved's scent glows.

Each of us has a unique personal odor as individual as our fingerprints and influenced by diet, gender, heredity, health, medication, occupation, emotional state, and mood. Personal odor communicates something about who we are and—instinctively and unconsciously, for better or for worse—is one of our criteria for choosing our friends and lovers. According to Susan Schiffman, MD, psychology professor at Duke University in North Carolina, "People who don't like each other's smell don't make it as a couple." North American cultures, however, may be too acutely aware of body odor. Given our constant attention to removing odor with deodorants and replacing it with synthetic scents, researchers speculate that we may have lost our innate ability to respond to natural sexual attractants.

The odoriferous substances manufactured by the apocrine glands—found in the axillae (armpits), face, nipples, anal and genital regions, and to a lesser extent in the ears, eyelids, and scalp—are called *pheromones,* from the Greek words *pherein* (to carry) and *hormon* (to excite). They become active at puberty, after which they play an interesting role in sexual behavior, puberty, menstruation, and menopause. (Before puberty, perspiration has no odor, which makes perfect biological sense: there is no need to signal or attract the opposite sex before we are able to reproduce.)

In Elizabethan times, lovers exchanged peeled "love apples," which were kept in the armpit until saturated with sweat, then presented to the lover so he or she could inhale the fragrance when they were apart. A similar custom was observed in parts of the Austrian Tyrol, where it was fashionable for a young man to dance with a handkerchief in his armpit and later wave it under the nose of the girl he admired to excite her sexually. Members of a tribe in New Guinea still say good-bye by putting a hand in each other's armpits, then rubbing themselves with the other's scent. In a similar custom in Australia, the Gidjingali people of Arnhem Land, upon departing, rub sweat from their own armpits on each other. To enhance their own scent, the Kallaway tribe of Bolivia boil the vanilla-like balsam of Peru in water to use as an underarm wash.

Humans cannot detect the scent of pheromones the same way we might notice a familiar perfume, but we may well sense them, and they may have an impact on how we act. One informal study found that when identical twins sat at a bar, the twin wearing (non-fragrant) pheromones attracted three times as many interactions from strangers over the course of an evening. Another study took manufactured pheromones and sprayed them on a chair in a doctor's waiting room; that was the chair consistently chosen by patients that day by more than four to one.

As far back as 1974, Lewis Thomas, PhD—who advanced the theory that mate selection can be traced to individual odor prints generated by a sequence of genes—suggested that a cluster of animal genes known as the "major histocompatibility complex" (MHC), which generates antibodies for protection, might be the key to the olfactory code. Immunologist Ted Boyse later proved the link between the sense of smell and the immune system by performing an experiment that demonstrated how MHC is influenced by smell. Working with strains of inbred mice, he was able to show that mice sniffed out genetically different mice with whom to mate, thus keeping the gene pool more diverse and establishing a more adaptable immune system. Mice even showed a preference to mate with those whose genetic makeup differed by only a single gene. A high variability in MHC is now thought to be essential for disease resistance.

Scents That Turn on Women

13%	licorice or cucumber
11%	lavender or pumpkin pie spice
4%	baby powder and chocolate
1%	women's perfume

Scents That Turn on Men

40%	lavender and pumpkin pie spice
31.5%	licorice and doughnut
20%	pumpkin pie spice and doughnut
19.5%	orange
18%	lavender and doughnut
13%	licorice and cola
13%	licorice
12.5%	doughnut and cola
11%	lily of the valley
9%	buttered popcorn
2%	cranberry

Courtesy of Alan R. Hirsh, MD.

Women's Sexuality

There have been many interesting studies on how the sense of smell affects women's menstrual cycles. One study, for example, showed that girls who had been separated from boys during adolescence (in a boarding school situation) generally started menstruating later than girls in a coeducational environment. This suggests that contact with boys' pheromones triggers a hormonal response that signals girls to become fertile. Studies also show that women produce a pheromone that causes their menstrual cycle to synchronize with that of nearby women after three or four months. Women's sensitivity to odor peaks at ovulation, when olfactory receptivity increases a thousandfold. Conversely, women's sense of smell is least keen at menstruation.

The male underarm scent can also regulate women's cycles, although merely being in prolonged, close proximity is not enough to trigger this effect; there must be intimate physical contact. Other studies show that women who have sex with a male partner at least once a week have more regular menstrual cycles, are more likely to have cycles of normal length, have fewer infertility problems, and experience a milder menopause than women who are celibate or who have sex in a "feast or famine" pattern. Scientists are trying to isolate the chemicals responsible for these phenomena to produce nasal sprays for scent-based birth control and cycle regulation.

Women have, in general, a keener sense of smell than men, even as infants. Research by Hilary Schmidt, PhD, of the Monell Chemical Senses Center, while suggesting that the same odor preferences occur in both children and adults, noted definite gender differences. Baby girls preferred a large selection of scented rattles while baby boys just went for the most pleasant scents.

Whatever the cause of these gender differences, it carries into adulthood. Women recognize scents, especially food-related ones such as cinnamon and coffee, much more readily than men. One study showed that women could guess the sex of a person more accurately than men just by sniffing a shirt the person had worn for twenty-four hours. In still another test, when puffs of fragrance were monitored by subjects, men performed better at simple mental tasks in unscented rooms while women did best in scented rooms.

Women take time to consider their preferences and label scents in much more detail. They can use a variety of different color hues, most often correlating pleasant scents with the color yellow and unpleasant ones with purple. Men, on the other hand, tend to automatically like or dislike a smell, but can offer little in the way of description. It's no surprise that researchers found that when women were given the male hormone testosterone, their ability to smell declined. Following menopause or a hysterectomy, women also begin to lose their ability to detect musk odors. The scent of musk is very close to human testosterone and can normally be detected in amounts as little as 0.000000000000032 ounces. (Twenty-five percent of people with smell disorders lose interest in sex; as part of their sex therapy, Masters and Johnson have helped couples learn to enjoy touching each other using scented lotion.) The ability to detect musk odors returns in women who go on hormone therapy. Fertile women who were exposed to a musk odor have shorter menstrual cycles, ovulate more often, and conceive more easily.

The effects of various aromas on sexual arousal have been measured in clinical studies by Alan R. Hirsch, MD, director of the Smell and Taste Treatment and Research Foundation. In a 1997 study, he used the increase in blood flow to the sexual organs as an indicator. What turned women on the most was the smell of either cucumber or licorice, as in the candy Good & Plenty (see opposite page).

Curiously, men's cologne lessened the women's sexual response (-1 percent). Even less appreciated were the scents of cherry (-18 percent) and barbecue smoke (-14 percent). However, maybe it's the type of cologne used in the study. The Kinsey Institute in Bloomington, Indiana, found that inhaling a traditional, ultra-masculine men's cologne did tend to increase physical stimulation in women.

Men's Sexuality

Although sex pheromones are produced in both men and women, the male sex pheromones seem to function mainly as aphrodisiacs for the female, whereas the female pheromones serve chiefly to announce her readiness. We found one reference to a scientist who lived in isolation for long periods on an island. By taking the dry weight of the hairs trapped by his electric razor every day, he discovered that his beard grew faster each time he returned to the mainland and associated with females.

Scent helps determine how you perceive other individuals. One group of male interviewers rated scented female applicants as less intelligent, albeit more attractive; when interviewed by women, fragrance-wearing female applicants were judged friendlier and more intelligent than those who wore no scent. When they sniffed a floral and spice combination, the men estimated that the women they viewed each weighed about four pounds less than the women who were viewed by men in rooms with no scents at all. Men who found the combination pleasant perceived women to be a full twelve pounds less than their actual weights.

Scent can also change how we perceive ourselves. A study at the College of William and Mary in Virginia showed that men and women who wear personal fragrances daily tend to perceive themselves as better than people who don't wear fragrance. They maintain higher self-esteem, self-acceptance, and social competence, and are more willing to take a stand on important issues. Men who frequently use cologne regard their body as more appealing than non-perfume wearers.

Napoleon was keenly aware of how scent affects sexuality. It is reported that he once sent a message to Josephine that read, "Home in three days. Don't wash." Goethe carried around the unwashed bodice of his lover so he was never without her fragrance. Studies done with men who smell the natural aroma in women's clothing have found that they tend to be most attracted to clothing that was worn by women described as "shy and retiring" compared to clothes worn by more dominant and aggressive women. It is assumed that men subconsciously associate the smell of testosterone with too much aggression. Conversely, most women prefer the clothes of men who are testosterone-rich.

All of the thirty scents presented to thirty-one men sexually aroused them, but it was a combination of lavender and pumpkin pie that they found most aphrodisiacal. Next in effectiveness were the scents of licorice and doughnuts. Yes, it's true that almost all of the top ten scents that aroused men are food! We can't help but wonder if the pumpkin pie and cranberry cancel each other on Thanksgiving—no matter, the tryptophan in the turkey will put them to sleep anyway. The most effective scents did vary according to the man's age. For instance, older men tended to respond strongly to vanilla more than the younger men.

It is really no surprise to learn that sperm smell their way to the egg, which researchers say could lead to advances in contraception and fertility treatments. *Science* magazine reports that German researchers, trying to work out how sperm find their way to their intended destination, have identified an odor receptor in testicular tissue, usually found in the sensory nerve cells of the nose. If successful, this could help fertility doctors identify the most mobile sperm, increasing the chances of conception.

Aphrodisiacs

Scents that have age-old reputations as sexual stimulants are jasmine, musk, patchouli, sandalwood, ylang-ylang, rose, and vanilla. Studies show that jasmine, musk, and ylang-ylang are both relaxing and stimulating to the brain. Although it may seem that these actions would cancel each other, they actually combine to produce a very enjoyable mood. The combination of relaxation and stimulation is probably one of the secrets behind most aphrodisiac scents. The state of being completely relaxed, yet at the same time stimulated, offers the perfect combination for an aphrodisiac, since stress and tension are strong deterrents to passion. Other aphrodisiacs include the stimulants cinnamon and coriander, which is the aphrodisiac mentioned by Sheherazade in the famous story *The Arabian Nights*. Aphrodisiacs are useful as part of a program to help overcome sexual dysfunctions.

APHRODISIAC BLEND

Lavender is not an aphrodisiac but is added to make the fragrance more mellow. It can be a relaxing and emotionally uplifting scent. If you love patchouli, try it in place of ylang-ylang.

  4 ounces sweet almond essential oil
  10 drops lavender essential oil
  10 drops sandalwood essential oil
  2 drops ylang-ylang essential oil
  2 drops vanilla essential oil
  1 drop each cinnamon and jasmine essential oils

Combine ingredients.

CHAPTER 4

Scent and Psyche

INTERNATIONAL Flavors and Fragrance (IFF) has found a way to create aromatherapy clothing, sheets, and other textiles. Technology developed in 2005 allows fragrance and even ingredients such as aloe vera and vitamin E to be impregnated into cloth so the scent will release over time. The same company also collaborated with the fashion and art publication *Visionaire* to have top artists in a variety of fields create visual interpretations of twenty-one original fragrances that were created by IFF perfumers. It is common to find clothing impregnated with insect repellent at outdoor equipment stores. Similar technology led the Japanese to develop panty hose that comes in the buyer's choice of a rose or lavender scent.

Air New Zealand and Virgin Atlantic airlines developed kits of floral-scented bath oils to reduce jet lag. The blended "After Flight Regulator" oils are named Awake and Asleep and are sold at Heathrow Airport's International Terminal in London. Developed by aromatherapist Daniele Ryman, they are intended to be used as bath oil or shower gel when the traveler arrives at his or her destination. England's Queen Elizabeth, and previously, Princess Diana, reportedly used them regularly in their jaunts around the world.

Today marketing has discovered that scents appeal in selling products. Realtors know that the aroma of a few freshly baked brownies, strategically placed, and the fragrance from a few drops of essential oil on lightbulbs improve the chances of selling a house. Used-car salesmen magically rejuvenate rundown autos with "new car" fragrance straight from a can. Bakeries and other food stores have long known that piping the scent of freshly baked bread around the front door will draw customers. Watch anyone buying body-care products. How do they make their final decision? They give the product a sniff, of course. One Australian mail-order company found their final notice bills were paid sooner when they were scented.

Fragrance is already being used experimentally in a few large U.S. department stores to see whether it will encourage people to spend more money. It definitely seems to cause shoppers to linger longer, although not necessarily make more purchases. The Marketing Aromatics group in Britain had Warwick University test stress-reducing scents in more than one hundred UK department stores and travel agencies. Their scientists also developed blends to reduce stress in the workplace and signature scents for the corporate world, including scented company stationery.

Author and director of the Smell and Taste Treatment and Research Foundation in Chicago, Alan R. Hirsch, MD, predicted, "It is probable that by the year 2000 managers will use perfumes in department stores the world over.... Odorants are potentially more efficacious than any other modality in increasing salability."

Hirsch is busy comparing how different odors change consumers' reactions as they watch commercials for Oldsmobile cars or look at Nike running shoes. In his study, 84 percent of people liked the shoes more and were more likely to buy them when they were in a scented room, even though many of them were not conscious the room had been scented. The scented air also made many participants willing to pay more. In another project, he piped appealing odors into the Las Vegas Hilton to see whether it would affect gamblers. Affect them it certainly did: people stayed longer, they spent more money, and revenues increased by 45 percent. A London nightclub found that sales of the drink Malibu more than doubled when there was a coconut fragrance in the air. Let's not forget the signature scents now being used to brand products in stores such as the well-known lingerie chain Victoria's Secret.

Aromatherapy has even had a role in the entertainment field. An "odor organ" in the early twentieth century emitted different scents according to which keys were hit. The annual 1993 Comdex computer convention in Las Vegas displayed every kind of new computerized device, including a fragrance dispenser computer programmed to match the music's beat (and mood) as thousands of convention-goers danced. In London, a 1993 production of Prokofiev's *The Love of Three Oranges* added fragrance to the performance. The audience was cued at certain times to release each of six odors on scratch-and-sniff cards.

Hollywood had a similar idea in the early 1960s, when the first Smell-o-Vision movie houses, outfitted in New York City and elsewhere for the premiere of Michael Todd Jr.'s thriller, *A Scent of Mystery,* ran pipes, which puffed out different scents as the plot progressed, along the backs of theater seats (unfortunately, they never got the timing right: the smell of perfume was apt to arrive long before the heroine, destroying suspense, and the premature smell of horses ruined at least one love scene.) Later director John Waters reinvented the scratch-and-sniff gimmick for his 1981 comedy *Polyester.*

Similar, more-developed scent technology is allowing displays in museums, science centers, galleries, visitor centers, theme parks, and historical sites to incorporate aromas into the public displays. The custom aromas, such as the scent of popcorn, a campfire, erupting volcano, a woolly mammoth, and even skunk are infused into corn kernel–sized resin pellets called "scent orbs" that are released electronically. They are being used by a number of museums, including the Smithsonian Institution in Washington, D.C., and entertainment companies such as Walt Disney Productions. Visitors attending a display at the Smithsonian tended to have memories similar to sound or visual cues, except their recall was especially vivid.

Medical Aromatherapy

"Science has proven beyond a doubt that scent modulates mood," says Avery Gilbert, PhD, former president of the Sense of Smell Institute and scent scientist in a consulting service for the development and marketing of scented products. Extroverts are believed to favor floral scents, while introverts go for heady Asian aromas.

Several scientific conferences exploring essential oil production and use take place on a regular basis. In this arena, it is usually identified by the more scientific-sounding name *aromachology.* Although aromachology is still considered a fringe aspect of psychology, interest is growing. The First International Conference on the Psychology of Perfume was held in 1986. The 1990 International Conference on Essential Oils and Aroma Chemicals in Malaysia generated approximately fifty papers on the actions of essential oils. At the 1991 conference of the prestigious American Association for the Advancement of Science, the largest U.S. science organization, aromachology researchers from major U.S. universities delivered papers. Conferences devoted to aromachology followed, such as the International Conference on Essential Oils and Aroma Trades and the International Conference on Essential Oils for Perfumery and Flavours.

Aromachology differs from aromatherapy in that its emphasis is completely on the scientific studies, although these are sometimes based on the historical use of the scent plant. It is also not concerned with using the pure essential oils derived from plants, as are aromatherapists. Thus, the research uses some synthetically derived scents such as apple and peach.

Much of the funding for medical research into aromatherapy in the United States comes from the Fragrance Research Fund, a nonprofit coalition of companies in the fragrance industry organized by IFF. Some top fragrance companies, such as Estée Lauder, Avon, and Chanel, as well as several high profile magazines, head the membership of this organization. They began collaborating with Yale University's psychophysiology department in 1982 to study aroma science, described as the effect of fragrance on human emotions. They have also funded grants for clinical research that resulted in seven psychologists studying how the sense of smell functions and how it affects mind and body. Researchers are particularly interested in discovering aromatic relaxants, stimulants, antidepressants, and pain relievers. Since these categories—"uppers" and "downers"—represent some of the most frequently prescribed drugs, the pharmaceutical industry may be in for a change.

Psychophysicist Craig Warren, PhD, is the scientific affairs director of the Sense of Smell Institute, a research and education division of the nonprofit Fragrance Foundation, which follows research and increases public awareness of the role the sense of smell plays. Thanks to the Fragrance Research Fund, Warren developed a program and a mapping system using modern psychological techniques to study odor's effect on behavior and mood. He was able to test more than two thousand subjects over a twenty-year period to better understand how smell can relieve pain, touch off deep-seated memories, and affect personality and behavior. He is particularly interested in mood-elevating odors that prevent insomnia.

Also sponsored by the Fragrance Research Fund, Gary Schwartz, PhD, former professor of psychology and psychiatry at Yale University and now at the University of Arizona, believes that fragrances may provide valuable complementary treatment for a host of problems related to the emotions, such as fatigue, migraine headaches, food cravings, depression, anxiety, schizophrenia, and irregular heartbeat.

People tend to prefer familiar fragrances—that is, unless past negative associations get in the way. Researchers have demonstrated that odors with negative associations evoke negative emotions. When students at Warwick University in England were told they had performed poorly on a simple test they had taken while smelling a certain odor, they became depressed the next time they smelled that odor. Those who had been told they were successful had the opposite reaction: their self-confidence was boosted.

Susan Schiffman, MD, professor of medical psychology at North Carolina's Duke University, sprayed food scents into New York City subway cars to observe the effect on passengers. After comparing the number of pushes, shoves, and nasty comments in scented versus unscented cars, she concluded that fragrances can reduce such aggressive behavior by as much as 40 percent. Medical aromachology may not only cure, but may also help to diagnose diseases. Researchers at the Illinois Institute of Technology in Chicago developed an electronic nose that can identify odor groups, from citrus fruits to aromatic spices. Even more important, it finds bacteria in the bloodstream faster and cheaper than current medical tests. The "e-nose" sniffs out diseases such as tuberculosis and those caused by food-borne bacteria such as *E. coli*. It also picks up biomedical hazards such as anthrax. Hundreds of specific fingerprints identify the distinct odors produced by chemical wastes that different bacteria excrete into the bloodstream. Electrochemical sensors "sniff" the sample, and specialized computer software analyzes the information. Since the human nose contains several million smell receptors, a good electronic detector needs at least a thousand channels for identification. The technology is already used to detect rotten fish and harmful levels of gases such as cyanide gases in new buildings. Another possible application is a "smart" refrigerator that can tell when food has spoiled. You even may be able to send smells by email in the future.

Health and Body-Care Products

Because the fragrance field is virtually married to the cosmetics industry, it should come as no surprise that modern aromatherapy was born of the quest for new and improved beauty products. A "Sleep for Beauty Kit" designed by IFF in 1984 came with a fragrant pillow and vials of thirty scents, such as valerian and the relaxing neroli and valerian.

Marina Munteanu, former vice president of IFF's Fragrance Technology, projected that one day it will be commonplace for people to choose everyday scented items, such as shampoo, according to their emotional needs. Redken, a large cosmetics company, has taken this marketing hint to heart and introduced its Shinsen hair line to "relieve stress and promote peace of mind" with rose, honeysuckle, tuberose, and musk, or to "lift the spirits"

with orange, tangerine, and peach, though many are synthetically derived fragrances.

The first major cosmetics company to produce an aromatherapy line designed to influence the emotions was Avon with its "Tranquil Moments" bath products. Scientists at the Japanese fragrance firm Takasago, on the Avon payroll, measured brain-wave patterns and found that jasmine is stimulating and lavender is relaxing—the same qualities attributed to these scents through centuries of folklore. Both relaxation and stimulation of the mind can lead to increased concentration. In a Takasago study, errors made by computer workers fell by 20 percent when lavender was diffused in the atmosphere, by 33 percent when it was jasmine, and 54 percent when the scent was lemon. Takasago is also investigating aromatherapy to relieve nausea, dizziness, and other physical ailments.

Following Avon's lead, the Estée Lauder beauty company formed Origins, an "aromatherapy" body-care line sold in exclusive department stores. Their "Green Principles" products emphasize botanicals and carry names such as Sleep Time, Stress Buffer, Muscle Easing, Energy Boost, and Peace of Mind. Now that Estée Lauder also owns Aveda, they are well ensconced in the organic aromatherapy business, since Aveda's entire line of beauty and hair products uses only plant-based essential oils to fragrance their products. Aveda's acne skin-care line, called Outer Peace, contains organic essential oils with strict attention paid to the functional benefits of the blend of essential oils on bacteria that is associated with acne. The product boasted a 92 percent improvement rate in one month.

The world's third largest cosmetics company, after Avon and Revlon, is a Japanese company called Shiseido whose name means "harmony among the natural forces that govern the world." Shiseido believes that beautiful skin must have balanced *chi,* or life energy, and has put together an acupressure and aromatherapy facial with effects that are more than skin deep. Researchers found that the brain waves of subjects receiving aromatherapy facials duplicate those achieved during meditation or deep relaxation. Thus, in addition to improving the complexion and reducing acne, the facial stabilizes blood pressure, moderating both high and low readings.

The Shiseido Life Science Research Center blended an aroma of orange, neroli, and iris to reduce menstrual period stress, which can lead to disorders of the nervous system and skin problems. Women with high stress scores had more stress during menstruation, more skin problems, and poorer general skin function. When forty-five of these highly stressed women used an aromatherapy fragrance and air freshener, it reduced their levels of the sex hormones estrogen and testosterone, as well as their negative emotions. It also improved the women's ability to concentrate and significantly lowered their stress response. They claim the face became more moisturized, oil production on the forehead was reduced, and there was improved skin function, such as reduction of the various negative effects that are caused by having skin that is too alkaline. As a result, the company is now using similar blends in their skin-care line.

Airborne Therapy

Aromatherapy has also made itself at home in the house. Sponsored by the fragrance company PPF/Norda, a study of living-room environments indicated that participants react more favorably to furniture and décor when a room is scented. Robert Baron, professor of psychology at the Rensselaer Polytechnic Institute in Troy, New York, found that people perform a variety of tasks more accurately and efficiently in scented as opposed to unscented rooms. Clerical workers in one study set higher performance goals for themselves in scented offices.

The Japanese in particular have embraced aromatherapy and are leaders in innovative aroma applications. A futon-dryer that leaves the bedding smelling like flowers encourages sleep. Japanese firms have also developed clothes impregnated with aroma beads, such as the lavender-and-rose scented panty hose currently being sold on the European market.

Even house paint has entered the aromatherapy arena. As part of a new concept that has been termed "sensory engineering," it also incorporates sound and color, along with scent. An organic, milk-based paint with aromatherapy scents to enhance your mood was developed by the progressive paint company Anna Sova. The fragrance is said to permeate a room for up to six months, after which it can be refreshed with a wall spritz. The selections include orange-clove to allay indigestion, vanilla for anger and frustration, cedarwood and lime for fatigue and stress, and lavender to inspire peaceful sleep.

DVD-like disks that fill a room with scent as they are played on a special electronic scent player have been in the works for over a decade. Some of these players have actually come and gone, still in need of refinement. One company produced forty different essential oil–impregnated disks with individual essential oil scents, while another had scented theme disks with blends titled Ocean Breeze, Christmas Tree, Roses, and English Garden. Eventually, we'll see scent incorporated into music DVDs and computer programs and games.

Aromatherapy Health Care

Numerous scientific articles have described the potential of aromatherapy to promote health and well-being in hospital patients through massage, inhalation, baths, compresses, creams, and lotions. One of the first of these was a 1992 issue of the *British Journal of Occupational Therapy* with an extensive list of potential uses describing how aromatherapy can diminish stress, sedate, relieve depression, invigorate, promote activity and alertness, stimulate sensory awareness, facilitate interaction and communication, treat certain medical problems, and provide pain relief.

By 2006, a Cochrane Group survey found over thirteen hundred references to aromatherapy massage alone in the scientific literature. After reviewing the studies, it determined that aromatherapy massage provides at least short-term benefits to a person's psychological well-being and reduces anxiety 19 to 32 percent. In many cases, it also helps treat depression and seems to reduce pain.

Aromatherapy can be found today in clinics and hospitals around the world. For years, anesthetics in many hospitals have used a strawberry fragrance on ether masks to calm children before surgery. A citrus or orange scent in the waiting room of a dental office relaxed patients, especially the women, in one Austrian study. The participants felt less anxiety and more calm, and they were in better moods than a control group. In a controlled trial, long-term patients in an Irish neurology hospital felt less emotional distress and had improved mood scores after receiving an aromatherapy treatment of lavender, tea tree, and rosemary.

In New York City, the prestigious Integrative Medicine Service at Memorial Sloan-Kettering Cancer Center offers individual therapies for pain control and relaxation in aromatherapy massage and other forms of bodywork, acupuncture, music therapy, and spiritual/energy therapies. They use vanilla scent to relax patients undergoing magnetic resonance imaging (MRI) scanning, in which they must lie perfectly still in a small cylinder, often for over an hour. Aromas have been found to reduce anxiety in well over half the patients undergoing MRIs.

In England, similar aromatic methods are proving successful when used in conjunction with orthodox treatments to help patients cope with the emotional problems that may accompany serious illness. Aromatherapy is also used to diminish the side effects of drug therapies. Wirral Holistic Care Services in Cheshire, England, for example, offers aromatherapy along with other complementary therapies to help cancer patients tolerate the side effects of chemotherapy. Aromatherapy is available at the clinic, and patients are taught how to use it at home. Psychology

professor Michael Carey, PhD, at the Center for Health and Behavioral Sciences (Syracuse University in New York), has comforted cancer patients with the scent of rose to help them overcome negative reactions to chemotherapy and also to help prevent nausea.

Anxiety and Fear

Feeling panicked about an approaching job interview or a speech? Then sniff an apple, says University of Arizona psychologist Gary Schwartz, PhD. He has studied how the sense of smell affects the area of the brain that regulates fear and anxiety in over four hundred people. Schwartz, who says he was inspired by the old saying "An apple a day keeps the doctor away," believes that our sense of smell directly affects the part of our brain that controls fear and anxiety. To put his theory to the test, he asked a group of forty-eight people provocative questions such as "What kind of person makes you angry?" As expected, the subjects tensed up—that is, until they sniffed the scent of apple, whereupon their breathing became slower and their muscles relaxed. They felt less anxious and embarrassed and reported that they suddenly felt much happier. Their systolic blood pressure rates fell a point, while diastolic rates went down three to five points—a sign of letting go of stress. Adding a little spice—clove and cinnamon—to the apple relaxed them even more. Schwartz noted that if scent can reduce blood pressure in healthy individuals, it should help someone with high blood pressure even more. Clinical studies have found that smelling peaches reduces panic attacks, epilepsy, and narcolepsy, a disorder in which people tend to suddenly fall asleep at inappropriate times. International Flavors and Fragrance researchers have studied and patented two essential-oil blends to diminish anxiety and stress in the workplace. One is a combination of neroli, valerian, and nutmeg; the other is from compounds found in essential oils: myristicin from nutmeg and elemicin and isoelemicin from elemi. Both blends, which are designed to be rubbed into the skin or inhaled, reduce stress and blood pressure. Individuals say they experience much less fear, tension, and anxiety after sniffing them. These blends can also lower blood pressure. Interestingly, they seem to act only when needed, in one study being effective in people who already had high blood pressure, but not with individuals whose blood pressure was normal. John J. King, MD, a psychiatrist at the Smallwood Day Hospital in Worcestershire, England, found that fragrance can break the feedback loop created during stressful times. When anxiety develops, heart and breathing rates increase, affecting brain chemistry, which in turn stimulates more anxiety. If this loop can be stopped by physical or psychological means, relaxation ensues. King used pleasant, natural scents in therapy sessions in conjunction with such tension-reducing techniques as deep breathing, visualization, sound, and heat. The patients learned to associate a particular fragrance with deep relaxation and could later use the fragrance to draw on the association. Some of Dr. King's favorite anti-anxiety scents were lavender, rose, bergamot, cypress, and balsam fir.

Positive programming with scent to relieve anxiety and stress has been around for a long time. In twelfth-century Arabia, the Muslim doctor Al-Samarqandi wrote that breathing the fumes of the rose and sandalwood would "quiet the heat of the brain." Myrrh and frankincense are also aids to induce sleep and relaxation. The famous Egyptian fragrance *kyphi*, a perfume of frankincense, myrrh, calamus, and spikenard, was used to encourage sleep, alleviate anxieties, and brighten dreams. To ease migraine headaches, Al-Samarqandi suggested sniffing violets. Aromatherapists use these same fragrances to help someone who feels lonely or rejected or undergoing a major life transition.

These fragrances along with other aromatherapy oils have long been used to help one overcome episodes of anxiety associated with grief and sadness. Ancient Egyptians and Greeks, followed later by Europeans, found that marjoram, cypress, and hyssop were useful for comforting grief and sadness, and for "strengthening" the brain so the bereft individual could get on with his or her life. Sixteenth-century herbalist John Gerard, who wrote the often-quoted *The Herball, or Generall Historie of Plantes,* recommended marjoram's fragrance "for those given to much sighing."

Hyssop was said to help clear the mind and help a person think more clearly during trying times. Several ancient cultures, including India and Egypt, used sandalwood to comfort mourners during funeral ceremonies, while Europeans turned to sage, clary sage, and rosemary to overcome this and other forms of grief. Rosemary (the herb of "remembrance") was carried to funerals, then thrown into the graves.

Depression

Mood swings are a normal part of life, and temporary states of depression are normal, but ongoing depression is a complex problem that limits the quality of life for more than thirty million Americans. Depression has been steadily increasing in North America since the beginning of the twentieth century. It affects general health by suppressing the immune system and can lead to insomnia and other seemingly unrelated problems by causing changes in the brain's chemistry. Aromatherapy can play a role in conjunction with other types of therapy. In fact, many professional therapists are beginning to incorporate aromatherapy into their practices.

International Flavors and Fragrance studies have found that orange and other citrus scents reduce stress and depression. Both orange and neroli measurably lowered both stress and blood pressure. A blend of neroli, valerian, and nutmeg was so effective in helping release tension that the company patented it. In a recent study with aromatherapy massage, a blend of lavender, marjoram, eucalyptus, rosemary, and peppermint given to forty people with arthritis not only decreased their pain but also their depression.

According to biochemist George H. Dodd, PhD, and psychologist Steve van Toller, PhD, at the Warwick Olfaction Research Group in England, the effect of fragrance on the brain is similar to that of some antidepressant drugs. The two expound on this in the book they edited, *Perfumery: The Psychology and Biology of Fragrance.*

The scent of orange, and probably other citruses, alters brain chemistry to lower blood pressure and probably counters mood changes such as depression and anxiety. Even smelling an orange as you peel it helps as minute amounts of essential oils are propelled into the air to cheer you up. As aromatherapists, we have observed that some citrus scents are more effective than others, depending on the diagnosis. For example, true clinical depression often responds better to the more refined scent of orange blossom, also known as neroli, than it does to orange peel. Lemon's "clean" fragrance helps maintain emotional balance. Bergamot helps overcome compulsive behavior, including eating disorders. Tangerine and grapefruit appeal to children subject to depression and mood swings and assist adults doing "inner child" therapy.

In the 1970s and 1980s, Paolo Rovesti, PhD, then director of the Istituto di Richerche sui Derivati Vegetali in Milan, turned to essential oils to treat depressed and anxious patients. He had success with fragrances considered "herbal" or "green," such as lavender, marjoram, violet leaf, rose, cypress, and opopanax. Lavender turns out to be particularly effective in lowering anxiety and stress in patients following heart surgery. To treat depression, he used a mixture of jasmine, sandalwood, orange, lemon verbena, and lemon. For anxiety, he chose bergamot, neroli, cypress, petitgrain, lime, rose, violet leaves, and marjoram. Rovesti noted that "patients felt as if transported by the perfume of the essential oil into a different, more agreeable and acceptable world, so that many of their reactive instincts are curbed and they gradually return towards normality."

Someday you may be able to get an aromatherapy prescription to treat depression. This has already happened at an experimental convalescent clinic in Baku, Azerbaijan. The clinic prescribed sniffing a fragrant herb plant for ten minutes twice a week in a special sunroom. Rose geranium was recommended to overcome neurosis, headaches, and insomnia brought on by worry and depression. Science has not yet investigated the use of aromatherapy to counter compulsive behavior that is associated with depression, including eating disorders. However, aromatherapists use bergamot and grapefruit.

In sixteenth- and seventeenth-century European herbals, clary sage and lemon balm were suggested to counter depression and to help with paranoia, mental fatigue, and nervous disorders associated with depression. Writing in his sixteenth-century *The Herball, or Generall Historie of Plantes,* John Gerard said that sniffing lemon balm was a sure way to "gladden the heart" and that basil "taketh away sorrowfulness . . . and maketh a man merry and glad." In India, the scent of holy basil, or *tulsi,* is traditionally used to prevent agitation and nightmares.

Stress and Nervousness

Previous IFF chairman Henry G. Walter Jr. foresaw more and more companies marketing perfumes designed to ease stress. In a 1985 *New York Times* interview, he emphasized that the whole point of relaxation is to focus, saying, "When people are under stress, it is usually because they have too many things coming at them at once and cannot decide what to do in what order." The use of sedative fragrances remained a part of health care into the nineteenth century, when W. S. Watson, MD, found that certain scents, especially rose, sedated mental patients. Attar of rose appeared in a nineteenth-century medical journal as a remedy for "nervous digestion." In 1954, Austrian perfumer Paul Jellinek, PhD, even classified rose as a "narcotic" scent.

In the early 1920s, Italian doctors and researchers Giovanni Gatti and Renato Cayola conducted research on essential oils and the nervous system, including their effects as antibiotics and on blood pressure, breathing frequency, and blood circulation rate. They concluded that "the sense of smell has, by reflex action, an enormous influence on the function of the central nervous system" after extensive experiments showed that certain smells relaxed psychologically disturbed patients. When these essential oils were inhaled (or ingested), pulse rate, blood circulation, and breathing changed. Most sedating were the citrus scents: melissa, neroli, petitgrain, chamomile, asafetida, valerian, and opopanax. Gatti and Cayola observed that while repeated or increased doses resulted in sedation, light initial doses were often experienced as stimulating. The seventeenth-century herbalist Nicholas Culpeper noted that chamomile "comforts both the head and brain." We have found it particularly useful for treating children who are anxious or hyperactive, as well as stressed-out adults. When W. Gray Walter, PhD, and his associates started to record the CNV brain waves in the 1960s, they found that such waves surged whenever a person looked forward to an event or ingested a stimulant such as coffee. When the subject felt drowsy or took a sedative drug, production of these brain waves was reduced. Fragrance also affects CNV brain waves, but unlike coffee or drugs, produces no change in heart rate, reaction time, or alertness. The most sedative scents tested (in order of effectiveness) were lavender, bergamot, marjoram, sandalwood, lemon, and chamomile—some of the same ones noted by the herbalists Al-Samarqandi, John Gerard, and later by researchers Gatti and Cayola. Modern-day aromatherapists regard these scents as among the most emotionally balancing, specifically helpful in the treatment of depression, anxiety, headaches, and strain from overwork.

Lavender is one of the most popular fragrances to alleviate stress and, as a result, has been extensively studied.

EEG readings show that lavender oil increases alpha waves when the scent is inhaled for only three minutes. Alpha waves are associated with relaxation, focus, a meditative state, and increased drowsiness. When lavender is tested with volunteers, they tend to have lower anxiety scores and be more relaxed and less depressed. Two compounds in lavender, linalol and terpineol, were found to relax the central nervous system. Adding lavender oil to acupressure sessions provided clients at the Telehealth Clinic in Hong Kong with increased relief from neck pain within three weeks. They could move their necks more easily, felt nearly a quarter less pain and stiffness, and their level of stress went down an average of 39 percent. Another compound, alpha-pinene, which is found in pine, spruce, fir, and hemlock tree oils, also increases the alpha state.

Insomnia

Clinical studies demonstrate how well aromatherapy aids sleep. Lavender helps people suffering from insomnia fall asleep faster and experience fewer sleep-related symptoms. Subjects in several different studies needed less time to get started when they woke up in the morning, feeling more satisfied and invigorated. The scent also relieved some initial feelings of depression. One way that lavender acts on the mind is to increase deep, or slow-wave sleep, as well as the lighter, stage two sleep. Although it sends both genders to dreamland, women have been found to have less rapid-eye movement (REM) sleep after first falling asleep, while men experienced more REM.

Researchers at the University of Leicester in England lulled elderly patients to sleep in a room scented with lavender, then measured their sleep patterns. The lavender put them to sleep as effectively as the sedative drugs they had previously been taking. Once they did fall asleep, they were much less restless. In a study by aromatherapist Robert Tisserand, author of *Aromatherapy: To Heal and Tend the Body*, an essential oil blend that included lavender, marjoram, geranium, mandarin, and cardamom effectively relaxed individuals when it replaced their regular pharmaceutical sedatives.

William S. Cain, MD, of the John B. Pierce Foundation Laboratory at Yale University found that aromatherapy helps him sleep by pulling him out of the repetitive cycles of anxiousness called looping that are linked to insomnia. When he wakes up early, instead of worrying about work deadlines, he simply burns scented matches and the aroma puts him back to sleep.

Fatigue

In a study conducted by researchers at Rensselaer Polytechnic Institute in Troy, New York, clerical workers set higher goals for themselves and were more efficient when their offices were pleasantly scented. The fragrance worked even when those taking the test did not think that the scent was influencing them.

Studies on CNV brain wave patterns identified peppermint, clove, basil, ylang-ylang, cinnamon, jasmine, and black pepper as stimulants, as well as the somewhat weaker rose, patchouli, lemongrass, and sage. Researcher Shizuo Torii, PhD, of the Toho University School of Medicine in Tokyo determined that these oils arouse the autonomic nervous system, which controls such involuntary activities as breathing and blood pressure. This prevents the sharp drop in sustained attention that typically occurs after thirty minutes of concentrated work, sometimes even earlier.

Torii points out that the way fragrance keeps us alert is much different from adrenal stimulants such as caffeine. Instead of stimulating adrenal glands, it arouses the autonomic nervous system that controls breathing and blood pressure. Aromatherapy actually helps counter the typical adrenal rush caused by caffeine, as well as the resulting physiological stress, strain, or boredom, reducing drowsiness, irritability, and headaches. Earlier investigation of

fragrant stimulation to counter fatigue was done in the 1920s by Gatti and Cayola. They came up with a similar list of stimulating scents: clove, ylang-ylang, cinnamon, lemon, cardamom, fennel, and angelica. Studies in conjunction with the Fragrance Research Fund also identified peppermint and eucalyptus as stimulants.

To test the effects of fragrance on alertness and stress, researchers William N. Dember and Joel S. Warm gave subjects at the University of Cincinnati the difficult and stressful task of identifying patterns of lines on a computer for forty minutes. Those working in scented rooms did the best, with 88 percent correct answers, compared to 65 percent from people in unscented rooms. In addition, their performance levels didn't decline as rapidly. Interestingly, when questioned later, most of the participants in the first group didn't believe fragrance had improved their performance. The rooms contained the natural scents of peppermint, sandalwood, forest, or the vanilla-like benzoin. Cinnamon spiced apple and lily of the valley were also used.

The Smell and Taste Treatment and Research Foundation in Chicago found that simply having the presence of a floral aroma in the room increased volunteers' speed and performance on mathematics tests. Proofreaders made fewer mistakes when a Good Housekeeping Institute study scented their rooms with peppermint or lavender. Lemon increased the production of typists in one study by up to 54 percent and cut their keyboard errors by half. In a similar study, rosemary improved the alertness, memory, and general performance of typists as they copied data. Lavender proved the best choice for increasing immediate recall, and it also relaxed and slightly enhanced their moods, although it did slow reaction time for both memory and attention. Both lavender and rosemary increased contentment, while jasmine was soothing.

In the heating and air-conditioning systems in buildings, Tokyo's Kajima and Shimizu architectural and construction companies install computer-controlled "Aroma Generation Systems" that release scent into the air every six minutes. The aromas they offer are based on the work by Shizuo Torii on how different fragrances affect brain waves.

Kajima has teamed with the Shiseido cosmetics company to offer over twenty "Scent Plan" varieties to suit different customers' needs. At Kajima, workers are experiencing aromatherapy firsthand. Lemon is the morning wake-up call, followed by rose, which has employees working contentedly through the late morning. After lunch, an invigorating waft of cypress keeps workers awake.

Shimizu, the third biggest construction company in Japan, disperses peppermint into conference rooms to set a positive mood, boost work efficiency, and dispel physical drowsiness and mental fatigue. Either peppermint or a calming, antistress blend such as lavender and rose goes into offices. Lounges and restrooms are scented with cinnamon, and a dash of lemon ends the workday on just the right scent. A bank designed by Shimizu diffuses lavender or rosemary into customer areas, while lemon or eucalyptus keep workers alert. One hotel's lobby contains the refreshing scent of lemon. Relaxing essences are recommended to calm train and bus passengers, and antibacterial aromatherapy is used for hospitals. Even the Tokyo Stock Exchange began invigorating the afternoon air with peppermint.

Aromatherapy in Tokyo does not end at work. On their way home, employees can stop downtown at one of several atomizer-equipped booths for an aromatherapy escape from the stress of commuter traffic. At Club Harry's, clients lie on couches in rooms that are filled with aromas such as their peppermint refresher. And just in case the relaxed business environment has you feeling so relaxed that you sleep in late the next day, a Hattori Seiko alarm clock from Japan puffs out the forest scent of pine and eucalyptus scent to rouse you seconds before your alarm goes off. But you don't have to wait for the future. Oxygen bars are springing up in many U.S. cities to provide a quick stop to change your mood when you're out and about. We've visited them in San Francisco; Boulder;

Kona, Hawaii; and Nevada City, California. Oxygen, said to boost the immune system, improve thinking, and aid digestion, is scented with the customer's choice of aromatherapy essential oils for relaxation or as an energy boost. Many of these bars also offer herbal "cocktails" with combinations of herbs and fruit juice to help the mind, immune system, and especially to increase energy.

Aroma assists people whose jobs are not only monotonous but also rely on their staying alert for the safety of others. The cosmetics firm Charles of the Ritz markets a fragrance to keep car and truck drivers alert while driving. Peppermint, lavender, and anise have been found to lessen weariness and lack of concentration in flight controllers at the end of a busy work shift. Some train conductors in Japan and Russia rely on an "odorphone" developed by Russian professor of biology and odorologist V. Krasnov. Depending on your preference, his little machine spews out hot whiffs of pine, cedar, rose, or even seaweed or mushroom.

Memory

We've all certainly had at least one experience in which an aroma has brought back long-forgotten but still distinct memories. Psychologists refer to the experience of smell stimulating memory as the "Marcel Proust phenomenon." When the French novelist dipped a madeleine cookie in his lemon-blossom tea, the aroma brought back a flood of childhood memories that filled him with "a feeling of inexplicable happiness." This formed the basis of his multivolume masterpiece *Remembrance of Things Past*, which was published in the 1920s.

In fact, scientists tell us that our memory retention is much stronger when linked to smell than to sight. A whiff of certain fragrances often brings to mind images and feelings that are associated with a particular event. Psychology professor Trygg Engen of Brown University in Providence, Rhode Island, and author of *Odor Sensation and Memory* and *Perception of Odor* found that the memory recall associated with scent is at least twice as potent as that of visual recall. That's why a whiff of a certain perfume or some other fragrance that you haven't smelled for years will propel you back in time. With that scent comes everything associated with the original aromatic experience: sights, sounds, and emotional impressions. Engen says that smells serve as "index keys" to quickly retrieve certain memories in our brain. He supports the "nurture" theory over "nature" argument, believing that all smells are initially perceived as neutral and that we each learn to regard scents as pleasant or unpleasant, then retain that information in our memories.

Not surprisingly, studies funded by the Fragrance Research Fund found that pleasant scents cause one to remember pleasant experiences much more so than unpleasant scents. However, unpleasant scents create a longer-lasting impression. In one study connecting the sense of smell with memory, seventy-two students smelled chocolate while they looked at a list of words and wrote down the corresponding antonyms. The next day, those who again smelled chocolate recalled an average of 21 percent of the words on the original list, while those deprived of chocolate averaged only 17 percent. Later studies showed the same results using unpleasant scents, such as the camphorous aroma of mothballs. Even day-old infants in a study at University of California at Irvine exposed to a citrus scent for ten minutes while being stroked remembered that fragrance the next day and turned to the source with increased activity.

Rosemary has a long history of increasing memory, concentration, and even creativity. In the last act of Shakespeare's *Hamlet,* the mad Ophelia declares, "There's rosemary, that's for remembrance." In the seventeenth century, herbalist Nicholas Culpeper wrote that rosemary "helps a weak memory, and quickens the senses." Modern research conducted in Japan confirms rosemary as a brain stimulant. As an antioxidant, it slows the breakdown of acetylcholine in the brain. This important neurotransmitter is found at low levels in Alzheimer's patients.

Other historic memory stimulants are sage, basil, and bay leaf. Sixteenth-century herbalist John Gerard said sage is good for the head and brain and "it quicketh the senses and memory." During the Renaissance, graduates were adorned with bay leaf crowns to symbolize a quick mind. A baccalaureate or "bay laurel" is still given today, although without a wreath! Next time you need help remembering an elusive fact, sniff some aroma as you memorize it, then inhale the same aroma when you need to trigger your memory. In fact, you might try keeping a sprig of rosemary next to your computer.

Fragrance has proved useful to therapists in encouraging patients to recall early memories and associated emotions. Psychologist André Virel, formerly of the Institute of Psychotherapy in Paris, encouraged his clients to sniff vanilla to recall childhood memories. Perhaps unsurprisingly, he found that pleasant odors tend to produce pleasant memories.

Aromatherapy Blends for Emotions

Here are some blends that act on the brain. Feel free to create your own blends using the information in this chapter and the charts in the back of the book. If an individual has more than one emotional problem at the same time, for example, if they are both tired and depressed, then combine some essential oils from each category. Refer to chapter 15 to select oils that seem most appropriate and then chapter 11 for tips on how to make your blend smell wonderful.

LIGHTEN-UP BLEND

- 4 ounces sweet almond carrier oil
- 10 drops lavender essential oil
- 10 drops orange essential oil
- 2 drops marjoram essential oil
- 2 drops cypress essential oil

Combine the ingredients.

HEART-GLADDENING BLEND

- 4 ounces sweet almond carrier oil
- 10 drops marjoram essential oil (or orange or grapefruit)
- 5 drops clary sage essential oil
- 5 drops cypress or rosemary essential oil
- 1 drop rose essential oil (expensive, so *optional*)
- 1 drop melissa (or lemon) essential oil

Combine the ingredients.

HAPPINESS-ABOUNDS BLEND

For children, replace petitgrain with grapefruit or tangerine essential oil.

- 4 ounces sweet almond carrier oil
- 10 drops bergamot essential oil
- 10 drops petitgrain essential oil
- 3 drops rose geranium essential oil
- 1 drop neroli essential oil (expensive, so *optional*)

Combine the ingredients.

HAPPINESS-ABOUNDS SMELLING SALTS

- 6 drops Happiness-Abounds Blend without the sweet almond carrier oil (see previous blend)
- 1 heaping teaspoon rock salt

Drop the essential oil onto the salt. The salt will quickly absorb the oil. Carry the smelling salts in a small container with a tight lid, and sniff as needed.

ENERGY-PRODUCING BLEND

- 4 ounces sweet almond carrier oil
- 15 drops lemon essential oil
- 4 drops eucalyptus essential oil
- 1 drop each cinnamon, peppermint, and benzoin (if available) essential oils

Combine the ingredients.

MEMORY-STIMULATING BLEND

- 4 ounces sweet almond carrier oil
- 10 drops lavender essential oil
- 10 drops lemon essential oil
- 5 drops rosemary essential oil
- 1 drop cinnamon essential oil

Combine the ingredients.

PART II

therapy

The smell of violets hidden in the green
Pour'd back into my empty soul and frame
The times when I remember to have been
Joyful and free from blame.

—Alfred, Lord Tennyson

CHAPTER 5

Guidelines for Using Essential Oils and Herbs

WE CANNOT overestimate the synergistic effects of combining herbal preparations and essential oils, especially for body care. These botanical powerhouses naturally coexist in plants, and employing both modalities in therapeutic applications is the best of both worlds.

Essential oils are very versatile, and you can use them in a number of ways. To do so effectively, however, you need to be aware of safety issues, recommended dilutions, and methods of application. This chapter also introduces you to the different ways to combine herbal preparations with aromatherapy treatments and the different carrier oils from which you may choose. Always keep a meticulous record of how you make your herbal preparations. Your notes should include ingredients and proportions, the date you started and completed the preparation, processing procedures, comments, and improvements to be made next time. Label finished products with the date you made the product, ingredients, and instructions for use.

Safety Precautions

Because essential oils are concentrated, highly potent substances, a working knowledge of how to use them safely is vital to the success of your efforts. The potential hazards of an essential oil depend on the compounds in the oil, the dosage and frequency used, the constitution of the person, and the method of application. One of the advantages of aromatherapy is that adding a few drops of essential oil to a carrier is fast and easy. However, you also take on the responsibility to play it safe. Since essential oils are so concentrated, it is far easier to overdose with them than with most herbal remedies. Think of just one or two drops as being the rough equivalent of an entire cup of tea.

Nontoxic essential oils used in very small amounts are extremely healing, but use too much and you're asking for trouble. The three main concerns with essential oil toxicity are irritating the skin, burning the skin, and even more worrisome, damaging the liver and/or kidneys or adversely affecting the nervous system. These latter concerns rarely occur with external application, but it is well worth being aware of these potential hazards.

The liver is the organ responsible for helping clear essential oils from the body. In our modern, polluted world, all of our livers are probably already working hard. Add the task of clearing an overdose of essential oils to the liver's job description, and it may have to work overtime. It can take years to develop obvious symptoms of liver problems, so damage that results from repeated essential oil overdose may not seem to be related. If you have a liver condition, drink a lot of alcohol, have had hepatitis or cirrhosis of the liver, or have been exposed to environmental toxins, go easy on or avoid the use of essential oils. We recommend cutting the suggested quantities of essential oils by half and, even then, using only the gentlest ones. In some cases, it is best to completely avoid them. Even more important, eliminate all exposure to synthetic fragrances.

Guidelines for Safe and Effective Essential Oil Use

Research oil purity. Use only pure essential oils derived from plants, not synthetics made in laboratories. The company selling them should indicate the botanical (Latin) name on the bottle or in their literature.

Do not use undiluted oils. Don't put undiluted essential oils directly on the skin. They can cause burning, skin irritation, and in some cases, photosensitivity (see description later in this chapter). There are a few exceptions to this rule: it is acceptable to use the nonirritating oils lavender or tea tree as spot treatments undiluted on burns, insect bites, pimples, and other skin eruptions—as long as you don't have extremely sensitive skin or have a sensitivity or allergy to the oil. While these oils are generally considered nonirritating, we've seen people experience skin reactions to both. If you ever experience skin irritation or accidentally get essential oils in the eyes, dilute with straight vegetable oil, not water. If you find any of the safe-to-use essential oils irritating but would like to use them, and if you have determined that the irritation is not due to an allergy, try massaging the diluted blend into the soles of your feet. The oil will not irritate the skin and will still enter the body.

Seek purity. Use only pure essential oils and carrier oils that have been derived from plants.

Watch for skin sensitivities. Test for sensitivities. Most people with sensitivities to synthetic fragrances are not usually sensitive to high-quality essential oils. Also, people who are allergic to chamomile tea, for example, will not necessarily be allergic to the essential oil. These types of allergies may be caused by the pollen and not the essential oil. If you are uncertain about an essential oil, do a patch test of a 2 percent dilution in the crook of an arm or on the back of the neck at the hairline (that's about 10 to 12 drops of essential oil per 1 ounce of a carrier). Twelve hours is ample time for a reaction to occur, although it will usually be obvious within half an hour. If redness or itching develops, you may want to try a less potent dilution or choose an appropriate substitute for the irritating oil.

Beware of photosensitivity. Use with caution those essential oils that result in photosensitivity. Citrus oils can irritate skin, and some of them cause uneven pigmentation of the skin upon exposure to sunlamps or sunlight. This is especially true of bergamot, which contains bergapten, a powerful photosensitizer that causes allergic reactions in some individuals (bergapten-free oil is available). Of the citrus oils, bergamot is the most photosensitizing, followed by cold-pressed lime, bitter orange, and to some degree, lemon and grapefruit. Of the lemon oils, California oil is the least photosensitizing, although labels do not usually include plant origin, so be equally cautious of all lemon oils. If you are using photosensitizing oils on your skin, do so at night, stay indoors, or wait at least eight hours before exposing your skin to ultraviolet light. Never use a tanning bed with essential oils on your skin. Citrus oils that are steam distilled as opposed to cold pressed are less concerning, but erring on the side of caution with all citrus oils is the best policy as not all labels will specify the extraction method used to obtain the oil.

Avoid mucous membrane irritants. Use with caution those essential oils that are irritating to mucous membranes (the lining of the digestive, respiratory, reproductive, and urinary tracts) and skin. Keep all essential oils away from the eyes.

Rotate essential oils. Vary the essential oils you use. Using the same facial oil blend for a long period of time is acceptable because it covers a small part of the body. However, if you use the same blend of essential oils in a body lotion or cream over your entire body every day, it is wise to alternate with a product that contains a different mix of essential oils (and thus contains different chemical constituents) every couple of weeks. This applies to any "leave-on" body product, such as lotion and massage oil, but less so for "wash-off" products, such as body wash, shampoo, and hair conditioner that you rinse off. Uninterrupted use of some of the more potent oils may expose your liver and kidneys to chemical constituents that may be harmful over time. Rotating the oils also allows each one to work in its own unique way.

Use caution for different needs. Use essential oils cautiously with those who are elderly, convalescing, or have serious health problems such as asthma, epilepsy, or heart disease. Be cautious about using essential oils during pregnancy, especially during the first trimester. Even oils that are generally safe during this time may be too stimulating for women who are prone to miscarriage. Because so many oils are best avoided in pregnancy, it is easier to list the safe ones: gentle floral oils such as rose, neroli, lavender, ylang-ylang, and chamomile, as well as the citruses, geranium,

sandalwood, spearmint, and frankincense. You'll find that aromatherapy books do not agree which oils are safe for use during pregnancy because there is no hard and fast rule to follow. Some aromatherapists are more conservative than others, with everyone taking their best educated guess. Hormone surges play havoc with pregnant women who often develop aversions to specific smells, previously favorite foods, or products containing strong essential oils, so pregnant women should be sure to follow their noses and stay away from any aromas that are unappealing, no matter how therapeutic they may be. It is especially important during pregnancy and while breast-feeding to avoid synthetic-scented products (see the section on synthetics in chapter 12). So, toss out that peach-scented body lotion and the bubblegum-scented bath salts.

SAFEST ESSENTIAL OILS DURING PREGNANCY

chamomiles

citruses (bergamot, grapefruit, lemon, lime, mandarin, orange, petitgrain, tangerine, although can be photosensitizing)

frankincense

geranium

lavender

neroli

sandalwood

spearmint

rose

ylang-ylang

Keep from young children. Keep all essential oils out of the reach of young children. Older children can be taught to respect and properly use essential oils, but they should nevertheless be supervised. In general, when treating children with essential oils, use one-fourth to one-half of the adult dosage, and select only nontoxic oils. The herbalist guideline is to adjust the dosage by weight. An adult is estimated to weigh 150 pounds, so give a child who weighs 50 pounds only one-third the number of drops as an adult. Among the best and safest essential oils for children are lavender, tangerine, mandarin, neroli, frankincense, petitgrain, and Roman chamomile.

Use caution with pets. If you're treating your pets with essential oils, be very cautious. Dogs, and especially cats, have much thinner skin than people, so essential oils absorb into their bloodstream more efficiently. You can also use the ratio designed for children. If an adult's formula calls for 2 drops, a five-pound cat would receive $1/15$ of a drop!

Avoid overexposure. Avoid overexposure to any essential oil, either through the skin or through inhalation. This may result in nausea, headache, skin irritation, emotional unease, or a "spaced-out" feeling. These are all warning signals that you've had too much, and the time required for each individual may vary greatly. Regard any of these as an early warning sign of toxicity, and immediately get fresh air to help overcome these symptoms. Try to avoid these conditions from occurring in the first place by working in a well-ventilated area, especially when you are pouring essential oils to rebottle them or to make aromatherapy blends. Use funnels and set up your aromatherapy blending area so you do not spill essential oils on your hands. If you can't adequately ventilate a small blending area or massage studio, then invest in a HEPA-type or other efficient air filter, and take a break whenever possible. Professional perfumers often work for fifteen minutes on and fifteen minutes off.

Concerning oral use. Essential oils are rarely administered orally by aromatherapists. It would likely burn the mucous membranes of your mouth. It is also easy to overdose because essential oils are so concentrated. Learning to safely ingest oils is not to be entered into lightly and requires clinical training. It is, therefore, not recommended for beginners. The contraindications, quality of oil, medical history, allergies, dosage, and many other parameters must be considered before taking essential oils internally. Remember, one of the beauties of using essential oil topically is that it can be applied over the problem area to saturate underlying tissues instead of its action being diluted as it is distributed throughout the body.

One exception is our suggestion of using essential oils to flavor foods (see chapter 10). The dosages per serving in these recipes are minimal and harmless. The other exception is commercially prepared capsules containing essential oils that are specifically designed to be swallowed. The essential oil capsules most often commercially available are diluted oregano to help eliminate intestinal parasites and peppermint oil in "enteric" capsules specifically designed to release in the large intestine to treat irritable bowel syndrome. These capsules are specially made to go through the digestive tract and not release the oil until reaching the intestine. Otherwise, the essential oil would be absorbed long before it reaches its destination. Capsules containing essential oils are also highly diluted in a vegetable oil base, or the dose would be far too strong. Even so, be careful how many you ingest, and never exceed the recommended dosage on the bottle. These doses in these capsules are too

SAFE USE OF ESSENTIAL OILS

- Use only pure essential oils derived from plants.
- Don't use undiluted essential oils on the skin.
- Test for sensitivities.
- Use with caution those essential oils that result in photosensitivity.
- Use with caution those essential oils that are irritating to mucous membranes.
- Keep all essential oils out of the reach of young children.
- If you treat your pets with essential oils, do so very cautiously.
- Vary the essential oils you use.
- Don't take essential oils orally for therapeutic purposes.
- Be cautious about using essential oils during pregnancy.
- Avoid overexposure to an essential oil, either through the skin or through inhalation.

high for children or pets, and you should follow the label instructions for use or call the manufacturer for questions on age-appropriate usage. Also, be aware that oregano essential oil is potent and must be used carefully. Read about any oil you use anywhere in or on your body in chapter 15, describing individual essential oils.

The following information is from *Essential Oil Safety: A Guide for Health Care Professionals* by Robert Tisserand and Tony Balacs, adapted with permission. We recommend this book to anyone interested in a thorough study of the safety and toxicity of essential oils. They pooled information from a variety of different types of scientific studies; however, it is not necessarily conclusive. Regard this information more as indications of these oils' toxicity ratings. We prefer to err on the side of being overcautious, so restrict your use of these essential oils until more facts are available. We often turn to using the whole herb instead since the minute amount of essential oil in the plants is already so dilute.

PHOTOSENSITIZERS

angelica	lime
bergamot	opopanax
bitter orange	rue
cumin	verbena
lemon	

MUCOUS-MEMBRANE IRRITANTS

allspice	savory
cinnamon	spearmint
clove	thyme (except linalol-type)
oregano	

SKIN IRRITANTS

cinnamon	pimento
clove	savory
dwarf pine	thyme (except linalol-type)
oregano	wintergreen

Toxic Oils

Some of the oils in the following list have limited external use; others are used for perfumery. We have included Latin names to avoid any confusion. How toxic these oils really are is controversial. Certainly, bitter almond, sage, and wintergreen are often added to aromatherapy salves and liniments for external use. Pennyroyal is used in natural bug repellents, including flea collars (never directly on fur). We think restricted amounts of "potentially toxic" oils are probably fine, except for anyone with liver or nervous system problems and young children. Until more information is available, we prefer to stick to the least toxic essential oils whenever possible. Instead, we use these as herbs instead of in their more-concentrated essential oil form. The essential oils are contained within the herbs, but are safer for use because they occur in minute amounts.

POTENTIALLY TOXIC OILS

bitter almond (*Prunus amygdalus* var. *amara*)
inula (*Inula graveolens*)
khella (*Ammi visnaga*)
mugwort (*Artemesia vulgaris*)
pennyroyal (*Mentha pelugium*)
sage (*Salvia officinalis*)
sassafras (*Sassafras albidum*) (except for safrole-free oil)
thuja (*Thuja occidentalis*)
turmeric (*Curcuma longa*)
wintergreen (*Gaultheria procumbens*)

We recommend not using the plants in the following list as essential oils at all. Keep in mind that most of these are safe when using the whole herb in herbal medicine or in the small amounts for cooking. So go ahead and flavor your food with chervil, horseradish, mustard, nutmeg, and parsley. It is only when certain compounds are concentrated in the essential oils that these oils become too strong for use. For example, the essential oils of deer tongue and tonka bean, both of which have a vanilla-like fragrance, are fine used in potpourri or any product that does not cause the oils to contact the skin. Small amounts of rue, wormwood, wormseed, and ajowan, a Middle Eastern plant, are used to treat lung problems. All of these can be used as herbal medicine but not as essential oils because they are too toxic in the oil form.

Arnica oil is a popular and effective remedy to treat bruises and sprains. In this case, the arnica plant, not the essential oil, has been infused into an oil or alcohol base. This technique releases tiny and relatively safe amounts of volatile compounds into the base, along with other components in the herb. Even so, arnica products are not recommended for use on broken skin or internally unless they are prepared homeopathically, which is based on the highly diluted energetics of the plant (liquid "mother" tinctures of arnica are made by homeopathic companies that contain the herb itself, so follow the directions on the bottle; these are not for internal use).

Camphor oil finds its way into many liniments and warming balms because it increases a sensation of heat. You'll see it in both drugstore and natural food store products. We avoid using it, especially the more toxic brown camphor, and turn to peppermint oil when we need to create the sensation of heat/cool in our products. You'll find more information in our section on making liniments (see page 79).

Beware of wormwood. The original liqueur, absinthe, a favorite of artists and writers such as Vincent van Gogh, Henri Toulousse-Lautrec, and Oscar Wilde, was flavored with wormwood (Artemisia absinthium), which must be used carefully even in its herb form. The large amount of toxic thujone in the wormwood's essential oil can cause tremors, convulsions, hallucinations, and paralysis, and it contributes to psychosis. As a result, France banned the drink in 1915, followed by other European countries and the United States. The reemerging popularity of the drink has led people to purchase the ingredients on the Internet to make it. The pure essential oil, also available on the Internet, has been purchased and used by mistake, which resulted in soreness, congestive heart failure, and imbalances in electrolytes, kinase (an ATP metabolism component), and creatinine in blood and urine. There has been one report of a death possibly from absinthe and a thirty-one-year-old man became agitated, incoherent, and had seizures.

VERY TOXIC ESSENTIAL OILS

ajowan (Prychotis ajowan, aka Carum ajowan)

arnica (Arnica montana)

boldo (Peumus boldus)

calamus (Acorus calamus)

cascarilla (Croton eluteria)

chervil (Anthriscus cerefolium)

camphor, brown and yellow (Cinnamomum camphora)

deer tongue (Carphephorus odoratissimus)

horseradish (Cochlearia armoracia, aka Armoracia rusticana)

jaborandi (Pilocarpus jaborandi)

mustard (Brassica nigra)

narcissus (Narcissus poeticus)

nutmeg (Myristica fragrans)

parsley (Petroselinum sativum, aka Carum sativum)

rue (Ruta graveolens)

santolina (Santolina chamaecyparissus)

Spanish broom (Spartium junceum)

tansy (Tanacetum vulgare)

tonka (Dipteryx odorata)

wormseed (Chenopodium ambrosioides, C. anthelminticum)

wormwood (Artemisia absinthium)

Methods of Application

There are various methods of applying essential oils and also different dilutions used in aromatherapy. Your choice depends upon how you intend to use the finished product.

DILUTIONS

The most effective way to dilute essential oils is in carrier oil. A carrier can be any high-quality vegetable oil, such as almond, apricot, hazelnut, olive, grape seed, walnut, or sesame.

A safe and effective dilution for most aromatherapy applications is 2 percent, which translates to 2 drops of essential oil per 98 drops of carrier oil, or about 10 to 12 drops per ounce. This is suitable for various types of aromatherapy. There is rarely any need to go beyond a 3 percent dilution for any purpose. In aromatherapy, more is not better; in fact, "more" may cause adverse or opposite reactions. Some oils, such as lavender, are sedating in low dilutions and stimulating in high dilutions. Use a one-half to one percent dilution on children, pregnant women, the elderly, and those with health concerns. We also recommend using 1 percent, or about 6 drops of essential oil, to an ounce of carrier for massage oil, since so much is used during the course of a massage. This lower dilution is not only better for the health of the client but also for the health of the person giving the treatment.

You can create a safe and effective remedy with one or more oils. When combining essential oils in a therapeutic blend, it is easiest for beginners to keep it simple, using three to five oils at a time in a blend.

STORAGE LIFE AND SHELF LIFE

Store essential oils away from heat and light to preserve their freshness and potency. When stored properly, they have a shelf life of several years. The citrus, fir, and pine oils have the shortest shelf life of all essential oils, so they are best used within one year, but you may extend this period by refrigerating them and by keeping them out of sunlight. The longest-lasting oils, which improve as they age, tend to be thick oils (such as sandalwood, vetiver, spikenard, and patchouli) and resinous oils (such as frankincense and myrrh).

Also store carrier oils away from heat and light to ensure their freshness. The addition of jojoba "oil" (it is actually a wax) as 10 percent of your carrier oil will extend the shelf life of your blend by slowing down oxidation, which leads to rancidity. Vitamin E oil is an excellent antioxidant; adding it to any aromatherapy blend will extend the shelf life of most vegetable oils. One or two capsules (200 to 400 IU) per 2-ounce bottle of carrier oil is adequate. It is recommended that you make only enough of a blend to last a few months. A refrigerated blend may keep six months or more. Refrigeration of all vegetable oils is highly recommended. If that is not possible, at least keep them in a cool, dark place.

CARRIER OILS

Seed and nut oils, commonly referred to as vegetable oils, are high in vitamins A, E, and F. These soothing, skin-softening, nourishing, and rich-in-nutrients oils feed the skin and are among the best carriers of essential oils. They are called *fixed oils* because their large molecules do not evaporate as do essential oils. This means that they are often extracted with heat or solvents. Whenever possible, choose either expeller-pressed or cold-pressed vegetable oils, which means they have not been exposed to temperatures above 110°F. Olive oil is a good example of a cold-pressed oil that is easily obtained. Organic oils are always preferred.

There is less difference between the various types of vegetable oils than body-care product marketers would have you believe. Unlike essential oils, vegetable oil molecules are large and do not easily penetrate the skin, making them an ideal carrier base and diluter for essential oils in cosmetic products. What distinguishes one oil from another is primarily whether it contains additional healing compounds, such as certain vitamins, and how thick it is. A few oils contain extra skin nutrients, such as gamma linoleic acid (GLA).

The "saturation rate" of carrier oils measures how thick they are. The more saturated the oil, the thicker it is, the longer it stays on the skin, and the longer its shelf life. On the other hand, unsaturated oils give the illusion that they are being absorbed into the skin when they are actually slowly evaporating. The most suitable oil depends on the application. Most body workers prefer saturated oil for massage so they have a continually oily surface on which to glide their hands, but many cosmetics use less-saturated oils that feel less thick and sticky.

Measurement Conversion Chart

10 drops	1/10 tsp.	1/60 oz.	about 1/8 dram	about 1/2 ml.
12.5 drops	1/8 tsp.	1/48 oz.	1/6 dram	about 5/8 ml.
25 drops	1/4 tsp.	1/24 oz.	1/3 dram	about 1 1/4 ml.
50 drops	1/2 tsp.	1/12 oz.	2/3 dram	about 2 1/2 ml.
100 drops	1 tsp.	1/6 oz.	1 1/3 drams	about 5 ml.
150 drops	1 1/2 tsp.	1/4 oz.	2 drams	about 13.5 ml.
300 drops	3 tsp.	1/2 oz.	4 drams	about 15 ml.
600 drops	6 tsp.	1 oz.	8 drams	about 30 ml.
24 tsp.	8 tbsp.	4 oz.	1/2 cup	about 120 ml.
48 tsp.	16 tbsp.	8 oz.	1 cup	1/2 pint
96 tsp.	32 tbsp.	16 oz.	2 cups	1 pint

DILUTION PERCENTAGES

1% dilution: 5 to 6 drops essential oil per ounce of carrier oil

2% dilution: 10 to 12 drops essential oil per ounce of carrier oil

3% dilution: 15 to 18 drops essential oil per ounce of carrier oil

People often ask, "How big is a drop?" This is a very good question, because the size of a drop varies depending on the size of the dropper opening, as well as on the temperature and the viscosity (thickness) of the essential oil. A drugstore dropper will probably be accurate enough for your purposes. Many folks use a pipette dropper from a tincture bottle.

Some people find it easier to use drops; others prefer measuring essential oils by teaspoons, which are more convenient when preparing large quantities. Whatever your preference, use the accompanying chart as a general guideline. We've rounded off the measurements for your convenience. Keep in mind that the ratios of drops to teaspoon were calculated using water, which has a medium viscosity, compared to the range of viscosities found in essential oils.

Other factors to consider are smell and color. The light smell and color of almond, hazelnut, and grape seed oils put them among the most preferred oils for cosmetics. We've found that you need to go easy on using unrefined oils, which can leave you smelling like food.

Suggested Dilutions for Various Methods of Applications

BODY OIL	2% dilution (10 to 12 drops per ounce of vegetable oil)
	1% for pregnant women, people with health concerns, and children (2 to 3 drops per ounce of vegetable oil)
MASSAGE OIL	1% dilution (6 drops per ounce of vegetable oil)
BATH	3 to 10 drops per tub, depending on the oil and its irritant potential
COMPRESS	5 drops per cup of water
INHALANT	3 to 5 drops in a bowl of hot water (never boiling)
	Caution: Never use an inhalant during an asthma attack.
DOUCHE	3 to 5 drops per quart of warm water
	Caution: Choose nonirritant oils only (such as lavender, geranium, or tea tree)
FOOT OR HAND BATH	5 to 10 drops per gallon of water
SITZ BATH	5 to 10 drops per sitz bath
FRAGRANT BODY MIST	5 to 10 drops per 4 ounces of water
ROOM SPRAY	1 to 2 drops per 4 ounces of water
GARGLE OR MOUTHWASH	1 to 2 drops per ¼ cup of water
LINIMENT	18 drops per 1 ounce carrier

Common Carrier Oils

Almond: Almond is an affordable, nourishing oil that is well suited for massage. It provides just the right slip and glide without wasting oil. This makes it very popular among massage practitioners and for use in body-care products.

Apricot: This oil is derived from the kernel of the apricot pit. Its cost is comparable to that of almond, but it has a lighter consistency. It is suitable for body oils and lotion.

Avocado: A deep green color with lots of skin-nourishing vitamins, this thick oil is very rich on its own but combines nicely with other oils. It is well suited for dry-skin conditions.

Canola: This lightweight oil is high in the unsaturated linoleic acid, making it resistant to rancidity. Easily absorbed by the skin, it is an inexpensive addition to massage blends. However, canola plants are highly sprayed with pesticides as they grow, and the seed is often genetically engineered (GMO).

Castor: Castor oil is very viscous and not often used in aromatherapy, although it may be helpful in small amounts in formulas for eczema or other dry-skin conditions. Herbalists use castor oil to make compresses, or "packs," that break down fibrous tissue, enhance immunity, and detoxify the liver. We often add essential oils to castor oil compresses to increase their effectiveness. See page 64 for instructions on how to prepare castor oil packs. The medical intuitive, Edgar Cayce, used this oil extensively. Sulfated castor oil is water soluble and often used for aromatherapy bath oils.

Cocoa Butter: Similar to coconut oil in consistency, cocoa butter is derived from cocoa beans and has a distinctive "chocolate" scent. It will overpower the odor of most essential oils, but you may use it in small proportions as a thickener in lotions and creams. When combined with neroli, the fragrance is reminiscent of an exotic, delectable dessert.

Coconut: Highest in saturated fats, coconut oil is solid at room temperature and is said to contain medium-chain fatty acids. Use it in conjunction with other oils for massage and in body lotion or cream recipes. Coconut oil has a long history of use in many tropical countries, and recent research shows that it is useful in reducing cellulite fat. It is often solvent extracted, and if so, can cause allergic reaction in sensitive individuals and is not recommended for use on the face. Seek out cold-extracted or pressed oil for use.

Corn: This oil is rarely used in aromatherapy. It comes from our familiar table corn, mostly from the germ found in the corn's kernel. Unless it is highly processed, corn oil is somewhat stable because it contains a large amount of vitamin E, which prevents oxidation. This is a relatively thin oil, which reduces its stability but also leaves the skin feeling less greasy. Another negative is that it is often sourced from genetically modified corn. The less-processed form is sold as "corn germ" oil, but it has a strong odor.

Grape Seed: Light in texture, this odorless oil is mildly astringent and useful for situations in which heavy oil is not suitable, such as a product for acne or oily skin. Unfortunately, the seed is often solvent extracted, causing sensitivity in some individuals.

Hazelnut: Light and mildly scented, this easily absorbed oil is useful in facial blends for those with a tendency toward oily skin. Hazelnut oil makes a great base for calendula infusions (see the section on herb-infused oils in chapter 5) and for all cosmetic purposes, including massage.

Jojoba: The carrier of choice for perfumery and products that require a long shelf life, jojoba is technically not an oil but a liquid wax. It's more expensive than vegetable oils, but it does not oxidize or become rancid. Use a small amount (10 percent) to extend the shelf life of all blends. Because jojoba is very similar to the sebum produced by our own skin, it is particularly beneficial in facial and body oils, and it is recommended for scalp and hair treatments. It is pressed from the seed of the desert shrub.

Kukui: The thinnest, lightest oil for the face, kukui provides just the right amount of lubrication without leaving a greasy feeling. The kukui nut, native to Hawaii, is high in linoleic and linolenic acids, and is rapidly absorbed into the skin. Hawaiians have long used it for skin conditioning after sun exposure (but it is *not* a sunscreen). Kukui nut oil has a low toxicity level, but it is a laxative and therefore should not be ingested. It has a distinct odor and is very expensive, so you may want to combine it with other oils.

Macadamia: Slightly more viscous than kukui and also from Hawaii, macadamia oil has a high concentration of oleic, palmitoleic, and palmitic acids, and it is very similar to both mink oil and sebum, our skin's own natural oil. Its lightness makes it ideal as a base for facial or hair-care products, and it combines well with kukui.

Mango: This oil is commonly referred to as *mango butter* because it is so thick and creamy. It contributes this characteristic to products that contain it. It comes from India, and unlike many fixed oils, is available as cold pressed.

Olive: This oil is a favorite for dry skin, but the odor is a little strong for some people. It may be blended with other oils and has a nice texture for massage. This is one of the best mediums for herb-infused oils intended for medicinal applications, such as in salves or rectal/vaginal suppositories. Pure olive oil has excellent stability and can be stored without refrigeration for a year. Greek olive oil, which is much greener, is more acidic than oil from Italy or California, so it is not as good for use on your face or on acned skin.

Pecan: From the edible nut of the pecan tree, this oil has a consistency that is similar to almond oil. The scent of pecan is faint, making this oil suitable to use in aromatherapy products.

Rice Bran: This oil is naturally high in mixed tocopherols (vitamin E) and ferulic acid, another natural antioxidant. It flows on smoothly and is moderately penetrating without being greasy or sticky, so it is good for massage or lotions.

VEGETABLE OIL STABILITY

The more saturated an oil, the thicker its consistency and the longer it can be stored without refrigeration. Also, the lower the iodine value, the better the oil will keep. Values can vary according to the source of the oil. Some oils also contain other ingredients that improve their preservation, such as the natural preservative found in sesame oil.

OIL	IODINE VALUE	% OF SATURATED FAT
coconut	9	91
cocoa butter	40	50
olive	84	20
peanut	92	20
rice	104	17
corn	124	17
wheat germ	125	18
walnut	138	16
soy	130	15
sesame	110	13
almond	100	5 to 10
apricot	100	5 to 10
sunflower	130	6 to 8
safflower	143	6
castor	84	3

The values are based on information from *Bailey's Industrial Oil and Fat Products,* edited by Daniel Swerm, and *Food Oils and Their Uses,* by Theodore J. Weiss, USDA research chemist.

Safflower: This oil comes from an herb that is cultivated in California and Arizona, where it turns fields aglow with its colorful flowers. Safflower oxidizes easily, especially the natural, unrefined oil, so it is rarely used in aromatherapy products. It can be used in massage blends, but don't count on having the oil around for long, even when refrigerated. Safflower is relatively thin, which can be an advantage when you don't want a product to leave a greasy feeling on the skin or stain clothing. It is one of the least expensive of the vegetable oils.

Sesame Seed: This oil contains sesomolin, a natural preservative. Sesame is readily available in India and is relatively easy to press, so it has been used in that country for a long time. It is used in Ayurvedic medicinal preparations and remains the preferred oil for Ayurvedic practitioners worldwide. It is said to be rejuvenating to the skin and body generally. The unrefined variety has a strong scent, which is the biggest drawback to using this oil alone as a carrier. However, it is a good oil as a base for herbal preparations. Sesame has some ability to refract ultraviolet rays, so it provides a small amount of skin protection from the sun.

Shea Butter: This oil comes from an African tree. It is commonly referred to as *shea butter* because it is so thick and creamy, and it contributes this characteristic to products that contain it. Shea butter can vary depending upon its origin, which is usually Ghana or the Ivory Coast, and especially whether it is refined or unrefined.

Soybean: First introduced from Asia to the United States, this oil was rarely used before 1950 but now accounts for more than 65 percent of all oil used commercially in the United States. Because of its low oil content (16 to 18 percent), it is often solvent extracted. Soybean oil is high in linoleic acid and susceptible to oxidation. Use as part of a massage blend, but it is best sourced from non-GMO beans.

Squalene: This is a fraction derived from natural oils. Vegetable sources of this oil product are olive, wheat germ, and rice bran, but squalene can also be derived from shark liver oil. It is used as a fixative in perfumes and as a bactericide, and it is very expensive; 5 to 10 percent in a carrier blend is sufficient. Human sebum is 25 percent squalene, so it is thought to absorb particularly well into the skin.

Wheat Germ: Too thick and rich on its own, this oil is a useful addition to any carrier blend. It is high in vitamin

B, and because it contains the antioxidant vitamins A and E, it will help extend the shelf life of your blends. Add 10 percent to your carrier oil blend.

Specialty Carrier Oils

These oils are very rich, thick, strongly scented, and have more therapeutic properties than the typical fixed or vegetable oils described above. Use the oils sparingly in a carrier blend (10 percent); because they are expensive, price alone will probably keep you from using too much. Many are taken orally.

Black Cumin *(Nigella sativa):* These seeds have been used as food and medicine since ancient times in their native Near East, North Africa, and South Eastern Europe. The oil is a combination of essential and fixed oils that contain GLA and seem to boost the immune system in several ways, including promoting activity of the natural killer cells. It's a respiratory stimulant that reduces spasms, dilates bronchioles, and inhibits histamine, so it is sometime used for asthma. It also helps destroy fungal and bacterial infections, inhibiting twenty-plus bacteria, including staph, *E. coli*, and salmonella, and it has been shown to increase the activity of antibacterial drugs when used together. Studies show that it relieves pain and is more sedating than the drug chlorpromazine, possibly by indirectly activating opioid brain receptors. Don't confuse it with the related love-in-a-mist *(N. damascena)* that is grown as an ornamental flower, with the black cumin *(Bunium persicum)* from Central Asia and Russia that is cultivated and distilled into essential oil in India for flavoring, or with cumin essential oil *(Cuminum cyminum)* itself. Nigella oil is strongly scented.

Borage, Evening Primrose, Black Currant: The oils in this group are high in GLA, an important fatty acid that helps maintain healthy skin and repair skin damaged by the sun. GLA has been shown to help control hormone-like prostaglandins responsible for menstrual cramps and probably responsible for arthritic pain and inflammation. It also enhances immunity and reduces allergic response.

Studies show borage oil, probably due to GLA, can help speed recovery from breast cancer. The rejuvenating effects are especially useful for treating mature skin. They also have a short shelf life.

Rose Hip Seed *(Rosa rubiginosa):* Another oil high in GLA, oil from the seeds in rose hip is the very best for regenerative skin care. Combine it with infused calendula oil to treat stretch marks, burns, or scars. It has a short shelf life, so make small amounts and keep it refrigerated.

Sea Buckthorn *(Hippophae rhamnoides):* Native to Russia and China, the oil is used in Traditional Chinese Medicine (TCM) to treat problems associated with mucous membranes. In clinical studies, the oil has been shown to reduce injury and inflammation from stomach ulcers and hasten healing. The seeds from the edible berries are a potent antioxidant that reduces redness, promotes skin repair, and, in one study, was shown to help people with dermatitis. In fact, this is one of the most beneficial oils for aging skin. However, it is not always easy to find.

Tamanu *(Calophyllum inophyllum):* This is a native of tropical Asia and used in many Polynesian islands; it is considered sacred. This oil is known as *kamanu* or *kamani* in Hawaii, *tamanu* in the South Seas, and *fetau* in Samoa. Another variety, *faraha,* is from Madagascar. It is nontoxic and nonirritating. Anti-inflammatory and pain-relieving properties make *Calophyllum* suitable for sciatica, rheumatism, and shingles. It is antibacterial and nonirritating to mucous membranes and can be used to treat vaginitis and cervical erosion, infected wounds, eczema, psoriasis, chapped skin, cracked nipples, chemical or heat burns, and anal fissures. Modern research shows that this oil is very effective in treating acne. Historically, it was used extensively to treat leprosy.

Other Seed Oils: New to the market, raspberry (red and black), pomegranate, and cranberry oils are highly therapeutic for both internal and external use.

Herbal Preparations

Never pass up the opportunity to use herbs in your aromatherapy formulations. When the essential oil of a plant is deemed too strong for a particular person or application, the herb itself in tea or tincture form is likely a safe and effective substitute. When used together, whole plants and essential oils often create a synergy with greater potential for healing than either used alone.

Herb quality is as important to herbalism as purity of essential oils is to aromatherapy. Growing your own herbs is ideal, but we realize that many of you will buy herbs from an herb or natural food store. The good news is that it is much easier to determine good herb quality by smelling, seeing, and tasting than it is with essential oils. Dried herbs should not be brown and lifeless; they should be fragrant, colorful, and, ideally, organically grown or responsibly and sustainably picked in the wild. Buying directly from the grower, wildcrafter (one who picks wild herbs), or local sources such as farmers' markets, where you can inquire about growing methods, is probably the next best thing to growing your own herbs.

The following recipes provide a useful basis for making basic herbal preparations. They can either be made with individual herbs ("simples") or a combination of herbs ("compounds"). So get creative! If you need more detailed information on the specific uses of individual herbs or how to grow them, consult a good herb book such as Kathi Keville's *Herbs: An Illustrated Encyclopedia,* or attend one of her classes.

You can also use massage oils, skin lotions, and some creams that you purchase already prepared as a base for your products. Many massage practitioners use water dispersible massage oil because it washes out and doesn't stain the massage table sheets. Simply stir in drops of essential oil as you would do with any vegetable oil base, using the same proportions, which are generally 8 to 12 drops per ounce. Creams may or may not work, depending on their ingredients and what type of emulsifier was used.

EXAMPLES OF HERB-INFUSED OILS

Alkanet: This is an infusion of alkanet root in vegetable oil. Because of its brilliant color, it is used as a pink to red coloring for cosmetic preparations such as lip balms or cheek tints. The color's intensity depends on the amount of alkanet used. We like to have some alkanet-infused oil on hand so we can add a rosy color to products.

Calendula: Very healing to the skin in all cosmetic applications, calendula is specifically recommended for burns and is also antimicrobial, making it suitable for the treatment of many types of skin infections. A carbon dioxide extract of calendula is very concentrated and tarlike. It can be diluted in vegetable oil and added to any essential oil preparation. Calendula contains a small amount of volatile oil. It is available for sale, though quite expensive. We make our own oil infusion from flowers picked from our gardens. Do not confuse it with marigold (*Tagetes species*) essential oil, which is irritating to the skin.

Neem: Derived from a tree native to India, neem is used to treat a number of skin diseases as an astringent, antibacterial, and antiviral. It is also a preservative. The oil has a long history of use in the treatment of hair loss, dandruff, excess sebum production, brittle nails, nail fungus, and gum infections. This herb is hard to find, but commercially prepared oil can be purchased.

St. John's wort: Excellent for bruises, inflammation, and nerve damage, St. John's wort is made from the fresh flowering tops of the plant to obtain the desired deep red oil that is high in the healing constituent hypericin. Use it on a damaged complexion or on injured skin. It can also help reduce pain when applied directly on or over the painful area and is said to help repair nerve damage. St. John's wort contains a small amount of essential oil. The essential oil is available for sale, although it is quite expensive. If you use St. John's wort as the base oil for a cream or lotion, it will lend a reddish color to the product.

Yarrow: For treating the genitourinary system (see chapter 6).

PREPARING HERB-INFUSED OILS

Oils made by macerating (steeping) herbs in vegetable oil are called *infused oils*. These oils can be used instead of plain carrier oils in all of your aromatherapy preparations.

Finely crush (or coarsely grind) 1 cup of dried herbs in a blender. Place the herbs in a wide-mouth jar, and add enough oil to cover. Check the mixture in a day or two; you may need to add a bit more oil. Keep the mixture in a warm place and shake daily. The ideal temperature is 70 to 90°F, but fluctuations in temperature will not harm the oil. Let the mixture steep for 1 to 2 weeks; by this time, the oil should have taken on the color, aroma, and healing properties of the herb.

Strain the oil through a fine kitchen strainer, or through cheesecloth, muslin, or a thin dishcloth. Most of the oil will drain out. To get every precious drop, press with the back of a spoon or wring out as much oil as possible. Compost the herbs and store the infused oil in the refrigerator.

There are many variations on this preparation. Choose a vegetable oil such as olive oil for medicinal preparations such as salves; choose hazelnut, kukui, macadamia, or other light oils for cosmetic applications or massage. It is difficult to give exact measurements for each herb, because they are different in texture, weight, and volume. To double the strength, you can add a new batch of dried herbs to the once-infused oil. This is called a *double infusion*.

Another way to make infused oils is on the stove top. Place the dried herbs in a pot, and cover them with oil. Gently warm the herb mixture over low heat (about 100°F) without a lid, stirring occasionally (be careful not to deep-fry your herbs)! After about 6 hours, strain, cool, and bottle. A preferred method and the safest way to protect and extract the herbs is to follow this same procedure in a double boiler (over heated water instead of directly on the stove).

Some people like to use fresh herbs, although the water in fresh plants may cause the oil to mold and spoil. However, some oils—St. John's wort for example—are best when made fresh. When using fresh plants, wilt the plant material overnight to eliminate some of the water, then finely chop or crush. Process as instructed above for dry herbs. Be sure that all the plant material is submerged and with no air bubbles. Stirring the oil and herb mix with a chopstick helps release all of the air.

When straining the oil, simply let the mixture drip; wringing or pressing will give you more oil, but also more water, which is undesirable. When the water from the fresh plant has settled in the bottom of the jar, pour the oil off the top and discard the water (be prepared to lose a little oil).

Don't confine yourself to making only medicinal or cosmetic oils. Experiment with creating culinary oils too. Try a combination of basil, oregano, rosemary, and garlic infused in olive oil. It's great on pasta or as a dipping oil for French bread!

Always keep a meticulous record of how you make your herbal preparations. Your notes should include ingredients and proportions, the date you started and completed the preparations, processing procedures, comments, and possible improvements for next time. Label your finished products with the date you made the product, the ingredients, and instructions for use.

HERBAL BOLUSES

Herbal boluses are vaginal or rectal suppositories used to treat chronic infections, nonspecific vaginitis, cysts, and hemorrhoids (see "Reproductive System" in chapter 6).

⅛ cup finely powdered herbs (about two tablespoons)

¼ cup cocoa butter

10 to 15 drops appropriate essential oil

Melt the cocoa butter over low heat, and add the powdered herbs to form a thick, pliable paste. Add the essential oil. Form a long, thin trough from aluminum foil, and pour the mixture into the trough. Refrigerate until firm. Remove the hardened mixture and use a warm knife to cut it into 1½-inch lengths. Date, label, and store the boluses in a container in the refrigerator.

For treatment, insert one bolus each evening for 7 days. You may want to wear a panty liner to avoid soiling clothes. Women may want to gently douche every couple of days when using vaginal boluses.

Alternative: Instead of making a foil trough, purchase a flexible candy mold that is the appropriate size and freeze the mixture in that. One student found little bear molds that were the perfect size!

HERBAL SALVES

1 cup herb-infused oil

¾ ounce beeswax, shaved

Warm the herb-infused oil in a pan and add the beeswax (more beeswax creates a salve with a firmer consistency that won't melt in summer temperatures). You can shave the beeswax with a wide-hole cheese grater (for a quick cleanup, heat the grater over the kitchen stove, and wipe it with paper towels). Add essential oils at the end, after the salves cool a bit, so that the oils do not evaporate. (You can also add the essential oils to the individual jars before pouring.)

Make lip balms the same way as salves, but use 1 ounce beeswax for a firmer consistency.

To check the consistency of your salve or lip balm before it cools and hardens, try this trick: Put a spoon in the freezer for 2 minutes, wipe it dry, and dip the cold spoon into your warm salve. Feel the consistency and decide if you need more beeswax or more oil.

HERB TEA: INFUSIONS AND DECOCTIONS

For infusions, pour boiling water over fresh or dried herbs, let them steep, and cover (to keep in the precious volatile oils) for five to ten minutes, strain, and drink.

Infusions are good for delicate plant parts (such as leaves, blossoms, or fruits) or seeds and roots that are high in volatile oils. The amount of herb varies, but the general rule is to use 1 teaspoon dried herb (or 1 tablespoon fresh herb) per cup of water.

For hard plant parts, such as roots, barks, twigs, and some seeds, decoctions are preferable. We prefer to soak the herbs in cold water overnight, bring the water and herbs to a boil, then lower the heat and simmer, covered, for at least fifteen minutes. Roots and seeds that are high in volatile oils, such as ginger and valerian roots, or fennel and anise seeds, should be infused.

To make tea with both the leaves and roots, start by soaking the herbs overnight in the refrigerator, then bring to a boil, remove from the heat, and steep for fifteen minutes. You can also decoct the roots first, remove from heat, add the leaves to the decoction, and steep.

Teas are a great addition to bathwater, especially for those with highly sensitive skin who don't want to risk irritation from essential oils. Almost any herb or essential oil, alone or in combination, will do. Refrigeration is acceptable for up to three days.

HERBAL TINCTURES

Tinctures are best made with single herbs, and you can then mix them together to make compounds or formulas. This helps avoid undesirable constituent interactions that can occur when herbs are tinctured together. It also allows more flexibility in blending tinctures into different combinations. Tinctures are taken orally, typically 15 to 30 drops three times a day, mixed with a little water or juice. One advantage that herbal tinctures have over teas is that they need no refrigeration, remain potent for many years, take up little storage space, and are fast and easy to use, fitting into any busy lifestyle. Tinctures are also quickly and easily absorbed by the body, and they are easy to travel with when making tea is not possible.

fresh or dried herbs

vodka to cover (called a menstruum)

Chop or grind top quality herbs before tincturing to expose more surface area of the plant to the vodka, which contains water and alcohol, which breaks down the plant matter and extracts its qualities. Put the herbs in a jar with a tight-fitting lid, and cover with the menstruum. The proportion of herb to vodka is hard to specify, because the weight-to-volume of each herb varies so much. Just make sure that the herb is completely covered (and check in a few days in case you need to add more vodka). Tightly cover the jar, and let the herbs soak for 2 weeks in a cool, dark place, shaking daily, and then strain. You'll be surprised to find how easy this is, and it costs much less than commercial tinctures.

HERBAL VINEGARS

This vinegar can be used to make the fourteenth-century "Queen of Hungary water," other facial toners, hair rinses, baths, and douches (see chapter 8). In tincturing, vinegar also can be used as a substitute for alcohol for those who are alcohol-intolerant, but it is not a good menstruum for extracting the resinous constituents contained in certain plants. Herbal vinegars are suitable in the kitchen.

fresh or dried herbs

vinegar to cover

Make sure the fresh or dried herbs are completely covered by the vinegar. Shake daily for 2 weeks and then strain. If using for cosmetic application, add essential oils to the vinegar after straining, but remember to shake well before use—essential oils do not mix with watery carriers.

CHAPTER 6

Therapeutics

IN THIS CHAPTER we explain how essential oils help to support healing the body. We have divided the chapter into sections dealing with the major systems in the body—the heart and circulatory, digestive, respiratory, musculoskeletal, nervous, glandular, urinary, reproductive, dermal, and immune systems—as well as a section on therapeutics and children. We suggest how to treat common first aid–type ailments, things you would normally treat at home without the care of a doctor: the common cold, headache, a bout of indigestion, PMS, simple burns, bites and stings, and muscular aches and pains. You may have formerly treated such disorders with over-the-counter drugs. The biochemical complexity of essential oils—most of which cannot be synthetically duplicated—allows them to act on many levels and gives them multiple healing potential. You will not only achieve health dividends but also financial savings.

As herbalists and aromatherapists, we are eclectic in our approach to healing, using whatever remedy seems most appropriate. In some cases, we use aromatherapy exclusively; in others, we find that combining aromatherapy with herbs is more effective. To help you integrate the two modalities, we offer "herbal adjuncts," which are generally taken several times a day in teas, tinctures, capsules, or tablets.

Because true holistic healing requires individual assessment and the formation of a blend specific to each person, we do not give many recipes for specific ailments. We understand that some guidelines are needed, however, so we give formula examples for general conditions in each section to get you started. Our goal is to give you the tools and confidence you need to develop your own blends as your understanding of working with essential oils increases. Refer to charts and chapter 15.

Essential oils are extremely concentrated. Most of them are at least fifty times more potent than the herb from which they are derived. In her book *Aromatherapy: The Complete Guide to Plant and Flower Essences for Health and Beauty,* Daniele Ryman states that one drop of essential oil often represents the potency of one ounce of plant material. This gives you an idea of their healing potential—and of the potential hazards of improperly using essential oils.

Only about 5 percent of the essential oils produced today are used in aromatherapy, but there are plenty from which to choose. In fact, if you become familiar with only ten to fifteen essential oils, you'll be able to treat many common problems (it is better to know a few essential oils well than to know a little about many oils.)

Essential oils can be used as muscle relaxants (marjoram and black pepper), digestive tonics (cardamom and mint), circulatory stimulants (rosemary and basil), respiratory "mucolytics" (eucalyptus and rosemary verbenone), and hormone modulators (clary sage and fennel). Many repair injured cells (lavender and helichrysum); others help carry away metabolic waste (grapefruit and juniper). In addition, a number of essential oils enhance immunity (niaouli and tea tree), working with the body to heal itself. They are capable of stimulating the production of phagocytes (white blood cells that attack invaders), and some (tea tree and lavender) are antitoxic for insect bites and stings.

Many essential oils have been proven effective against fungi and yeast (tea tree, lavender, and geranium), parasites (bergamot), and viruses (cinnamon, thyme, and *Eucalyptus radiata*). Others fight infection with amazing effectiveness, killing bacteria by disrupting their life cycles. According to Jean-Claude Lapraz, MD, a specialist in essential oils, most essential oils slightly lower the pH of the blood, creating an inhospitable environment for bacteria, which thrive in alkaline environments.

Unlike conventional antibiotic drugs, which may cause undesirable side effects, essential oils are "probiotic": they not only kill pathogenic bacteria, but they also tend to leave beneficial bacteria (intestinal flora) intact. This seems to be an exclusive prerogative of natural remedies and remains a mystery to the scientific community. Also, bacteria typically do not acquire a resistance to essential oils, as they so often do to antibiotic drugs.

Essential oils act quickly in the body. Some are detectable in the breath within minutes after skin application and are eliminated from the body within several hours. Repeated applications may be required, especially when treating acute disorders that require a constant level of

Kit of Ten Basic Essential Oils

LAVENDER	overall first aid oil, antiviral and antibacterial, boosts immunity, antidepressant, anti-inflammatory, antispasmodic
CHAMOMILE	anti-inflammatory, antiallergenic, antidepressant, digestive, relaxant
MARJORAM	antispasmodic, anti-inflammatory, antiseptic
ROSEMARY	relieves pain, decongestant, circulatory tonic
TEA TREE	antifungal, antiyeast, antibacterial
CYPRESS	astringent, circulatory tonic, antiseptic
PEPPERMINT	digestive, clears sinuses, antiseptic, decongestant, stimulant
EUCALYPTUS	decongestant, antiviral, antibacterial, stimulant
BERGAMOT	antidepressant, antiparasitic, anti-inflammatory
GERANIUM	balancing to mind and body, antifungal, anti-inflammatory

essential oil activity in the body. Remember that less is more when it comes to aromatherapy. Consistent, low doses are safest and the most effective.

One advantage of aromatherapy treatments is that they don't need to work their way through the entire body to treat a particular area. Most of the essential oils suggested in this section are intended for dilution in carrier oils. You can massage these diluted oils directly over the area that needs treatment—on the chest, for example, to treat congested lungs, or on the stomach for cases of indigestion. Application by inhalation or bath is also appropriate for many treatments.

Essential oils are perfectly safe when used in the suggested dilutions, although applications complicated by pregnancy, epilepsy, serious health problems, and some medications do call for caution. A patch test is recommended before using any formula (see "Safety Precautions" in chapter 5 for further information on safety, applications, dilutions, and carrier oils; please also note the various "considerations" in chapter 15).

Health and vitality depend on the harmonious and collective functioning of each organ in the body. Therefore, the identification and separation of systems and their association with various oils is a simplification, albeit a necessary one. Also, because most plants have multiple actions, many are listed below for more than one system or symptom.

Heart and Circulatory System

The circulatory system transports blood throughout the body. It includes the heart and the blood vessels, as well as the lymphatic system, which supplies nutrients and moves cellular fluid through the system, cleansing the body of waste. Lymph nodes located throughout the body—but particularly in the throat, groin, breasts, and under the arms—act as centers for filtering the blood.

One of the best essential oils for a lymphatic massage is true bay *(Laurus nobilis);* lemon and grapefruit are also good. (A good carrier oil for these essential oils is herbal infused oil of calendula.) Use infused oils from the herbs basil, rosemary, thyme, marjoram, and clove to improve general circulation. Stress-related heart problems respond well to a sedating massage of the essential oils of melissa, neroli, lavender, and ylang-ylang. Along with marjoram and ginger, these oils also help normalize high blood pressure. Studies show that just sniffing neroli can lower high blood pressure.

Chamomile, myrtle, and cypress ease the inflammation and pain of varicose veins, phlebitis, and hemorrhoids; frankincense constricts distended veins. All of these oils are especially effective in an infused oil St. John's wort. If the skin is ulcerated and broken, apply a compress of carrot seed essential oil. Add a few drops of oil to about 2 cups of water, soak a cloth in the water, wring it out, and place over the area.

FORMULA FOR VARICOSE VEINS

6 drops cypress essential oil

3 drops myrtle essential oil

3 drops German chamomile essential oil

2 drops frankincense essential oil *(optional)*

1 ounce St. John's wort–infused oil

Combine ingredients. Apply externally. You can also make this into a salve by heating the oil and adding ½ teaspoon shaved beeswax before adding the essential oils.

Herbal adjuncts: Among the herbs that strengthen heart and reduce blood pressure are hawthorn flower and berry and motherwort. Lymphatic cleansers include echinacea, cleavers, and Oregon grape root, which may be taken as teas, tinctures, or capsules.

The kitchen cupboard supplies many spices whose essential oils enhance circulation, make blood vessels more elastic, and inhibit blood clotting. These include garlic, onion, cayenne, and ginger. Ginger has a normalizing effect; it can either raise blood pressure by restricting external blood flow or lower it by dilating surface blood vessels. Garlic and onion also lower high blood pressure. Lemongrass contains five different compounds that inhibit blood clotting.

Digestive System

Our well-being is largely influenced by how effectively we process and assimilate nutrients and how thoroughly we eliminate waste. What we eat is important, but so are how and when we eat. Creating a peaceful environment, eating fresh whole foods in season, and proper elimination constitute a good start toward digestive harmony.

Aromas signal the brain that food is on the way, so simply sniffing a pleasant food aroma, such as pasta sauce or baking bread, begins a chain reaction that sets the stomach grumbling in anticipation. The response is almost immediate, as digestive fluids are released in the mouth, stomach, and small intestine.

The essential oils found in common culinary herbs—such as rosemary, basil, cumin, anise, coriander, ginger, and cinnamon—not only make food tasty but also help digestion. In addition, some spices have special applications: cumin relieves indigestion-promoted headaches, rosemary improves poor food absorption, and basil helps overcome nausea, even from chemotherapy or radiation treatments when conventional antinausea drugs have had little effect. Lemongrass is used in Southeast Asia to relieve indigestion. To decrease appetite, try dill and fennel.

If you are plagued by ulcers or stomach acidity, try chamomile and sandalwood. Fennel seed and melissa relax the stomach muscles while soothing irritation and inflammation. Try a small amount of honey flavored with one of these oils in a cup of herb tea (see chapter 10 for instructions on how to make this honey).

Poor digestion can also result from too little hydrochloric acid, which is needed to break down protein. Improperly digested protein is thought to be a cause of certain food allergies. Black pepper and juniper berry both increase stomach acid. Use these essential oils in a massage blend over the stomach, add fresh-ground pepper to your meal, or chew a couple of juniper berries before eating.

As an herb, ginger is one of the best remedies for nausea—especially motion or morning sickness—with peppermint tea running a close second. The British medical journal *Lancet* reported that ginger is more effective than the popular antihistamine drug Dramamine for preventing motion sickness, and unlike the drug, ginger doesn't leave you feeling sluggish. You can also use these essential oils in a 2 percent massage blend, although herb teas are both effective and tasty. Even eating ginger cookies, a piece of crystallized ginger (sold in Chinese food stores), or peppermint candy can help.

TUMMY SOOTHER MASSAGE OIL

For kids, use half the number of drops in the recipe.

   5 drops chamomile essential oil
   3 drops dill essential oil
   2 drops ginger essential oil
   2 drops peppermint essential oil
   1 ounce carrier oil

Combine the oils and gently massage the abdomen.

DIGESTIVE TONIC HERBAL TEA

   1 teaspoon fresh ginger root (or ½ teaspoon powdered)
   ¼ teaspoon cinnamon bark
   1 teaspoon peppermint leaf
   ¼ teaspoon anise seed
   ¼ teaspoon cardamom
   3 cups water, boiling

Mix the herbs together, pour water over them, cover, and steep. Drink a cup 30 minutes after your meal. The hot water will naturally extract the essential oils from the herbs.

NATURAL GINGER ALE

   3 cups digestive tea (see previous recipe)
   ¼ cup honey
   1 cup carbonated water
   1 lemon slice

Stir the honey into warm tea. Add carbonated water and lemon just before serving.

BOWEL PROBLEMS

The bowels can become irritated or infected by tainted foods. Even excitement or stress can agitate the bowels. Ginger, peppermint, fennel, coriander, and dill help counter gas. Peppermint is specific for irritable bowel syndrome. For constipation, use rosemary or black pepper.

For diarrhea, use cypress, cinnamon, and myrrh. These herbs can be used as teas, or substitute oils of choice and follow the directions for "Tummy Soother Massage Oil" in the previous section.

Garlic is one of the best ways to eliminate worms for the whole family, including pets. Eat fresh garlic during meals or take it in capsules. Rosemary, thyme, tea tree, and chamomile kill many types of worms; chamomile also decreases the resulting intestinal inflammation. Researchers have discovered that all forty-two components in ginger oil that is used in East Africa to kill parasites will also, in isolation, kill roundworms in the intestine (in studies, some of these compounds actually worked better than the commonly prescribed piperazine-citrate preparations). These oils can also be used in a massage over the abdomen area as a part of a more inclusive treatment.

LIVER TONIC

The liver is also involved in digestion, and its health affects the entire body.

  3 drops chamomile essential oil

  3 drops lemon essential oil

  3 drops carrot essential oil

  3 drops helichrysum essential oil

  1 ounce carrier oil

Combine ingredients (or use any of these oils alone). Massage the oil over the liver, or use it in a bath.

Herbal adjuncts: Use at least one aromatic herb with any remedy for diarrhea or constipation to prevent intestinal cramping. Turn to herbal "bitters," such as gentian, Oregon grape root, barberry, and dandelion root to treat long-term digestive problems such as chronic diarrhea, constipation, indigestion, and certain food allergies. These bitter tonics are best taken before meals. Laxatives include the mild-acting yellow dock or the stronger cascara bark and senna leaf.

To treat diarrhea, use blackberry root tincture. For stomach ulcers or overacidity, use soothing slippery elm and marshmallow, antispasmodic chamomile or wild yam,

the natural antacid meadowsweet, and licorice, which helps diminish ulcers.

To eliminate worms, eat raw carrots, garlic, and pumpkin seeds as well as fibrous vegetables, and restrict carbohydrates and milk products (worms thrive on their sugars). Then flush everything out with an herbal laxative. Repeat the treatment in a week to kill any newly hatched parasites.

Respiratory System

Afflictions of the respiratory system include irritation and infection of the ears, nose, and throat. Respiratory problems also may involve congestion, which can be decreased by inhaling rosemary (especially the verbenone type), hyssop (use var. *decumbens* only), tea tree, eucalyptus, lavender, or peppermint. Cypress helps dry up a persistent runny nose; peppermint, tea tree, and eucalyptus reduce sinus infections; and anise and cypress help reduce coughing.

Many asthma sufferers wage a constant battle with low-level congestion. It is difficult to use essential oils during an asthma attack, but better to treat asthmatics between attacks with a chest rub of German chamomile, frankincense, or lavender (you can use hyssop, but be very careful to only use var. *decumbens,* as it lacks the harmful ketones present in regular hyssop oil). During an asthma attack, you can treat the *feet* with these oils, but never use them directly on the chest or back because such a direct application can be too strong. One technique for treating babies with asthma is to hold them over steaming water with a few drops of lavender oil added. Put a few inches of hot water in a bathtub or sink, add lavender, and then hold the baby so he or she can breathe in the steam (be careful not to let the baby touch the steaming hot water). Severe episodes require medical attention.

ESSENTIAL OILS AS INHALANTS

It is theorized that the compound called *chamazulene* in chamomile releases cortisone from the adrenals to act as an anti-inflammatory during an asthma attack. We disagree with the herb books that recommend against using chamomile to treat hay fever and also asthma. Erroneous reports started circulating in the 1980s that if you had allergies to ragweed and similar plants, you were probably also allergic to chamomile. Not so. In fact, studies have shown chamomile to be very safe and to have a low potential to cause allergies, likely because most people are allergic to the pollen of many plants, which is not in the essential oils. We always recommend patch testing with highly allergic people, however.

The source of 90 percent of respiratory ailments is a virus. Many essential oils are antiviral so you can use them as an effective treatment. Also, turn to essential oils as preventatives to fend off illness when the cold and flu season arrives, the kids start school, or you will be traveling.

Oils of sandalwood, rosemary, peppermint, ravensara, tea tree, eucalyptus, bergamot, black pepper, melissa, and hyssop help inhibit most flu viruses. Lemon and eucalyptus oils are effective against bacteria that cause staph, strep, and pneumonia infections. A few drops in a basin of hot water make an effective vapor steam; a couple of drops in water is sufficient as an antiseptic gargle or inhalant.

Steam treatment carries essential oils directly to sinuses and lungs, and it provides warm, moist air to help open nasal and bronchial passages. To do a steam, boil a pan of water, turn off the heat, and cool for 1 minute. Add 3 to 6 drops of essential oils to the water, and use a towel to corral the steam around your head as you breathe deeply. Essential oils can also be used in many humidifiers or as an ingredient in steamy hot bathwater.

If steaming is impractical—at the office, say, or while traveling—inhale a handkerchief or tissue scented with your choice of one or a combination of these essential oils. We know people who carry a scented nose and mouth mask—they now come in designer colors!—when they travel to certain countries. You can scent any of these items with a drop or two of a single oil. If you enclose them in a plastic bag, they will retain their scent for days. As needed, apply more oil. Or you can use a natural-products nasal inhalant, which is sold in natural food stores, or you can make your own very simply.

HOMEMADE NASAL INHALANT

    2 drops eucalyptus essential oil
    2 drops rosemary essential oil
    1 drop peppermint essential oil
    1 tablespoon rock salt

Combine ingredients. Place a few pieces of rock salt in a vial and add the oils. The salt will quickly absorb the oil. Inhale as needed.

An aromatic diffuser—a glass piece (often hand-blown) connected to a small electrical air compressor—disinfects the atmosphere by releasing droplets of essential oil as a cool, micronized mist. One advantage to using a diffuser is that the essential oil vapor can be directed near (not directly into) the nose, throat, or even ear passages. It can be turned on in a sickroom for 10 to 15 minutes every hour to clear airborne bacteria.

Do not use thick oils such as vetiver, sandalwood, vanilla, myrrh, or benzoin in a diffuser unless you first dilute them with thin oil—such as the citruses, eucalyptus, or rosemary—or mix them with alcohol. If oils sit too long in a diffuser, they oxidize and thicken, clogging your apparatus. Expressed citrus oils may clog a diffuser due to sediment. To clean or unclog it, soak the glass unit in alcohol, and unplug the opening with a pin or toothpick. Rinse and air dry.

Diluted essential oils can also be used as a throat spray through "nebulization." A nebulizer sprayer, with a long spout that reaches to the back of the throat, used to be a standard item in the home medicine cabinet. A perfume atomizer or spray bottle will work just as well to mist toward the back of a sore throat with oil diluted in water.

If you don't have a diffuser, simply combine water and essential oils in a spray bottle. Studies show that a 2 percent dilution of eucalyptus oil kills 70 percent of airborne staph bacteria (about 10 to 12 drops of essential oil per ounce of water.)

DISINFECTANT ROOM SPRAY

The following combination is also suitable as a chest rub to ease congestion. Just replace the water in the recipe with carrier oil.

> 3 drops eucalyptus essential oil
>
> 1 drop peppermint essential oil
>
> 2 drops pine essential oil
>
> 1 drop tea tree or rosemary essential oil
>
> 2 drops bergamot essential oil
>
> 1 ounce water

Combine ingredients and shake well before using.

THROAT SPRAY/GARGLE

Generations of Europeans, especially singers, have gargled with sage, thyme, or marjoram herbal tea sweetened with honey to relieve laryngitis and tonsillitis. A few drops of cypress or lemon essential oils diluted in two ounces of water may also do the trick. In case of a sore throat, gargle frequently, at least every half hour.

> ½ cup warm thyme or sage herb tea
>
> 2 drops cypress essential oil
>
> 2 drops lemon essential oil
>
> 2 drops tea tree essential oil

Before each use, shake well to disperse the oils. For a gargle, dissolve half a teaspoon of salt in the solution.

VAPOR BALM

For lung congestion, you can rub a salve or a massage oil containing essential oils over the chest, back, and throat. The oils will be absorbed through the skin and lungs as the vapor is inhaled. Place a piece of flannel fabric on the chest after rubbing in the oil to increase warmth. Commercial "vapor balms" still use derivatives of essential oils (or their synthetic-oil counterparts)—such as thymol from thyme and menthol from mint—in a petroleum ointment base. Natural alternatives are also sold in natural-food stores.

> 1 teaspoon peppermint essential oil
>
> 1 teaspoon eucalyptus essential oil
>
> ½ teaspoon thyme essential oil (chemotype linalol is best)
>
> ½ cup olive oil
>
> ¾ ounce shaved beeswax

Melt the beeswax into olive oil over very low heat. Cool a bit, add essential oils, and stir (be sure to keep your face away from the oils as you stir them in). Allow the mixture to harden. Store at room temperature. Note: This is a higher than normal amount of essential oils, since the mixture is used over a small area rather than the whole body.

POULTICE

Poultices are an age-old remedy for chest congestion. A ginger or onion compress on the chest breaks up lung congestion and makes breathing easier. Onions also help curb asthma and allergic reactions.

> 1 onion, chopped
>
> ¼ cup grated ginger
>
> water

Lightly cook the ingredients together in a little water until soft. Cool slightly, mash, and apply to the chest while still warm. Cover with a soft cloth.

Herbal adjuncts: Herbs that loosen mucus from the lungs include elecampane, horehound, and mullein. Respiratory relaxants, such as wild cherry bark and wild lettuce, are used in cases of extreme spasmodic coughing. Demulcent herbs, which soothe inflamed mucous membranes, include flaxseed, marshmallow root, and licorice. Use these herbs in teas, tinctures, pills, or syrup.

Ears and Eyes

Antiseptic essential oils such as lavender and tea tree can be diluted in olive oil and rubbed around the outside of—never in—the ear and over the lymph nodes on the side of the neck. If the ear problem is caused by a throat infection, be sure to also use an antiseptic gargle. Hot compresses soothe pain in the ears. Always treat both ears, even if only one hurts, and continue treatment for several days after the pain is gone to make sure the condition does not return.

EAR RUB

> 3 drops lavender essential oil
>
> 3 drops tea tree essential oil
>
> 6 drops Roman chamomile essential oil
>
> 1 ounce carrier oil

Rub around the ear and down the side of the neck. Apply 1 drop to a piece of cotton, and place it in the ear. For children, use ½ this dilution (6 drops of essential oil in 1 ounce carrier oil). Never drop this oil directly into the ear; you can use the next formula directly in the ear, since it is strictly herbal infused oils with no essential oils added.

HERBAL EAR OIL

Garlic is antibacterial, eases the pain and inflammation of simple ear infection, and is the remedy of choice for the fungal infection called "swimmer's ear," a condition that typically creates lots of itching. Mullein is a tried and true remedy for ear inflammation. Calendula also relieves inflammation. All three are antiseptic. We like to combine them into a super ear oil. Many ear oils containing garlic and mullein are available in the natural food store.

> ½ ounce garlic-infused oil
>
> ½ ounce calendula-infused oil (optional)
>
> ½ ounce mullein blossom–infused oil

Use olive oil as the carrier for this infusion. Warm the oil before dropping it into the ear: Heat a spoon under hot water, dry it, and drop the oil into the warm spoon; now draw the drops back into the dropper, and place 2 drops in each ear.

For eye problems such as sties or inflammation, use a compress soaked in anti-inflammatory hydrosols such as lavender, chamomile, or rosewater, which was a popular eyewash in the Middle East. Just make sure to use a pure hydrosol without added essential oils. If hydrosols are not available, tea bags of chamomile or regular black tea provide a quick compress. Steep them in warm water for a few minutes, cool, place a tea bag over each eye, and cover with a cloth.

Musculoskeletal System

Bones and muscles give form to the body and permit physical movement. Unless damaged by injury, the health of this system depends on the overall health of the body. With degenerative conditions such as arthritis and rheumatism, the entire body must be treated, especially the digestive and eliminative systems. Use anti-inflammatory essential oils that stimulate the circulation and eliminate toxins such as grapefruit, juniper, and helichrysum. Pain relievers such as birch are also useful. A commonsense diet—avoiding foods that create acidic reactions, such as red meat, eggs, and dairy—is also helpful. Refer to chapter 7 for additional suggestions for the treatment of muscular aches and pains.

Some aromatherapists use rosemary and lemongrass to ease stiffness. According to Dietrich Gumbel, PhD, they help remove the lactic acid buildup in the muscles that causes stiffness. Also use the following formula for arthritis:

PAIN FORMULA

6 drops helichrysum essential oil

4 drops marjoram essential oil

2 drops juniper essential oil

4 drops birch or wintergreen essential oil

3 drops chamomile essential oil

3 drops lavender essential oil

3 drops ginger essential oil

2 ounces of carrier oil

Combine ingredients. Use this formula as a massage or add 1 tablespoon to a bath oil.

Herbal adjuncts: Anti-inflammatory herbs include meadowsweet, willow bark, and devil's club, or add cayenne, ginger, mustard, and horseradish to food. Dandelion, sarsaparilla, burdock, celery seeds, parsley, and yarrow help eliminate toxins through the kidneys. Pain relievers include valerian and St. John's wort.

Nervous System

The nervous system provides the intricate connection between mind and body. As a result of mental or emotional responses, a problem in one area of the body may affect another.

For stress in general, try bergamot, chamomile, lavender, melissa, clary sage, neroli, rose, or jasmine. For insomnia due to mental agitation or overwork, clary sage, marjoram, ylang-ylang, and neroli can help you unwind. Headaches due to nervous tension are also helped by these oils, but keep in mind that headaches can result from many causes—from indigestion to hormonal problems—and should be treated accordingly.

RELAXATION/ANTIDEPRESSANT FORMULA

2 drops lavender essential oil

2 drops neroli essential oil

2 drops marjoram essential oil

2 drops ylang-ylang essential oil

2 drops chamomile essential oil

2 drops clary sage essential oil

1 ounce carrier oil

Combine the ingredients. Use this formula as a massage or bath oil.

NEURALGIA RELIEF

Neuralgia, or nerve pain, is best remedied by treating the cause, although essential oils can alleviate the pain, especially when used in conjunction with massage.

5 drops helichrysum essential oil

3 crops chamomile essential oil

2 drops marjoram essential oil

2 drops lavender essential oil

1 ounce carrier oil

Combine ingredients and use for massage.

Herbal adjuncts: Herbs can stimulate or relax the nervous system. A number of plants are relaxing, including California poppy (completely safe, with no addictive alkaloids), hops, valerian, passionflower, and catnip.

One of the best tonics to repair the nervous system is wild oats (even eating oatmeal does some good); others include skullcap and vervain. St. John's wort repairs damaged nerves and helps overcome depression. Tinctures and capsulated extracts of these herbs made from the fresh plant are probably the best way to take them and are easily obtained.

Glandular System

In his book *The Holistic Herbal*, David Hoffmann states, "It is in the complexities of our inner control systems that mind meets body most closely. If consciousness is seen as a faculty of the brain, then the partnership of nervous system and endocrine glands acts as a bridge linking consciousness and body." The glandular system includes the pituitary, thyroid, parathyroid, adrenals, pancreas, pineal, thymus, and gonads (ovaries or testes). Endocrine glands secrete and release hormones directly into the bloodstream.

Receptor sites for different hormones in each cell trigger changes or reactions in the cell's metabolism. Fatigue is probably the biggest complaint of North Americans and often results from overworked adrenals. Jobs, family, noise pollution, and the stresses of today's busy lifestyles all contribute. Drinking coffee and other caffeine beverages puts an extra burden on already overworked adrenal glands.

ADRENAL SUPPORT

Pine and spruce oils help revive adrenals. A massage or bath with the following blend supports adrenal function—but don't forget to schedule time to relax!

    4 drops pine essential oil (Pinus sylvestris)

    4 drops spruce essential oil (Picea mariana)

    2 drops lavender essential oil

    1 ounce carrier oil

Use this blend in the bath or as a massage oil. For extra stimulation, add 2 drops rosemary.

Herbal adjuncts: Regulating the thyroid with essential oils alone may not be enough. Use an eclectic approach of herbs, diet, and exercise for best results. For underactivity, some aromatherapists use seaweed absolute diluted to 3 percent and applied to the thyroid, although eating seaweed itself is more often recommended.

Digestive bitters—roots of goldenseal, dandelion, and yellow dock, for example—are useful here, acting through reflex stimulation. Beneficial herbs for the adrenals include ginseng and licorice. Add garlic, onions, and seaweeds such as kelp, dulce, hijiki, and wakame to your diet to boost an underactive thyroid.

Urinary System

The urinary system, consisting of the kidneys and bladder, regulates the body's water content and salt balance and eliminates waste. The kidney determines what to eliminate and what to recycle. It is also involved in regulating blood pressure.

Antiseptic diuretics to treat bladder infections include oils of cedarwood, tea tree, bergamot, and fennel. Unlike some urinary herbs used to treat infection, such as uva-ursi, these essential oils work well in both acid and alkaline environments, which means they can be used in conjunction with cranberries to acidify the urine. Use these oils preventatively in a regular bath or a sitz bath.

BLADDER INFECTION ADJUNCT RELIEF

There is a big difference between a minor bladder irritation and a full-blown infection. Be sure to see a medical professional if it does not resolve quickly after using the following blend.

    6 drops tea tree essential oil

    2 drops thyme essential oil (linalol type only, or substitute with sandalwood)

    2 drops juniper essential oil

    2 drops clove essential oil

    2 drops oregano essential oil

    1 ounce carrier oil (calendula is one of the best choices)

Mix the oils. Use as a massage over the bladder area twice per day. This is also safe to use externally if you are taking antibiotics.

Herbal adjuncts: Use essential oils as part of a more comprehensive healing program that includes herbs and diet. The use of soothing herbal teas is a welcome adjunct to any treatment. Examples are plantain, marshmallow root, and corn silk (yes, the hairy stuff under the husk; eat the inner green threads fresh—they taste just like corn—or make them into tea).

"Kidney stones" are mineral deposits most often composed of crystallized calcium and uric acid (or the amino acid cystine). Diet seems to be the primary cause, but excess weight, an inherited tendency, and previous kidney infections are all potential contributing factors. Studies in Paraguay, where rosemary is an important folk medicine, found that this herb inhibits 95 percent of urease (found in alkaline and infected urine) and probably inhibits the formation of some urinary stones. Lemon and grapefruit help reduce the size of kidney stones and help prevent infection.

To treat a bladder infection, use herb teas including uva-ursi, yarrow, and goldenrod flowers. A good urinary tract tonic consists of a tincture or tea of dandelion and nettle leaf, wild oat, and rose hips. Hydrangea root, stone root, wild yam, cramp bark, corn silk, and plantain leaf help eliminate kidney stones, but this condition may require professional help. Use these regularly if you are prone to bladder problems; they are good preventative aids.

Reproductive System

Among the most common problems for women are those involving the reproductive system. As women with personal experience in this area, we will focus first on several female problems, the topic of which has been the subject of some good books. We recommend Kathi Keville and Christopher Hobbs's book, *Women's Herbs, Women's Health* (see bibliography for further recommendations).

PMS AND MENSTRUAL CRAMPS

The more researchers learn about hormonal substances called *prostaglandins,* the more obvious it becomes that they can cause premenstrual syndrome (PMS) and menstrual cramps. Certain prostaglandins called PG2 can be responsible for headaches, bowel changes, nausea, breast tenderness, joint pain, and water retention, and they may contribute to moodiness, irritability, and alcohol cravings—all common PMS symptoms. Ginger, cinnamon, cloves, thyme, and garlic lower PG2, and you can add these herbs to foods. Relieve menstrual cramps with essential oils of chamomile, lavender, marjoram, and melissa. For depression associated with PMS, nothing is better than clary sage, but you may also try neroli, jasmine, and ylang-ylang. If you experience water retention, use

grapefruit, carrot seed, and juniper. Any of these essential oils (except garlic) can be used as a massage or bath oil. If headaches are among your PMS symptoms, try inhaling lavender, marjoram, or melissa. (For best results with any PMS or menstruation remedy, begin using it a couple of days before symptoms are expected.)

For problems related to hormonal imbalance, treat the liver with carrot seed, rosemary, helichrysum, and rose. To encourage menstruation, use clary sage. Most women's conditions benefit from the use of the balancing blend of lavender, geranium, and rose oils.

MENSTRUAL CRAMP OIL

4 drops lavender essential oil

2 drops marjoram essential oil

2 drops chamomile or clary sage essential oil (see considerations in chapter 15)

3 drops geranium essential oil

1 drop ginger essential oil

1 ounce carrier oil (infused oil of yarrow)

Combine ingredients. Apply to abdomen, hips, and lower back.

YEAST INFECTIONS

Many women have experienced at least one bout of yeast infection, which is usually easy to control. In laboratory experiments, chamomile, lavender, bergamot, and tea tree inhibited about 70 percent of candida growth. Although opinion varies among gynecologists as to whether common yeast infections can be transmitted between sex partners, it's safest to treat both individuals.

Douching has met with criticism in recent years because some practitioners believe it can upset the normal vaginal balance of a healthy woman or spread infection into the uterus. If done gently, however, douching is one way to treat vaginal infection. Be sure to suspend the bag no higher than hip level so that the flow of water isn't too strong.

An appropriate essential oil blend can also be applied to the abdomen or used in a bath. Another recommendation is to soak a tampon—or better, a small, soft natural sea sponge—in water containing essential oils. Use two sponges and alternate, sterilizing sponges between use by gently boiling or soaking in vinegar with a few drops of lavender oil (rinse well before using). Whichever you choose to use, remove and replace two to four times per day.

Tea tree or lavender is very effective for vaginal yeast. For carrier oils, we recommend tamanu *(Calophyllum inophyllum)* oil or yarrow infused into oil.

YEAST RELIEF

If you don't have the chemotype linalol or geraniol, don't replace it with any other thyme—most are too irritating.

- 1 drop thyme essential oil (chemotype linalol or geraniol only)
- 1 drop German chamomile essential oil
- 1 drop lavender essential oil
- 2 drops tea tree essential oil
- 2 drops palmarosa essential oil
- 1 drop geranium essential oil
- 2 cups warm yarrow tea

Combine the ingredients. For a simpler recipe, use 4 drops each geranium and palmarosa oils. Gently douche two times a day. You can also mix the essential oils in ½ ounce of an infused oil of calendula or in tamanu oil. Insert one dropperful morning and night. A panty liner is recommended during the day.

VAGINAL BOLUS

Boluses (see chapter 5) are effective treatments for a host of vaginal problems, especially cervical dysplasia (irregular cell growth on the cervix, which may be precancerous). *Eucalyptus polybractea* (cryptone type) is one of the best remedies. The following recipe can be customized to treat specific infections:

Nine Essential Oils for Women's Health

ROSE	universal female tonic and balancer, suitable for all gynecological problems
CLARY SAGE	depression, PMS, menopause, postpartum blues (avoid long-term use if you have fibrocystic breasts or uterine fibroids)
MARJORAM	antispasmodic, headache, menstrual cramps, constipation
CHAMOMILE	anti-inflammatory, soothes frayed nerves, PMS, migraine
LAVENDER	overall equalizer, skin care, shock, stress
GERANIUM	hormone balancer, menopause, PMS, yeast
TEA TREE	antibacterial, herpes, the best yeast remedy, cystitis
BERGAMOT	widely antiseptic, water retention, yeast, depression
NEROLI	insomnia, depression, anxiety, stretch marks

BOLUS RECIPE

If *Eucalyptus polybractea* (cryptone type) is not available, replace it with lavender or use 16 drops of geranium essential oil.

- 2 teaspoons dried and powdered calendula blossoms
- 1 teaspoon goldenseal root powder
- 1 teaspoon dried and powdered yarrow leaves or flowers
- 8 drops geranium essential oil
- 8 drops *Eucalyptus polybractea* (cryptone type)
- ¼ cup cocoa butter

Run all powdered herbs through a sieve to remove any chunks. Combine the ingredients. For use, see "Herbal Boluses" in chapter 5.

POOR CIRCULATION

Many female complaints are due to what TCM calls "blood stagnation." This basically means poor circulation in the abdomen, which contributes to problems as varied as hemorrhoids, menstrual cramps, and pelvic inflammatory disease (PID). Use castor oil packs and sitz baths with essential oils (see the following) to stimulate circulation. (For an understanding of TCM, we recommend Leslie Tierra's book *Herbs for Life*.)

Sitz bath: A sitz bath can decrease menstrual cramps, PID, and hemorrhoids. The bath requires two tubs large enough to sit in with water covering the abdomen. Fill one tub with hot water, the other with cold. Switch back and forth between the hot and cold tubs about four times. We find that four minutes in the hot and one minute in the cold is tolerable and actually feels good after a few rounds (you will soon want the hot water hotter and the cold colder!). When you get out, your midsection will be bright red with healthy blood circulation. This remedy provides great relief from pain. Repeat this routine as often as possible during the day.

Castor oil pack: Getting results from a castor oil pack requires dedication, is a bit messy, and can take weeks or even months to produce results. Still, it can work wonders on pain from internal scar tissue, ovarian cysts, fibroids, and even infection. You will need enough cotton flannel—several layers thick—to cover the abdomen, and about two cups of castor oil. Warm the oil, then dip in the flannel to thoroughly soak it. Wring it slightly to remove excess oil (it shouldn't drip). Place the flannel over the abdomen, and cover with a piece of plastic and then a heating pad. Leave the pack on for thirty minutes to one hour. When done, wrap the flannel in a plastic bag. After removing it from the bag, you may reheat it in a low 200°F oven. Replace every two weeks or so, depending on how much you reuse it.

We like to add essential oils to the castor oil pack. You can do this in two ways: by mixing a few drops of appropriate essential oils into the castor oil right after you warm it or by rubbing a body oil containing the essential oils on the skin before the castor oil pack is placed on it. The essential oils that are most often used with these packs are ones that are anti-inflammatory, enhance the immune system, and facilitate healing, such as lavender and tea tree.

MENOPAUSE

Menopause symptoms can include hot flashes, bone fragility, confusion, depression, and a dry, less-elastic vagina with a thinner lining—all caused by erratic hormone activity. Both dry skin and vagina need a rejuvenating massage oil or cream. The hormone balancers geranium and lavender help menopausal symptoms. Pharmacologist Tony Balacs states that many essential oils have hormonelike activity and speculates that their structure is so similar to hormones that they interact with the same receptors. Estrogenic oils include clary sage, sage, anise, fennel, angelica, coriander, cypress, and niaouli (a relative of tea tree oil).

Herbal adjuncts: Beneficial uterine tonics include raspberry leaves, false unicorn root, and motherwort. Herbs that help promote a normal menstrual flow are blue cohosh and partridge berry. Herbs that slow excessive menstrual flow or bleeding after birth include shepherd's purse, sage, and lady's mantle.

Good remedies for PMS or cramps are GLA (found in evening primrose, black currant, and borage seed oils), vitex, wild yam root, red raspberry leaf, licorice root, and cramp bark.

The best hormonal normalizer is the herb vitex, suitable for almost any reproductive-system condition, and that is especially useful for treating PMS, irregular menstruation, cervical dysplasia, uterine fibroids, and menopause. Vitex is now available as an essential oil, either from the leaf or the seed (stronger activity). It can be used externally, but start out slowly as women report differing results of activity levels. Herbs for balancing menopausal hormones are black cohosh, ginseng, dong quai, Siberian ginseng, licorice, fenugreek seed, and hops. Vitamin E is often useful.

PREGNANCY

Inhaling spearmint helps alleviate morning sickness (don't use peppermint as a substitute, it is too strong); neroli and lavender can be very soothing throughout pregnancy and during labor. See chapter 7 for a recipe for massage oil for pregnant bellies (see chapter 5 for contraindications in pregnancy and for information about which oils are safe to use).

Herbal adjuncts: In the first trimester of pregnancy, use gentle herb teas such as chamomile and lemon balm to deal with the usual maladies, but avoid strong emmenagogue (menstrual flow-inducing) herbs such as pennyroyal, rue, wormwood, goldenseal, juniper, sage, and tansy. Recommended herbs for threatened miscarriage include black haw, cramp bark, and false unicorn root. Toning and nutritive pregnancy herbs include raspberry, rose hip, chamomile, wild oat, nettles, and partridge berry. For morning sickness, try an herbal tea of meadowsweet, spearmint, ginger, and chamomile.

LACTATION

Use oils of anise, dill, and fennel in a bath or massage to help ensure a healthy supply of milk for your baby. The herbs themselves can also be added to food or made into tea. Drinking these herbal teas can not only increase the quality of your milk but also increases the fluids you need in your body to create it. Sage helps decrease lactation when you are ready to wean your baby (drink at least two cups of tea per day).

PROSTATITIS

Aromatherapy can help prostatitis (inflammation of the prostate) when combined with herbs and nutrition. An herbal sitz bath with chamomile and rosemary teas reduces inflammation, stimulates circulation, and relaxes muscles in the pelvic region. Although it is not quite as effective but more practical for some men, apply a warm compress or massage oil behind the scrotum. Research has shown that muscle relaxation is vital in relieving a prostate that is chronically inflamed because of hormone imbalance. Be sure to have a doctor check this condition before attempting self-treatment.

PROSTATE OIL

 5 drops lavender essential oil

 3 drops pine essential oil

 3 drops German chamomile essential oil

 1 ounce calendula-infused oil

Mix oils and apply to the area near the prostate twice daily to help reduce inflammation.

MALE HORMONAL TONIC

 2 drops niaouli essential oil

 5 drops pine essential oil

 3 drops sandalwood essential oil

 2 drops myrtle essential oil

 1 drop patchouli essential oil *(optional)*

 1 ounce St. John's wort–infused oil

Combine ingredients. Use daily in the bath or as a massage or body oil.

Herbal adjuncts: For an inflamed prostate, drink a tea (or take a tincture or pills) of saw palmetto berries, nettle root, sarsaparilla root, uva-ursi leaves, and echinacea root.

VIRAL SKIN INFECTION

Genital warts are caused by the human papillomavirus (HPV) and affect both men and women. They're difficult to detect at first, but turn white when dabbed with a half vinegar, half water mixture. Essential oils offer one of the most effective antiviral treatments for common or genital warts. Apply oils with a glass-rod applicator, dropper, or a cotton-tipped swab two to four times daily—and apply only to the wart itself, as the oils can burn sensitive skin. Protect the surrounding area with salve. Have genital warts removed by a doctor if the oils don't eliminate them. They can be passed to sexual partners and can cause cervical dysplasia and possibly even cancer.

GENITAL WART OIL

The vitamin E facilitates healing and can be obtained by opening two 400 IU capsules.

5 drops thuja essential oil

10 drops tea tree or *Eucalyptus polybractea* essential oil

¼ ounce castor or *Calophyllum* (tamanu) oil

800 IU vitamin E oil

Combine the ingredients.

HERPES

Herpes is a viral infection common among both men and women. *Herpes simplex* manifests around the mouth (cold sores) or the genitals. The painful shingles *(Herpes zoster)* is caused by the chicken pox virus. Both strains can lie dormant in the nervous system and are often triggered by stress.

HERPES FORMULA

4 drops *Eucalyptus citriodora*

4 drops MQV (niaouli)

1 drop geranium essential oil

2 drops tea tree essential oil

2 drops bergamot essential oil

1 ounce carrier oil (calendula-infused oil is best)

Combine ingredients. Apply to the infected area 2 or 3 times a day.

Integumentary System (Skin)

A spray of diluted essential oils makes an excellent antiseptic for skin conditions. The germ-killing abilities of essential oils high in terpenes, such as tea tree, pine, eucalyptus, and lemon, are effective when a 2 percent solution is sprayed through the air. The antiseptic quality of tea tree is said to increase in the presence of blood and pus. Superficial cuts, scrapes, and burns may also be treated with a salve. Although studies show that oils are antiseptic when diluted in an alcohol base instead of oil, this may sting in cases of an open wound. Tea tree, lavender, helichrysum, cistus, eucalyptus, rose geranium, sandalwood, and rose repair skin damage and encourage new cell growth for faster healing.

ANTISEPTIC SKIN SPRAY

15 drops tea tree or eucalyptus essential oil

10 drops helichrysum essential oil

5 drops lavender essential oil

2 ounces distilled water

½ ounce grain alcohol or goldenseal tincture

Combine and shake well before each use to help disperse the oils. Spray as needed on minor cuts, burns, and abrasions to prevent infection and speed healing.

FUNGAL INFECTION

Treat fungal infections with tea tree, lavender, eucalyptus, myrrh, palmarosa, and geranium. Small amounts of peppermint help relieve itching. Soak a compress in these essential oils diluted in vinegar, which also deters fungus, and apply to the affected area. A fungal powder is also appropriate to keep the area as dry as possible.

ANTIFUNGAL POWDER

¼ cup bentonite clay

1 tablespoon goldenseal root powder

12 drops tea tree essential oil

12 drops clove essential oil

12 drops geranium essential oil

Combine all the ingredients, and liberally powder the affected area. For fungal conditions, such as athlete's foot, an aromatic footbath is a great treat.

SOAK THOSE PUPS

5 drops tea tree essential oil

5 drops sage or rosemary essential oil

2 drops peppermint essential oil

Fill a portable basin or tub with hot water—or, better yet, sage tea. Add essential oils to water, and soak feet for at least 15 minutes. For feet that sweat excessively, finish with a foot powder.

RASHES CAUSED BY POISONOUS PLANTS

The menthol in peppermint relieves the painful burning and itching of poison oak, ivy, or sumac. A 2 to 3 percent dilution (12 to 24 drops per ounce) in vinegar or witch hazel provides blessed relief to nerve endings. You may also add 4 cups of quick-cooking oats (they dissolve best) wrapped in a muslin cloth and/or 1 cup Epsom salts to a lukewarm bath, or mix a smaller amount and sponge on. Lavender and a few menthol crystals added to a tincture of jewelweed or sassafras is also helpful during the first stages of a reaction. Oil-based products aren't usually recommended, although some people find that a lotion relieves itching during the later, dry stage of poison oak, ivy, and sumac.

POISON OAK / IVY / SUMAC REMEDY

3 drops lavender essential oil

3 drops helichrysum essential oil

3 drops Roman chamomile essential oil

3 drops geranium essential oil

3 drops cypress essential oil

½ teaspoon salt

1 tablespoon water

1 tablespoon vinegar

½ teaspoon menthol crystals

1 ounce calendula tincture

Combine ingredients. Apply externally as needed. When healing begins, externally apply 6 drops of Spanish lavender and 6 drops of cistus (diluted to 2 percent) in aloe gel or juice.

Herbal adjuncts: Take liver herbs such as milk thistle, burdock, and dandelion; avoid sweets and fruits. Take extra vitamin C and pantothenic acid.

INFLAMMATION AND BURNS

For inflammation, immediately apply a cold herbal compress with an anti-inflammatory oil, such as chamomile, lavender, or marjoram. The first step in treating burns and sunburns is to quickly immerse the area in cold water containing a few drops of one of these essential oils, or apply a cold compress that has been soaked in the water with essential oil or cold green tea. Lavender oil and aloe vera juice promote new cell growth, reduce inflammation, and stop infection. Aloe, which is so healing it has even been used successfully to treat radiation burns, also contains the natural "aspirin," salicylic acid.

SUNBURN SPRAY

50 drops (½ teaspoon) lavender essential oil

4 ounces aloe vera juice

1 teaspoon vitamin E oil

1 tablespoon vinegar

Combine ingredients. Store in a spritzer bottle, and shake well before using. Use as often as needed to reduce pain and speed healing. Keep the bottle in the refrigerator for extra cooling relief.

INSECT BITES AND OTHER CRITTER ATTACKS

For mosquito or other insect bites that don't require much attention, a simple dab of essential oil of lavender or tea tree provides relief. Chamomile and lavender essential oils reduce swelling, itching, and inflammation, and together with external application of tinctures of echinacea and plantain, they often prevent an allergic response (if an allergic reaction does occur, take 1/2 teaspoon of echinacea tincture orally).

FIRST AID REMEDY

This remedy is excellent for skin irritation, bites, stings, burns, inflammation, bruises, or scrapes.

3 drops lavender essential oil

3 drops tea tree or peppermint essential oil

3 drops German chamomile essential oil

3 drops helichrysum essential oil

1 ounce calendula-infused oil

Mix together.

CLAY POULTICE

Adding essential oil and tinctures to clay keeps the medicine reconstituted, preserved, and ready for an emergency. As the clay dries, it pulls toxins from stings and bites to the skin's surface to keep them from spreading, while helping to draw out pus and embedded splinters.

12 drops lavender essential oil

1 tablespoon bentonite clay

½ teaspoon tincture of echinacea root

½ teaspoon tincture of chamomile flowers

distilled water

Put clay in the container to be stored. Slowly add the tinctures, stirring as the clay absorbs them. Add lavender oil, stirring to distribute it evenly. Add enough distilled water to form a paste (about the consistency of toothpaste). Store poultice in a container with a tight lid to slow dehydration; it should stay soft at least a couple months. If the mixture does dry out, add distilled water to reconstitute it.

INSECT-ASIDE BUG REPELLENT

Nothing is more annoying than trying to enjoy the outdoors while shooing away pesky insects. Many people don't care for the smell of citronella, a traditional repellent, but this formula smells great.

5 drops eucalyptus essential oil

2 drops orange essential oil

4 drops lavender essential oil

2 drops lemon essential oil

8 drops cedar essential oil

1 drop peppermint essential oil

1 drop clove essential oil

1 drop cinnamon essential oil

2 ounces carrier oil

Mix together and apply liberally. Keep out of eyes.

COOTIE OIL

Few "creepy crawlies" can survive the following blend. Use for skin fungi, scabies, or other nonspecific critters.

> 10 drops thyme essential oil (linalol type)
>
> 3 drops lemon essential oil
>
> 5 drops lavender essential oil
>
> 5 drops rosemary essential oil
>
> 1 drop clove bud essential oil
>
> 1 drop cinnamon bark essential oil
>
> 2 ounces carrier oil

Combine ingredients. Apply as needed.

Herbal adjuncts: Jewelweed leaves, garlic, black walnut hulls, and the lichen usnea are all specific against fungi and can be used as an external wash or soak. For other herbal adjuncts, see chapter 9.

Immune System

Natural remedies can correct the terrain and increase the body's resistance to disease by improving its ability to fight infection. Using a single essential oil alone may not heal a person, but many plants have confirmed immune-modulating properties. As with any natural healing modality, essential oils should not be solely relied upon in case of serious illnesses—but they may be integrated into any therapeutic program.

Lavender, lemon, bergamot, thyme, chamomile, pine, sandalwood, myrrh, and vetiver stimulate production of infection-fighting white corpuscles. The antiviral action of specific essential oils is one of their most valuable attributes—especially since allopathic medicine has little to offer. Essential oils with terpenoid compounds are very specific, notably the citruses and pine oils, as well as some oils in the phenol group. (See chapter 13.)

Building health is the best insurance against contracting illnesses. The following blend helps build the body's natural resistance.

BASIC IMMUNE TONIC BLEND

> 3 drops lavender essential oil
>
> 3 drops tea tree essential oil
>
> 2 drops bergamot essential oil
>
> 2 drops ravensara essential oil
>
> 2 drops eucalyptus essential oil
>
> 10 drops tamanu oil (*Calophyllum inophyllum*)
>
> 1 ounce calendula-infused carrier oil

Use daily as a body oil in the bath as part of a health-maintenance program or to treat acute conditions such as a cold or flu.

Herbal adjuncts: Adaptogens are defined as safe, beneficial herbs that have a balancing and toning action. There is controversy over which herbs fit the criteria, but there is little argument against the *Panax* ginsengs (Korean and American) or Eleuthero ginseng. The immune tonics echinacea, myrrh, calendula, garlic, wild indigo, astragalus, shiitake and reishi mushrooms, schizandra berries, and ligusticum all help build resistance.

Therapeutics and Children

Care must be taken in treating children with essential oils, although there are a number of safe ones. Use a third to a half of the adult dose: a 1 percent dilution (5 or 6 drops of essential oil per ounce of carrier oil), and don't forget that citruses may irritate the skin. See chapter 5.

Chamomile, melissa, and fennel used as massage oil, or taken as herb tea, soothe a variety of tummy aches—and the problems that can lead to stomachaches, such as frayed nerves, anxiety, and overexcitability. Colic, gas pains, nausea, and food allergies are also good candidates for these remedies. A study from Israel found that a chamomile, fennel, and melissa herb tea with licorice helps stop crying and fussing in infants with colic. Researchers think the essential oils naturally present in the tea relieve muscle spasms caused when babies swallow air as they eat. Nineteenth-century parents gave colicky babies a "gripe water" of dill, fennel, or anise, and East Indian and Lebanese mothers still use dill to ease colic. A European carminative water contains fennel, chamomile, caraway, coriander, and bitter orange peel, which are all known to kill bacteria and relieve flatulence.

TUMMY RUB OIL

Most digestive woes are helped by a simple tummy massage.

> 2 drops Roman chamomile essential oil
> 1 drop fennel essential oil
> 2 drops dill essential oil
> 1 drop melissa essential oil
> 1 ounce carrier oil

Mix together and gently massage the tummy.

A relaxing treatment for children before bedtime is a warm lavender and chamomile essential oil bath. Most children love taking aromatherapy baths, particularly if they have their own personal blends, and may want to get involved in choosing and blending scents. Popular fragrances include orange, grapefruit, and tangerine—all antidepressants and relaxants (see the baths section of chapter 8 for proper dilution guidelines for kids). Nature's gentle relaxant teas such as melissa, linden, lavender, and chamomile can calm a nervous, overstimulated cranky child, make headaches go away, or gently induce sleep—as well as help soothe a worn-out parent!

A child suffering from a headache, sleeplessness, or overexertion will find relief in a cool compress of lavender placed on the forehead. Frankincense used in a vaporizer or as massage oil is safe and effective for respiratory congestion or infection, even for infants. Other safe essential oils for children include mandarin, marjoram, neroli, jasmine, and petitgrain. Treat a fever, measles, chicken pox, or mumps with a tea of yarrow, catnip, peppermint, and elder flower; ginger with a touch of lemon juice and honey is also effective. The soreness of mumps is relieved by syrups and gargles made from teas of thyme, rosemary, or

sage. Antiviral oils of melissa and bergamot have proven effective against the mumps and chicken pox virus (if you use melissa, be sure it is the real thing and not the common adulterants citronella or lemongrass; these don't have the same healing properties). Use these essential oils in a steam, or make a tea from the herbs.

For teething pain, give the child chamomile tea, and rub the outside of the cheeks with a little diluted German or Roman chamomile oil.

NECK WRAP

Use the following formula for swollen tonsils, mumps, or other lymphatic swelling in the neck area.

> 2 cups warm water
> 8 drops lavender essential oil

Mix the water with the essential oil. While the water is still warm, soak a soft cloth, preferably flannel, in the water and wring it out. Wrap the cloth around the neck. Cover with a towel to hold in the heat, and remove it before it gets cold. Repeat as many times as you wish.

DILLY PILLOW

European children were once given "dilly pillows," filled with aromatic herbs such as lavender and dill, to send them off to dreamland. The scent was also considered a digestive. Add chamomile and thyme to prevent nightmares.

> *1 cup total:*
> lavender flowers
> hops strobiles
> lemon balm leaves
> chamomile flowers
> dill seeds

Fold a 5 by 10-inch piece of cloth in half, and sew up the edges, leaving just enough room to stuff the herbs inside. Combine the herbs in equal parts to make 1 cup. Stuff the herbs into the material, then finish sewing it up (you can add a few drops of lavender oil to the herbs). Place beside or under the child's regular pillow.

CHAPTER 7

Massage

AS HIPPOCRATES SAID, "The way to health is to have an aromatic bath and a scented massage every day." Aromatherapy enhances any type of bodywork by positively influencing the subject's moods and increasing relaxation. Essential oils are absorbed through the skin into the blood system for therapeutic actions, so simply rubbing the body oil into the skin directly over the problem—say, an upset stomach or headache—puts the oil right where it is needed.

If you've ever given a massage, you know that it often takes the person receiving the treatment some time to relax fully. Slowly, but very slowly, the breathing slows down and deepens. Tense muscles begin to relax. When you use aromatherapy massage oil, you will be surprised how quickly the person slips into a deep relaxation state that usually takes at least an hour of massage to achieve. The longer you work, the deeper he or she goes.

As professional masseuses, we have both had wonderful experiences using the two techniques together, but don't think that you must be a trained masseuse or masseur to qualify to use body oils with massage. Even if you aren't familiar with massage techniques, you can still give a therapeutic rub that will make the recipient feel good. Even treat yourself to a massage: rub your own tight shoulders, sore feet, or cellulite thighs twice daily with aromatherapy oils.

Among the best oils to relieve stress and muscle pain are bergamot, clary sage, chamomile, jasmine, lavender, marjoram, neroli, rose, rosemary, sandalwood, and ylang-ylang. Liniments made with warming oils such as peppermint, cinnamon, and cloves relieve or inhibit muscle soreness. You can also specifically design oils for foot massage, babies, headache relief, pregnant women, and even for helping reduce cellulite. We've provided a variety of simple formulas to get you started.

For any type of massage, make sure that the oils are lightly scented. Too strong a smell quickly overwhelms both the person getting and the person giving the massage. The most therapeutic action occurs when the scent is very faint, just barely detectable (you'll find people that actually like lighter versions of oils they otherwise wouldn't care for). The amount of massage oil depends on the style of massage. Some massage schools teach methods that use a lot of oil. In this case, use less essential oil in the base or vegetable oil. We suggest a 2 percent dilution of essential oil in carrier oil for a standard massage oil.

When doing a lymph-drainage massage or other type of bodywork requiring lots of oil, lower dilutions may be more appropriate. For a liniment, which must be more concentrated to work properly (it is used in spot treatments), a 3 percent dilution is generally sufficient.

If you are working as a professional, you need a well-ventilated room; otherwise, you'll be dizzy from all the oils by the third client of the day. Nothing fancy is needed; airing out the room between clients by opening the windows or by using a fan is usually sufficient. If that's not possible, use an air filter to remove scent from the air. Monitor the room to check how strong it smells: walk outside, stroll around, take a few deep breaths, and then come back inside. You may be surprised how accustomed you've become to the scent and how strong the room really smells.

Essential oils are versatile and can treat many common problems. Oil blends are ideally custom designed for individuals. This demands some blending skill—chapter 11 should be enough to start you out—and some skill in choosing the most appropriate oils. Until you have enough expertise, stick to simple problems and focus on relaxation, which is healing in itself. Custom blending is beneficial if you have the time, but it is not always necessary.

We like to keep a selection of aromatherapy body oils on hand to treat the most common complaints. If you're going to do much bodywork, make a series of blends. Use the various charts in this book for ideas on designing body oils for individual needs.

LEGAL IMPLICATIONS AND SAFETY PRECAUTIONS

In the United States, certified bodyworkers are allowed to give relaxing massages, but treating internal problems, diagnosing, and prescribing go beyond the boundaries of the law, especially when you charge for your services. However, you may give specific treatments to your family and friends with their consent. Professional bodyworkers may give an aromatherapy massage treatment as long as they are just providing relaxation, instead of diagnosing and treating physical or emotional disorders. Just keep a few safety precautions in mind:

- Don't treat beyond your scope of knowledge.
- Make pleasing aromatherapy blends, not medicinal formulas.
- Use words such as "balance," "nourish," "assist," "tone," "uplift," and "relax."
- Don't try to come up with a medical "diagnosis" or "prescription."
- Know when and where to refer those with severe problems.
- Don't massage strenuously near varicose veins, bruises, or other types of broken veins.
- Watch out for sensitivities to the essential oils.

An Aromatherapy Massage

Receiving aromatherapy along with massage is simultaneously receiving two treatments. It deepens the effects of your massage, and we guarantee that your clients will come back for more. We've both found that adding aromatic treatments sends the massage far beyond an unscented massage. You'll find yourself being able to listen to clients' complaints and addressing them while you work.

There are many ways to approach the use of aromatherapy on the massage table. The simplest technique is to have one favorite scented massage oil, but why not be prepared with at least a few premixed blends so you can select the one that is most appropriate for each client? Or expand your practice to include a variety of different aromatherapy techniques. In the same way that you adapt your massage techniques for different individuals, customize your aromatherapy work. Most people enjoy being pampered, especially when they are getting a massage.

Use special treatments to address special needs. Massage oils that are made for spot treatments can have a higher concentration of essential oil than regular massage oil. They need to be used on small areas of the body instead of as an all-over massage oil, or it can be too much essential oil for the body to handle. For example, a spot therapy oil could be 12 to 20 drops essential oil per ounce instead of 6 to 10. Try to arrange your time so you work on the problem area, such as a tense neck or leg cramps, early in the massage, giving the oil time to do its magic. Return to the same place at least a couple times during the massage, reapplying the special oil each time. Refer to the formulas and charts in this book for ideas on specific aromatherapy products you can use. In the United States, a Certified Massage Technician (CMT) offers one of the best certifications for using aromatherapy. Keep in mind that having a CMT certification extends to relaxing, relieving pain, and making the client more comfortable, so use these special techniques in this context.

Most massage schools suggest always maintaining physical contact while working on a client. This can become complicated when you use several different products during the same massage, so make sure the various bottles are easily within reach. Practitioners have found different ways to do this. Use a small, rolling cart that moves smoothly without squeaky wheels, have a small table under the massage table, or position the massage table close enough to shelves that hold your products. No client ever complains if you do briefly need to turn away to get a heating pad, compress, or hot rocks. They also won't mind if you need to wash aromatherapy oils off your hands before working on the face. It is all part of the extra pampering.

Be sure to make notes on all the oils and techniques you use on your client and how the person responded to follow up on their next visit. It seems appropriate to follow a course of successive healing by altering the client's formula with each visit. However, people often become attached to their personal blend and look forward to having it used on them again. When that occurs, you may want to make only slight variations or leave it the same. An advantage of using the same massage oil is that the association the clients build with relaxation and the oil's particular scent will enhance their ability to relax with each visit. You can also send some home with them to use between visits; the aroma will remind them of the relaxation that took place during the therapeutic massage.

Whatever your technique for working with aromatherapy, if you see massage clients, it's a good idea to display a selection of the aromatherapy products you use. This proclaims your experience in using aromatherapy and sets you apart from other practitioners who rely on a single bottle of scented massage oil. If you have a waiting room, this is an excellent place to do so. That way, clients will know they are in store for something special. You might even provide them with a checklist of favorite oils while they wait; then you will know their preferences when you blend a customized formula.

Choose one or a few aromatherapy techniques to custom design each body treatment, because it demands coordination to incorporate several methods into one massage. Start slowly and slowly incorporate more techniques. If you use sprays or briefly need to leave the client's side to wash your hands, also tell them this so there are no surprises while they are in deep relaxation. Before the massage, be sure to explain that you will incorporate several essential oils. We guarantee the person will get off the table feeling like she had a longer, more complete, and quite possibly the best massage she ever had.

BEFORE THE MASSAGE

Scent the waiting area. An electric plug-in or a more elaborate glass diffuser that pumps out unheated fragrances will scent the room. For a very light scent, add a few drops of essential oil to a lightbulb ring, and turn on the bulb just before the client arrives. Lightly spray furniture where people will sit with a fine mist of scented water (avoiding silk pillows and any fabric that reacts to water).

Spray scent on the sheets. Lightly mist the massage table sheets with scented water. It will dry and be ready for the client in a few minutes.

DURING THE MASSAGE

Get misty. Lightly misting a floral water or hydrosol over the person receiving the massage gives a special touch in any type of bodywork. Spray the mist a couple feet above the client. Just be sure to do it high enough in the air so the droplets don't chill the subject's skin. This is especially nice on a hot day or anytime you want to introduce an additional light scent into your treatment. You can also spray a light mist below the head cradle during the massage when the client is lying on their stomach. This is certainly not up toward their face, but close enough so a light scent will rise up and they can smell the aroma. An excellent time to use this technique is when you feel the person needs to relax or breathe more deeply. Have the appropriate sprays on hand.

Mix it up. Switch oils during the massage to delightfully confuse your client, and send them into even deeper relaxation. Plan ahead of time how many different massage oils to use and their order, or once you're experienced working with aromatherapy, determine this as you go along.

Use a sticky solution. Tape a scented strip of paper or fabric under the massage table near the head cradle. That scent will only be apparent when the client is lying facedown. When clients are uncomfortable due to sinus congestion, peppermint or eucalyptus helps them breathe. Some practitioners attach a permanent strip of Velcro to make it easy to change strips. This is a good technique for chair massage or when you aren't using massage oil.

SPECIAL TREATMENTS

Ease muscle cramps. Choose a massage oil to relieve tight muscles; when heat is appropriate, you can relax a person before you begin a massage by placing a hot pad or a warm herbal compress over the tight muscles. During or after the massage, place the pad or compress over the tight muscle after applying the oil. Simply add a few drops of an appropriate essential oil to very warm water. Any essential oils suggested for massage are suitable for a compress. Submerge a soft cloth into the water, swish it around, wring it out, and place it on the skin for two to five minutes (or even longer if you have time). Just don't let the cloth cool and become uncomfortable. For an extended treatment, place a towel, hot rocks, or a heating pad over the compress to keep it warm. After removing the compress, pat the skin dry with a warm towel.

Use hot rock therapy. Apply penetrating massage oil on the areas where you will put the hot rocks to intensify the treatment. Or add a few drops of essential oil to the water in which you heat the rocks.

Heat it up. Warm tight muscles with liniment to increase the warmth and relaxing power. The more you rub a liniment, the warmer the area becomes.

Relieve joint pain. Turn to a deeply penetrating oil that relieves pain and inflammation.

Get the point. Use a high strength massage oil (15 to 20 drops essential oil per ounce of vegetable oil) directly on acupuncture, acupressure, or reflexology points to activate them before working. After working the points, the essential oils in the massage oil will continue to work.

Focus on problem areas. There is no reason to abandon problem areas that you cannot directly massage, such as varicose veins. You can still give a full body massage by applying, without using pressure, special oil that is designed to treat the specific condition.

Help a headache. A drop of diluted eucalyptus or peppermint on the temples can relieve headaches and sometimes even migraines (combine 10 drops of one or both essential oils in 1 teaspoon vegetable oil).

Alleviate eye strain. Placing a hot, or sometimes cold, scented pad over strained eyes; a small flax pillow works well and eases frontal and back-of-the-eyes headaches. One may prefer to place a hot pad on the back of the neck and a cool one on the forehead. Use a small heating pad. You can also make a compress by swishing a soft wash cloth in water that contains about 3 drops of essential oil, and wring it out before applying—be sure to remove the cloth before it feels cold and clammy on the skin. Use gentle herbs such as chamomile or fennel. Avoid oils such as peppermint that can burn sensitive eyelids. Or mist cotton pads with rosewater, and apply gently to closed lids. You can also use true hydrosols as an eye compress or to gently mist the face, but make sure they are not water with essential oils added.

Address injuries. If you wish to address these, use the appropriate treatment. For example, use a burn spray on burns and an antiseptic spray on wounds. Impact injuries without broken skin or bruises respond well to calendula oil with chamomile or helichrysum.

Special Types of Massage

Aromatherapy can be used in other types of bodywork and special types of massage. For acupressure or other methods that don't normally use massage oil, a small amount of massage oil can safely be applied to the fingertips. Use the oil with or without acupressure to "spot" and activate certain areas. Other methods of aromatherapy, such as an essential oil diffuser or a potpourri cooker filled with water, can be used in bodywork that does not require massage oil. A few drops of essential oil will fill the room with the fragrance and encourage relaxation.

CELLULITE MASSAGE

Cellulite, which is really just a fancy word for puckered fat, has been characterized as "orange-peel skin" (textured and lumpy) and is found most often in the thighs and buttocks. Cellulite affects women more than men and does not necessarily result from being overweight. The following recipe, used in a bath or as massage oil, is most effective if combined with other weight-loss activities—exercising and restricting bad sources of dietary fat, such as refined and hydrogenated oils. There is a lot of evidence that consuming good fats including fish oil and coconut oil in your diet will help reduce cellulite. Geranium and fennel both balance hormones and, along with grapefruit, have historically been used to facilitate weight loss. Cypress and juniper stimulate circulation, and juniper is a diuretic.

CELLULITE OIL
10 drops cypress essential oil
10 drops geranium essential oil
10 drops grapefruit essential oil
5 drops juniper essential oil
5 drops fennel essential oil
4 ounces carrier oil

Combine the ingredients.

PREGNANCY MASSAGE

A pregnant woman's expanding belly needs massage and aromatherapy oils to help the skin expand and thus prevent stretch marks. To massage a pregnant woman, support her on her side with pillows to make her as comfortable as possible, and select only the safest essential oils (see chapter 5). The important consideration is that she be comfortable, not strained or compressed anywhere. If lying down is impractical or uncomfortable, she can sit facing the back of a straight chair for a back massage. Common sense and thoughtfulness are really all you will need. A pregnant woman will probably also want her lower back massaged. Although it's always a pleasure to have someone else give you a massage, the belly is fortunately in a handy location to self-massage. Apply the appropriate oil to the belly at least twice a day. The following belly oil formula is suitable for the whole body. If you want to use a carrier oil that is infused with herbs, a good choice is calendula flower. This same belly oil is also suitable for giving the new mom a massage after giving birth. Add a couple drops of clary sage to help counter postpartum depression.

PREGNANT BELLY OIL

Rose and neroli are both expensive, so you may make this oil with just lavender.

> 15 drops lavender essential oil
>
> 5 drops neroli essential oil
>
> 2 drops rose essential oil
>
> 800 IU vitamin E
>
> 4 ounces carrier oil (calendula is good)

Combine the ingredients.

Many women also appreciate some massage during labor to promote relaxation. Lavender is an old standby in the birthing room. As mentioned in chapter 4, lavender flowers traditionally were heated, pounded into a poultice, and placed on the woman's lower back. Lavender was chosen because it is a muscle relaxant that "opens up" constricted areas. Old texts talk of its ability to "raise the spirit" of both the people attending the birth and the child who is coming into the world.

It would be nice to see lavender return to the birthing room, even though poultices are messy to make and use, especially during birth when a pregnant woman is likely to be changing positions. The perfect alternative is a lavender massage oil, such as the belly oil described earlier, which can be rubbed into a tight back or anywhere the woman feels tension. The light scent imparted into the air will serve the ancient purpose of raising the spirit even better than a poultice.

MUSCLE MASSAGE

Everyone has at least a few tight muscles. The shoulders and neck are favorite places for storing tension, but muscles anywhere in the body can become cramped. Muscle cramping, including menstrual cramps, is greatly relieved by massage with a muscle relaxing oil. You may not think that stomachaches and gas pains need external treatment, but these problems are often caused by muscle cramping and are thus helped by gentle massage.

MUSCLE MASSAGE OIL

The following recipe contains a lot of essential oil and is not designed for an all-over body massage. Instead, rub it directly over areas where there is soreness or pain.

> 30 drops lavender essential oil
>
> 10 drops marjoram essential oil
>
> 5 drops frankincense or Boswellia essential oil
>
> 2 ounces carrier oil

Combine the ingredients.

FACIAL MASSAGE

Did you know that more muscles are concentrated in your face than anywhere else in your body? These muscles allow you to smile, cry, and pout, but all of that movement leads to some very tired face muscles. Facial tension contributes to wrinkles and poor blood circulation in your face.

A facial massage makes a good accompaniment to the aromatherapy facial described in chapter 9, and is a nice way to introduce someone to massage (a good facial massage takes much less time than a body massage and is unusually relaxing for the whole body). Always use very lightly scented oils around the face, and be sure to keep oil well away from the eyes. We recommend a 1 percent dilution (about 5 to 6 drops per ounce). Choose a light carrier oil as well.

A good sequence for a facial massage is to begin at the chin and work up, against gravity. If there's time, give the tight shoulders and neck a quick rub. Be sure to use gentle, light strokes on the face—kneading the face too much only contributes to more wrinkling. Because you're working on such a small area with so many different planes, tiny circular motions are good for most of the face. A light tapping motion with the fingers, as though you're typing, gives a stimulating massage without being at all abrasive. Don't forget to work around the ears and the jaws, areas that frequently hold tension.

BABY MASSAGE

Most babies love massages, and because they are so expressive, it's easy to tell what a baby likes and dislikes. Listen and observe and use the reactions as your guide to the amount of pressure (begin very gently) and the best types of strokes. Baby massages tend to be short. Watch for a response; when the baby begins getting fussy or bored, it's time to stop.

You don't need many guidelines, and you certainly don't need to know any fancy strokes to simply rub in an oil. Do make sure, however, that your hands aren't too rough (or your nails too long) for the child's tender skin. Also avoid putting oil on a baby's hands or face, because it can easily get into the eyes (babies tend to dislike facial massage anyway).

In Europe, massage is widely used as a treatment for colic. Colic is caused by stress and indigestion, two of the problems helped most by massage. In the late 1980s, the Danish physician Jan-Helge Larsen's clinic prescribed belly massage for colicky babies. With the baby facing away, support the baby under the arms and place one hand under the stomach. Starting at the navel, use that hand to work in a clockwise direction around the abdomen (the way the intestines normally flow) for at least 15 minutes after a feeding. This helps expel the gas pains that result in colic. It's easiest to do this sitting down, although you may want to do it while walking and gently swinging the baby if he or she needs to be calmed.

Another colic-relief method is to lay the baby on its back, gently rotate the legs, then massage the belly. Don't try this right after a feeding, because this position makes burping difficult, and insufficient burping contributes to colic. Of course, even a baby who doesn't have colic will still appreciate the massage.

Baby oil blends are designed to protect the skin and provide an enjoyable and relaxing massage. Babies are new to our environment, so ingredients that appear mild to us sometimes cause reactions on their delicate skins.

The best baby-care products are made with pure natural ingredients. Avoid standard commercial baby oil and ointments, which are typically made from mineral oil (petroleum), a good machinery lubricant but questionable for use on skin. Mineral oil, which is made from petroleum, robs the body of important skin nutrients. Vitamin E (800 IUs) can be added for its skin-healing properties. For an easy source of vitamin E, pierce a few vitamin capsules. The following formula is an extra-gentle ½ percent dilution (5 drops per 2 ounces of carrier).

Massage isn't just for babies. Older children enjoy a massage with baby oil (providing, of course, you give it another name). Because essential oils are absorbed through the skin, massage oils treat problem areas without children having to swallow anything. Ask your little patient what feels good and how hard to press. Most children prefer gentle, light strokes, but not too light—some kids are *very* ticklish.

THE AROMATHERAPY MESSAGE: KATHI'S STORY

Many years ago, my interest in aromatherapy was sparked by my massage practice. I was fortunate to live on an herb farm and as I led tours through the fragrant herb garden, I noticed that each patch produced a different reaction in the visitors. Most interesting was that each group responded again and again in the same way to certain plants. Passing by the rows of lavender always resulted in smiles and raised voices, which dropped as the group approached the chamomile bed. Mint never failed to liven things up again; visitors began talking excitedly as they sniffed the pungent leaves. And the honeysuckle—ah, the honeysuckle. It's fragrance found us all reminiscing. I guessed that the source of their reactions was the herb's fragrance and imagined how I might transfer the reaction onto the massage table.

Lavender seemed a logical beginning because it initiated the strongest responses and was already my favorite. So I cut a handful of its fragrant flowers, placed them in a canning jar, and covered them with almond oil. After a few days in the sun, the almond oil in the jar smelled strongly of the lavender, so I strained out the flowers. I awaited my next massage client with a bottle of lavender massage oil close at hand. Because this was in the early 1970s and I hadn't heard the term *aromatherapy*, I asked if the client would like a "fragrant therapy" massage. Of course, the response was positive. I'm sure the client wasn't sure what I meant, but it sounded pleasant enough to try. That massage, more than thirty-five years ago, was my initiation into a journey of using fragrance for healing.

My first experiment proved so successful that I couldn't wait to give my next massage. The lavender sent the clients into deep relaxation faster than massage alone. At the same time, it soothed sore muscles and headaches and seemed to produce a sense of peacefulness. Certainly, this was one perfect massage oil, but I couldn't resist exploring other fragrant plants in my herb garden. I found that peppermint gave a spark to anyone who felt exhausted after a long day, that chamomile revived the depressed. As long as the smell was pleasant, the fragrances harmonized. Thus, a relaxing chamomile could blend with a touch of spearmint, and the client would feel both relaxed and revitalized.

I produced my first commercial aromatherapy oil, "Herbal Blossom Calming Massage Oil," in 1975. It contained infused lavender flowers, chamomile flowers, and rose petals in almond oil. It was soon followed by the spicy "Warm Glow Stimulating Massage Oil," containing cinnamon, orange, and peppermint. Now that I look back on those first formulas, I realize they were quite simple, but they certainly worked well.

The next step was to create body oils from the essential oils themselves. Good-quality essential oils were not so readily available then, but I found some sources and began building up a collection. After much experimentation, I developed seven generic blends so I could offer my massage clients a selection from which to choose.

I had to ask clients how they felt before initiating the massage. I quickly learned the importance of qualifying this request, because my intention was to give an aromatherapy massage, not to listen to a litany of problems. I also asked my clients to take a sniff before I applied the oil. This request might seem simple, but many people are too polite to criticize your creation, especially after you choose it especially for them.

I began to custom design oils for each client. First, I would take into consideration the client's brief description of his or her emotional and physical state. As the client prepared for the massage, I quickly blended something special just for the occasion (my good nose and years of working with fragrant plants came in handy). I had a selection of about forty different essential oils from which to choose, and I added the oils to a base that I had already prepared by mixing several of my favorite vegetable oils. If the preparation took a few extra minutes, no one minded. After all, what a treat to be massaged with your own personal blend, designed for that moment in time. When the massage is complete, I offer a bottle of the client's own special blend to take home for use as a bath oil.

HERBAL BABY OIL

    4 drops lavender essential oil

    1 drop Roman chamomile essential oil

    2 ounces carrier oil (calendula oil is good)

Combine the ingredients.

BABY TUMMY-RUB OIL

You can use lavender instead of dill or melissa, which is quite expensive.

    3 drops melissa (lemon balm) essential oil

    2 drops chamomile essential oil

    2 drops dill seed essential oil

    2 ounces vegetable oil

Combine the ingredients. Rub on every hour or as needed.

SPOT MASSAGE AND LINIMENTS

Spot massages, using liniments, are good for particularly painful areas. Liniments are used externally to warm or to reduce inflammation and as disinfectants for spot treatments on wounds or pimples.

Liniments reduce muscle and joint pain. Like body oils they are rubbed into the skin, but contain a higher concentration of warming essential oils, which are potentially irritating (use no more than a 3 percent dilution—about 18 drops per ounce of carrier oil; the idea is to warm the skin, not burn it). Liniments are designed for spot massage on particularly painful areas, not for an overall body massage. Fitness experts currently suggest applying a liniment before exercise, not afterward. The liniment's warming action is like a mini-warm-up, relaxing "cold" muscles and allowing them to stretch better. Warm-ups are still a good idea, but you will get a lot more out of them when you use a liniment.

Liniments perform two functions. They are primarily heating agents that warm the skin over the muscles or joints, which actually plays a trick on the brain. The brain registers "heat," which equals "burning," which equals "major problems," and concentrates its attention on the skin's surface where it senses a potential emergency, instead of on the painful muscle. This breaks the cycle between brain and pain, whereby the painful muscle says, "Oh, this really hurts," and the brain confirms that by signaling with pain responses, such as further tightening. With the liniment, the focus switches to a dialogue between the perceived "burning" skin and the brain. Thus the painful muscle has a chance to relax while the brain concerns itself with the burning sensation.

A liniment may also have a penetrating action, depending on which essential oils you choose. Liniments containing actual muscle-relaxing essential oils, such as rosemary, marjoram, and lavender, penetrate the skin to work directly on the muscle. If you prefer, make a penetrating liniment that does not heat up the skin.

Now that you understand the principles behind liniments, you are ready to choose the best carrier. You have your choice of alcohol or oil for a base. Both work fine. The difference is that alcohol emphasizes the cooling nature of the liniment and quickly evaporates, leaving the essential oils to penetrate the skin. When using alcohol as a base, we prefer vodka to rubbing alcohol, which is toxic internally. Add a 3-percent dilution of essential oils to the vodka (about 15 to 18 drops essential oil per ounce of alcohol). If you do use rubbing alcohol, be sure to mark the solution "For External Use Only."

On the other hand, an oil-based liniment stays on the skin longer, so it heats up faster. It doesn't work immediately, but it has a time-release type of action, making it last longer. Oil-based products are also easier to massage into the skin, although they leave an oily residue.

Experiment to discover which type of liniment you prefer, depending on the situation. You can even get fancy and mix alcohol and oil liniments together. Just be sure to shake the mixture before using. To make an herb-infused liniment, follow the directions for making a tincture or an oil. Generally, this type of oil isn't hot enough by itself, but infused vegetable oil or alcohol can be used as the carrier base that has essential oils added to it.

LINIMENT FORMULA

12 drops eucalyptus essential oil

12 drops peppermint essential oil

6 drops ginger essential oil

6 drops cinnamon essential oil

2 ounces carrier oil or alcohol (either rubbing alcohol or vodka)

Mix ingredients. Shake or stir a few times a day for 3 days to disperse the essential oils in the alcohol.

Adjunct Therapies

There are a number of other ways to extend the benefits of massage.

Diet: Eating lightly and drinking a lot of water are two of the simplest ways to continue the cleansing process that massage initiates. A Swedish-style or lymphatic drainage massage is best supported by a light diet of steamed vegetables or fresh fruit. Fresh-squeezed juices such as carrot, beet, and parsley are well known in a cleansing regimen. Deep-tissue massage needs protein to help rebuild connective tissue that has been heavily worked. With any type of massage, one should avoid stimulants, sweets, and fatty foods and drink plenty of fluids afterward. You need a minimum of 1 quart of water or herbal tea, but 2 quarts is best. Drinks with electrolyte replacement are also beneficial.

Herbs: The physical manipulation of massage can stir up toxins; drinking herbal teas that are lymphatic cleansers, such as cleavers leaves and calendula flowers, are very helpful in continuing the detoxification process. Also useful is supporting the involved organs, such as the kidneys and the liver, with burdock root, dandelion root, parsley leaves, yarrow flowers, and celery seed. Nervine tonic teas such as wild oat, vervain leaves, chamomile flowers, linden flowers, or passionflower leaves can help one sustain a calm interior for a sane life in this world of stress and high tension. Sore muscles can benefit from circulatory stimulants, such as ginger and peppermint, or a cayenne- and rosemary oil–infused liniment. The antispasmodic activity of cramp bark, black haw bark, and kava root is useful for cramped muscles.

Let's not forget the benefits of fragrant plants in the form of essential oils. A scent alone is enough to trigger a memory association in the brain, taking you back to that massage table and state of relaxation. Lavender oil itself also has many benefits beyond the memory association. Its healing attributes for the body include nervine benefits for sore muscles, insomnia, stress, and depression. It heals burns, bites, or skin abrasions, slows the aging process with antioxidant and anti-inflammatory properties, and is pleasingly fragrant.

Bath: Both herbal teas and essential oils can be used in the bath for their healing benefits and skin detoxifying properties. Start with five to eight drops in a full tub; do not exceed 15 drops of even the safest oils such as lavender or geranium; you will merely waste money and precious resources. If using peppermint, lemon, or other citrus-scented oil such as lemongrass, do not exceed three drops of these skin irritant oils. Essential oils can be added to vegetable oil prior to adding it to the bath to help moisturize the skin and reduce any irritant effects of the essential oils for those with sensitive skin. A cup of Epsom salts can also be added to the water; the magnesium chloride provides nutrients for further muscle relaxation. Soak for about 20 minutes and languish in the memory of the massage. Using the same oil blend provided by the massage therapist will trigger the memory of the relaxation experienced during the massage.

If you absolutely must be active after your massage, a bath of stimulating essential oils can help restore your vigor.

POST-MASSAGE HERBAL DETOX TEA BLEND

- 1 ounce dandelion
- 1 ounce cleavers
- 1 ounce parsley
- 1 ounce linden
- 1 ounce peppermint
- 1 ounce ginger

Mix together 1 ounce of each herb in a jar. Use 1 teaspoon per cup of water, and steep for 10 minutes. Strain and drink.

POST-MASSAGE MUSCLE-RELAXING BLEND FOR THE BATH

- 3 ounces yarrow
- 3 ounces burdock
- 3 ounces calendula
- 3 ounces cramp bark
- 3 ounces black haw

To make an herbal bath blend, mix the dried herbs to make 1 cup of dried herbs to 2 quarts of water. Bring the water to a boil, remove from heat, add the herbs, cover, and steep for 30 minutes. Strain the tea into a full tub of water.

POST-MASSAGE ESSENTIAL OIL BLENDS FOR THE BATH

There are a total of 8 drops in each of the following blends—enough for one bath; you can also add them to 1 teaspoon of vegetable oil for a moisturizing soak. Add to a full tub of water or water with herbal tea. Soak for at least 20 minutes.

RELAXATION

- 4 drops lavender essential oil
- 2 drops chamomile essential oil
- 2 drops orange essential oil

MUSCLE RELIEF

- 5 drops marjoram essential oil
- 2 drops eucalyptus essential oil
- 1 drop lemongrass essential oil

STIMULATION

- 5 drops rosemary essential oil
- 2 drops fir essential oil
- 1 drop peppermint essential oil

MAKING MASSAGE BENEFITS LAST: MINDY'S STORY

There I was, lying on the massage table, basking in the afterglow of an hour of totally relaxing bliss. Do I really have to get up now? The reality of daily life was slowly creeping in. How can I make the most of this experience and carry the calmness of this moment throughout my day, my week? Anyone who has ever had a great massage has likely had these thoughts. There are a number of things one can do to maximize the physical and emotional benefits of the post-massage experience.

- Consider scheduling your massage at the end of the day to avoid making a mad dash back to the office for that afternoon appointment or picking the kids up from school to chauffeur them to their myriad of activities.

- Try to break the routine of drinking coffee to keep you revved up for the next thing on your list of accomplishments for the day.

- Savor this moment for yourself, and make the most of extending your massage time by enjoying a cup of tea in a quiet atmosphere or taking a nice long bath accompanied by candlelight and soothing music.

We are all aware of relaxation techniques such as meditation or deep breathing to sustain that inner peace, but we can also do things to help our physical bodies garner the maximum benefits of massage.

Using Herbs in Your Bathtub or Teacup

If you add herbs to your bath, it helps to keep them contained so they don't end up in the drain and all over you. Tie them in a porous bag or piece of fabric, or use one of the large tea strainers designed just for this purpose.

	DESCRIPTION	TEA	TUB
LYMPHATIC HERBS	**CALENDULA** This anti-inflammatory flower is demulcent, antiseptic, and well known for a variety of skin complaints (including bruises, sprains, and strains), but it also supports detoxifying through the lymph system. This is a good choice for the bath since it contains a small amount of essential oil and other beneficial compounds that are water soluble when used in the bathwater.	X	X
	CLEAVERS One of the best lymphatic tonics; has alterative (blood-cleansing) and diuretic properties; supports the detox process when glands are swollen	X	
RELAXING NERVINE HERBS	**CHAMOMILE** Of its endless list of benefits, this humble flower is best known for its calming effects in treating insomnia and anxiety and its anti-inflammatory action on tired and inflamed muscles. This antispasmodic is a strengthener for the nervous system that promotes relaxation from stress and tension.	X	X
	LINDEN A calming nervine, linden flowers help remove cholesterol deposits and prevent further buildup. It has a long history of use in France for bathing.	X	X
	PASSIONFLOWER The leaves of this sedative, antispasmodic, pain-relieving herb are one of the best choices for insomnia and neuralgia.	X	
	WILD OAT Perhaps the best herbal nerve tonic, the fresh seed is specific for nervous debility and exhaustion, partly because of the richness of calcium and silica it contains.	X	X
DETOXIFYING HERBS	**BURDOCK** These roots encourage digestion, liver and kidney functions, and promote toxin elimination.		X
	CELERY SEED This antirheumatic, diuretic, and digestive herb reduces uric acid levels and supports countering arthritic conditions.	X	X
	DANDELION An important diuretic, this root has the benefit of preventing the elimination of potassium.	X	
	PARSLEY The leaves of this culinary garnish are also an effective diuretic and digestive aid as well as a source of vitamin C.	X	
	YARROW A urinary antiseptic and diuretic, yarrow flowers stimulate digestion with their bitter flavor and tone the blood system.	X	X
MUSCLE-RELIEVING HERBS	**CRAMP BARK AND BLACK HAW BARK** These relaxers of muscle tension and spasms have sedative effects that reduce blood pressure by relaxing peripheral blood vessels.	X	X
	GINGER An anti-inflammatory root (actually a rhizome), it is useful for sprains, muscle spasms, and fibrous muscle conditions. It increases peripheral blood circulation, which promotes perspiration.	X	X
	KAVA This popular South Pacific root is known for its relaxation benefits for muscular relief, mental or physical anxiety, and bladder spasms, though some research has put its safety into question.	X	X

CHAPTER 8

Body and Hair Care

THE CONDITION of our hair and skin reflects our inner health and beauty. Nature's gifts of herbs and essential oils offer many body-care benefits. A century ago, women made their own personal care products to keep their skin and hair healthy, using common ingredients from recipes handed down through generations.

The beauty industry is becoming aware of the healing implications of pure essential oils in rejuvenating the skin and treating common complaints such as acne, rosacea, overly dry or oily skin, and aging concerns. Holistic practitioners recognize that essential oils can also provide support in conditions such as eczema, wound healing, burns, and other skin concerns that are beyond cosmetic applications. Since stress is the main culprit of many skin conditions, essential oils provide both physical and emotional support by addressing both issues through soothing aromatic treatments. Such treatments can be expensive in a spa setting, but you can create this nurturing environment in your own home with adherence to some simple, yet important guidelines. Let's start by looking at the function and physiology of the skin.

Skin Sense with Scents

Your skin is the largest organ of absorption and elimination in the body; it accomplishes many vital functions, but people often neglect or misunderstand the skin. It is responsible for most of our sensations, protects our internal organs, and adjusts our body temperature. To achieve this, every inch of your skin contains about nine million cells, one hundred sebaceous glands, six hundred and fifty sweat glands, and thirteen hundred nerve endings. In this small area, there are also nineteen yards of blood vessels that supply nourishment to the skin, an important job since more than half of the body's total blood supply goes to the skin. You may not consider the skin an organ of elimination (the liver or kidneys seem more likely candidates), but the skin helps rid the body of toxins through sweating.

A cross section of skin reveals three layers. The top layer is called the *epidermis.* Next comes the *dermis,* and underneath these, the fatty *subcutaneous* layer provides body contours and insulation. Looking more closely at these layers, we see that the outermost epidermal layer is divided into four levels of its own. New skin cells are formed in the deepest basal layer of the epidermis, called the *stratum germinativum.* These cells reproduce rapidly and undergo many changes as they gradually rise to the surface. One important change is an increase in the amount of protein (called keratin) they produce. In a process called *keratinization,* cells grow, mature, and die as they reach the outermost protective layer, the *stratum corneum.* Ideally, the epidermis is composed of tightly packed cells. These cells are continuously shed (at the rate of five billion a day!), making room for a new underlying skin layer every fourteen to thirty days, depending on your age. However, if keratinization occurs too quickly, the outer skin becomes thick, cracked, and vulnerable to infection. If the regeneration process is too slow, the immature surface skin is raw and tender.

The next layer down, the *dermis,* has two layers of its own—the *papillary* and the *reticular* layers. The dermis is highly sensitive and contains many other components, including nerve endings, sweat glands, oil glands, fat cells, hair follicles, and lymph vessels (part of the body's filtering system). A veritable skin factory, the dermis depends on a good supply of oxygen and nutrients from the blood to manufacture cells, which is one reason why decreased circulation (from lack of exercise, poor health, or aging—especially after age 50) adversely affects the appearance and health of the skin. The dermis is composed of 70 percent collagen fibers arranged like the meshwork of woven fabric. It is collagen, not muscle that is responsible for giving skin strength, form, and stability, and it contains flexible and resilient elastin (elastic) fibers. Together elastin and collagen keep skin toned, firm, and unwrinkled. However, as time goes by, they eventually lose their strength, and the skin wrinkles and sags without its underlying support to help it bounce back.

The most important element for the skin is water. Healthy skin contains 50 to 75 percent water, which keeps skin cells soft and supple, decreasing flakiness, dryness, and wrinkles. Unfortunately, the skin constantly loses water through sweat and evaporation. To help retain this precious commodity, sebaceous glands (tiny coiled structures next to hair follicles) secrete sebum, which is oil that coats the skin. Sebum, water-attracting compounds, and beneficial bacteria combine to create Natural Moisturizing Factors (NMFs); these also help to hydrate and protect the skin. Keratin protein is one of the skin's best friends because it increases the amount of water the skin can hold.

Another important factor to consider is the skin's acid/alkaline balance. Healthy skin is slightly acid, with an approximate pH of 4.5 to 5.5. The pH scale ranges from acid to alkaline: 0 to 14 respectively, with 7 being neutral. This "acid mantle" is a protective barrier that keeps out harmful bacteria and other potential pathogens. Test the pH of any cosmetic product in the 4.5 to 7.5 range with nitrazine paper, available from most pharmacies.

Essential Oils in Skin Care

Though very little clinical research exists on the effects of essential oils on skin, such as sebum production and wrinkle prevention, there is some data about essential oils and other skin problems, such as healing wounds and burns. Most aromatherapy practitioners have had to rely on anecdotal evidence, personal experience, and historic use for other skin ailments.

We do know that essential oils enter the skin because of two critical factors—they are oil (lipid) soluble, and they have a small molecular size (low molecular weight). They penetrate into the deep dermal layer of the skin and affect the physiology of the body through lymphatic vessels, capillaries, and nerve endings located in this region. It is in this critical layer that new cells are formed and the health of the skin is most affected. The rates of absorption and elimination of essential oils vary from person to person and depend somewhat on the constituents found in the oil and the amount of fat cells and metabolic rate of the individual. In an average healthy adult, absorption can be detected in twenty minutes and eliminated in ninety minutes.

The Aromatic Bath

What better way to enjoy the therapeutic benefits of essential oils than in a bath. Aromatic baths help insomnia, colds, premenstrual syndrome, muscular aches, and anxiety—while the warm water promotes additional relaxation.

You can add essential oils to the bath in undiluted drops, but they are typically *hydrophobic* (they don't dissolve in water) and *lipophilic* (they are drawn to oil). In the bath, therefore, where your skin is the only oil medium, undiluted essential oils are drawn into your body much more quickly than those diluted in a vegetable oil base. Hot water also causes your skin to be especially receptive to absorbing essential oils. We recommend that you use 3 to 10 drops of essential oil per tub, depending on the particular oils that are selected and the bather's skin sensitivity.

Oils that are irritating or stimulating, such as basil, lemongrass, citruses, and peppermint, are better mixed in minute amounts with other essential oils than used alone in a bath oil formula. With nonirritating oils such as lavender, sandalwood, and geranium, 10 drops are not only safe but they are also delightful.

Some essential oils will slightly disperse in the water, but many oils will remain in little droplets, forming a fragrant film on top of the water. For best results, fill the tub with water and add the oils just before you get in. Be sure to agitate the water well to distribute the oils. If you do experience any skin irritation in the bath, rinse with cool water, get out of the tub, and apply straight vegetable oil to the skin to disperse and dilute the activity of the essential oils.

FLOATING AROMATIC BATH OILS

Floating aromatic bath oils are wonderful! While bathing, you receive an aromatherapy fragrance treatment, and when you get out, your entire body will be lightly coated with a fragrance that will waft around you for hours. The vegetable oil base dilutes the essential oil, helping it to disperse and float over the surface of the water. As you emerge, the oils cling to your skin, scenting it like a body perfume.

Have you ever noticed how your skin shrivels up like a prune after you have been in the water for a long time? The surrounding water actually draws moisture out of your skin. It is a loss of water more than a loss of oil that makes skin feel dry. If you have dry skin—or love to take long soaks in a hot bath—be sure to use an aromatic bath oil. Some people with very dry skin find they can't take baths because their skin itches and feels even drier afterward. Their problems will likely disappear when they use an aromatic bath oil, especially one formulated with essential oil suited for dryness and itching skin.

Although an aromatic bath oil may seem like some exotic fragrance concoction, it is extremely easy to create and makes a wonderful aromatherapy gift. Simply dilute essential oils with vegetable oil. We recommend a 4 percent dilution in oil—about 20 to 24 drops per ounce of carrier (keep in mind that this dilution represents all of the oils in the blend combined, not 4 percent of each oil). This is double the strength of a massage oil, but add just 1 teaspoon to a full tub.

Try some blends from our suggested aromatic combinations, listed later in this chapter, for the bath. If you feel creative, make your own combination. With information from chapters 11 and 15 you can enhance your bath oil with herbs and treat special problems.

An aromatic bath is a perfect way to slow children down, especially at bedtime. Use a little extra precaution when using essential oils in a tub for a young child. Unlike adults, who may add essential oils directly to bathwater, you must be careful with undiluted oils with children, especially so undiluted droplets do not get rubbed into sensitive eyes. Suggested dilutions for a child's bath oil is 1 percent (only about 5 to 6 drops); add ½ to 1 teaspoon of bath oil to a full tub. Bubble baths are another option for diluting essential oils for children. Use a pH-balanced shampoo as the soap base.

Part of the elegance of bath oils comes from their containers. Beautiful bottles add glamour to the oils you display in your bathroom or give as gifts. Import stores or mail-order catalogs are a good source of fancy bottles, though we've obtained some of our favorite containers at garage sales and flea markets. Decorate your creations by inserting a few sprigs of dried flowers or herbs in clear bottles, or use colored glass containers with a few herbal sprigs tied to the container with a ribbon.

Instead of introducing skin-drying soap into your bathwater—especially when you plan to spend some time relaxing in your tub—treat yourself to an oat scrub by filling a porous piece of cloth with ½ cup ground oats (grind oatmeal or whole oats in a coffee grinder or blender). Tie the mixture into a bag, and use it for scrubbing. It works nearly as well as soap and is great for your skin. If you wish, add a few drops of an essential oil or a tablespoon of fragrant, chopped herbs, either fresh or dry.

FLOATING AROMATIC BATH OIL

25 drops (¼ teaspoon) essential oil
1 ounce vegetable oil

Shake to mix. Use 1 teaspoon per bath. For babies, mix only 6 drops of essential oil with 1 ounce carrier oil, and use ½ to 1 teaspoon per bath, taking care to choose only gentle oils.

DISPERSING BATH OILS

Scented oils that disperse throughout the bathwater produce a hint of fragrance without leaving a coating on the skin—perfect for those with oily skin or who find a floating oil bath too rich. To get an essential oil to disperse rather than float on top of the water, you need an emulsifier. Commercial bath products use coconut oil or chemically based emulsifiers, but a single egg yolk is an excellent home emulsifier. Another alternative is sulfated castor oil, which is water soluble.

Hydrous lanolin, another water-soluble substance, makes a richer, more emollient bath oil. *Hydrous* (meaning "with water") lanolin is easier to work with than sticky, thick anhydrous (without water) lanolin. Lanolin, derived from sheep's wool, is moisturizing to the skin.

FRAGRANT DISPERSING BATH OIL

2 ounces sulfated castor oil
25 drops (½ teaspoon) essential oil
½ teaspoon hydrous lanolin *(optional)*

If you use lanolin, warm it with the castor oil until it melts completely. Add the essential oils after the other oils cool. Use 1 teaspoon per bath.

PROTEIN-RICH DISPERSING BATH FORMULA

1 egg
12 drops essential oil

Separate the egg, saving the egg white for kitchen uses. Mix the essential oil into the yolk, and add the mixture to a full tub. The water will be a bit cloudy, but the essential oil will be distributed evenly. Substitute 2 tablespoons of heavy cream, if you prefer.

AROMATIC BATH VINEGAR

Another variation on aromatic bath oils is aromatic vinegars, which are well suited for oily skin, fungal skin infections, or for anyone with sensitivities to the alkalinizing effects of soap. Any type of vinegar will do, but for an attractive bathroom display, use red wine vinegar—which imparts a beautiful color—and put it in a clear bottle, of course. Instructions for making herbal vinegars are provided in chapter 5.

For dramatic flair, make a vinegar-and-oil dressing (body salad, anyone?). Fill the bottle with equal parts of

ANTIBACTERIAL SOAP CONTROVERSY AND AROMATIC REMEDIES

We have all seen the dramatic headlines warning us of the overuse of antibiotics and their failure to treat infections that they once effectively eradicated. In spite of commonly held assumptions that all bacteria are bad, optimal health requires that we maintain a symbiotic, health-enhancing partnership with many types of bacteria. For example, many different bacteria live within our digestive system and are essential for proper digestion and long-term health. Every time we use an antibiotic, we undercut this bacterial partnership. By indiscriminately killing off all bacteria, we create an environment that may be filled by health-compromising pathogens or antibiotic-resistant bacteria that now have no competition for growth. This encourages the production of harmful microbes against which the immune system has no defense, such as the current spread of methicillin-resistant *Staphylococcus aureus* (MRSA). Continued reliance on antibiotics has ominous future implications, given the increase in antibiotic-resistant bacteria. There is a very real possibility of producing new strains of drug-resistant bacteria and mutant viruses from genetic mutations.

TRICLOSAN

Triclosan is a chemical that is often used for its antibacterial properties. It is found in many cleansing products, such as detergents, dishwashing soap, and the increasingly popular antibacterial liquid soaps. It is also used in cosmetics as a preservative and in antimicrobial lotions and creams, toothpaste, and deodorant. In addition, it is an additive in various plastics and textiles. It is approved for all these uses, yet triclosan's safety has been questioned. The U.S. Environmental Protection Agency (EPA) registers it as a pesticide and gives it high-risk scores as both a human health and an environmental risk. Toxic exposure can possibly occur when food items such as utensils or countertops are disinfected. In fact, some news broadcasts have warned against overdisinfecting such areas because using strong antibiotic agents such as triclosan for everyday use also destroys beneficial bacteria.

Triclosan is a phenol (chlorophenol) compound that is highly corrosive and can cause injuries to the eyes, skin, mouth, and gastrointestinal area. It can also produce nausea, vomiting, and diarrhea, and can damage the liver, kidneys, heart, lungs, and nervous system. There is some evidence that this class of chemicals also promotes cancer in humans. Externally, the chemical phenol irritates skin, but since it temporarily deactivates sensory nerve endings, it may produce little pain. Taken internally, even small amounts can lead to cold sweats, circulatory collapse, convulsions, coma, and death. Additionally, as a chlorinated hydrocarbon, triclosan is related to the toxic dioxins and PCB plastics and accumulates in body fat. Virtually every creature on earth has some of these pollutants in their body fat. Long-term exposure seems to suppress the immune system and disrupt hormones, at least in frogs exposed to high doses. Even more worrisome, when mixed with chlorinated water, triclosan goes through a chemical reaction that produces carcinogenic substances. It is assumed that municipal city water does not contain enough chlorine to be problematic, but this has not been proven.

TURNING TO ESSENTIAL OILS

Aromatic medicines are gaining attention in the treatment of many disease states, but none so much as when antibiotics have lost their effectiveness on infections. The University of Manchester and many other medical institutions have carried out clinical trials on the effectiveness of essential oils against "superbugs" that are unresponsive to conventional antibiotic therapies. According to many researchers, studies reveal specific essential oils that kill MRSA, *Shigella*, and *E. coli*, as well as many other bacteria and fungi, some within minutes of contact. Most essential oils have some degree of antibacterial, antifungal, and antiviral properties, but they also exhibit physical and emotional effects such as stimulation, relaxation, stress reduction, pain relief, and healing, depending on the chemical constituents of each individual essential oil.

bath vinegar and bath oil for a two-layered bath dressing. The only trick is to make sure the scents of the bath oil and the vinegar blend pleasantly. Use your imagination to add contrast between the different shades of vegetable oils and vinegars. Keep it in a fancy bottle, and shake well before using.

AROMATIC BATH VINEGAR

25 drops essential oil

4 ounces vinegar

Combine ingredients. Let the essential oil sit in the vinegar for a week, shaking the bottle every day. Use 2 tablespoons per bath.

TWO-LAYERED BATH OIL

2 ounces prepared bath oil

2 ounces prepared bath vinegar

Combine and shake well before using.

AROMATIC BATH SALTS

Simple-to-make bath salts are a luxurious addition to bathwater and are always a welcome and exotic gift. They make the water feel silky, remove body oils and perspiration, soften the skin, relax the muscles, and soak away the stresses of the day.

Most water in the United States is naturally "hard" because of the minerals it contains. Hard water presents no problem until you use it for washing. Then the minerals in the water chemically combine with the free alkali in soap to form an insoluble compound that bears the unattractive name *soap scum* (also known as *bathtub ring*). Having nowhere else to go, this compound also deposits itself in a fine film on your skin and hair, leaving them dull and rough.

One solution is to add sodium salts that react with hard minerals to soften water, which makes the water feel silky and smooth and helps soap work better by creating more suds and preventing it from leaving a filmy residue. An example of this is the addition of washing soda to laundry to prevent hard water from making clothes feel stiff.

Bath salts are made from very simple ingredients. Any sodium salt will work, but one of the gentlest is common table salt, sodium chloride. Other sodium salts include baking soda, which absorbs odors and relieves itching, and borax *(sodium borate)*. Many companies that make commercial bath salts list these together as "mixed salts," but it is possible to make quality bath salts using just plain salt.

For fancy bath salts, the addition of ground seaweed (if you don't mind the smell) or clay increases the mineral content and makes your creation seem more like a treatment at a mineral spa. Using sea salt also contributes tiny amounts of minerals to the bath.

Epsom salt is another type of bath salt but is magnesium sulfate and therefore not a water softener. In fact, it is a water hardener, but it works much better than other salts to soothe sore muscles, sprains, and stiff bodies in general. All salts, especially magnesium, are dehydrating, so use them sparingly if you have dry skin.

AROMATIC BATH SALTS

1 cup borax

½ cup sea salt

½ cup baking soda

50 drops (½ teaspoon) essential oil

Mix the dry ingredients together, and add the essential oils, mixing well to combine. Use ¼ to ½ cup of bath salts per bath. For muscular aches and pains, the addition of ½ cup Epsom salts to this recipe is very helpful.

AROMATIC COMBINATIONS FOR THE BATH

The following are some suggested essential oil combinations for the previous recipes. Be creative and have fun—the proportions are up to you. Use the recipe blends to make stock bottles of concentrates, which you can later use to create bath oils, bath salts, massage oils, and so on. The proportions and amounts are up to you.

RELAXATION BLEND

neroli	Roman chamomile
marjoram	lavender

STIMULATION BLEND

rosemary	grapefruit
peppermint	

BALANCING BLEND

lavender	orange
geranium	

APHRODISIAC BLEND

sandalwood	jasmine
ylang-ylang	

STEAM BATHS

The Scandinavian steam bath or sauna and the Native American sweat lodge both traditionally employ fragrant plants. The herbs are either placed directly on the hot rocks or infused in the water that is poured on the rocks. Cedar leaf and sage are traditionally used for sweat lodges, while eucalyptus is the most popular essence for steam baths. You can also use essential oils of Atlas cedar and fir, or place a small amount of the resins frankincense or myrrh directly on the hot rocks. However, never pour essential oils directly on the heating unit of a sauna. They will quickly burn or ignite and could injure some types of units. First add essential oils to water, and then pour it on the hot rocks to create scented steam.

Each of these methods encourages sweating, which aids circulation and helps to flush out the system and revitalize the skin. This type of bath ritual was used by many different cultures in the treatment of disease, with some adopting it as part of their spiritual practices. Never use citrus oils in steam and then expose your skin to sunlight or tanning beds.

FOOT OR HAND BATH

You may be surprised to learn that foot and hand baths with herbs and essential oils are effective ways of treating problems in other parts of the body. The famous French herbalist Maurice Messegue and aromatherapist Madame Maury did much of their healing work with these baths. Use 5 to 15 drops of essential oil per treatment, depending on how much water you use and which essential oils

AN AROMATIC BATH EXPERIENCE

Follow these steps to bliss to escape from the world for 40 minutes:

1. Light some incense, or put a few drops of your favorite essential oil in an electric cooker with a little water, to create a fragrant environment.

2. Play some soothing music.

3. Arrange the needed bath materials: a thick, scented towel, warm robe, slippers (impart the fragrance of your favorite essential oils to all of your linens by tucking small scented cloths or empty essential oil bottles in your linen closet).

4. Draw a hot bath.

5. Drink a soothing cup of chamomile tea as the tub fills.

6. Add half a cup of scented bath salts to the bathwater.

7. Add 1 drop of exotic oil, such as rose or jasmine, and swirl to disperse it.

8. Light a candle and turn off the lights.

9. Step into the bath and relax for 30 minutes with no thoughts of the outside world.

10. Emerge, dry off, and either dust with fragrant powder or apply a moisturizing cream to your entire body.

11. Wrap up in a warm robe, carry the candle to the bedroom, and place a fragrant herbal dream pillow under your bed pillow.

12. Slip into bed, blow out the candle, and enjoy fragrant dreams and a restful slumber.

you choose. The soles of the feet and the palms of the hand are much less susceptible to the irritating potential of many essential oils. Water temperature can vary depending on the condition you are treating. Warm or hot water usually feels best, but cool to tepid temperatures are more appropriate for sprains or fevers. Follow your instincts and listen to your body.

Aromatic Body Powders

Arrowroot, cornstarch, and white clay all make good bases for natural aromatic body powders for babies or adults. Commercial powders are usually made with talc (magnesium silicate). In *A Consumer's Dictionary of Cosmetic Ingredients,* Ruth Winter cites studies identifying talcum powder as a possible carcinogen. A 1972 study by the FDA Office of Product Technology showed that 39 out of 40 talc samples tested contained up to 1 percent asbestos, a proven human carcinogen. Even without asbestos, talc fibers are similar enough in composition to asbestos to pose a potential hazard, especially in the lungs. Winter also refers to a 1982 article from the journal *Cancer* that links ovarian cancer with talc use. She reports that gynecologist Daniel Cramer found that women who used talcum powder on their genitals and sanitary napkins had more than three times the risk of ovarian cancer and that the use of talc on latex gloves in surgery contributed to inflammation of the internal organs. Winter further states that it has been reported to cause coughing, vomiting, or even pneumonia when it is inhaled by babies.

The addition of finely powdered herbs to a cornstarch- or arrowroot-based body powder can be an added bonus. To evenly blend the essential oils into the powder, put everything through a sieve, mix well, and let the mixture sit for a few days so the scents mellow and evenly permeate the powder. When using any powder, avoid creating a cloud of dust that can be inhaled, especially by babies.

AROMATIC BABY POWDER

- ¼ cup arrowroot
- ¼ cup cornstarch
- 1 to 2 tablespoons fine white clay
- 1 teaspoon goldenseal root or myrrh powder (both *optional*), for diaper rash
- 3 drops lavender essential oil
- 3 drops Roman chamomile essential oil
- 3 drops neroli essential oil

LAVENDER SUNRISE BODY POWDER

- ½ cup powder base
- 2 tablespoons finely ground and sifted dried lavender flowers
- 3 drops lavender oil
- 5 drops rose oil
- 5 drops orange oil

MEN'S BODY POWDER

- ½ cup powder base
- 2 tablespoons fine sandalwood powder
- 5 drops sandalwood oil
- 3 drops jasmine oil
- 3 drops lime oil

"OOH! AH!" FOOT POWDER

- ½ cup powder base
- 5 drops geranium oil
- 5 drops lavender oil
- 1 drop cinnamon or clove oil
- 3 drops rosemary oil

Natural Deodorant

Sweat is sterile until it contacts airborne bacteria; byproducts created by that interaction produce underarm odor. Our culture tends to regard a person's natural scent with some disdain, so antiperspirants are popular. Most are made with potentially toxic aluminum compounds that have recently raised suspicions for some major health concerns. The underarm area is especially sensitive, and it is notorious for its susceptibility to irritation and rash. Blocking the sweat glands may also be detrimental to the normal process of eliminating toxins from the body. It is theorized that once the effects of an antiperspirant wear off, the underarm sweat glands increase their production of perspiration to make up the difference. Even the simplest deodorants are often loaded with questionable ingredients and synthetic fragrances. Natural deodorants (that don't stop perspiration) offer the concerned consumer an alternative. The most important action of any deodorant is to kill bacteria, and natural brands do so with essential oils and plant extracts. Coriander essential oil has been found to be effective in inhibiting underarm bacterial growth and is used in some natural deodorant products. Roman chamomile oil is also used in a number of natural deodorants, and its anti-inflammatory action is helpful for those with sensitive skin. Sage extracts also reduce moisture production.

If you want a completely pure natural deodorant, why not make one yourself? Some people who don't perspire much find that a simple aromatic body powder will do, but many prefer a liquid that can be sprayed or sponged on.

UNDERARM DEODORANT

15 drops ho or sandalwood essential oil

5 drops cypress essential oil

5 drops sage essential oil

5 drops coriander or lavender essential oil

2 ounces aloe vera juice or witch hazel

1 tablespoon alcohol

Combine all the ingredients in a spray bottle. Shake well before every application.

Nail Care

Neglected, chewed, or abused nails just don't get the attention they deserve. Gentle shaping, moisturizing, and buffing encourage healthy growth and strengthen the nails. Brittle nails that crack easily indicate possible dietary problems: Are you getting sufficient calcium/magnesium, protein, and silica? Detergents, nail polish, glue for artificial fingernails, formaldehyde-based nail hardeners, and household chemicals are just a few of the substances that can be tough (and toxic) on fingernails. It is not unusual to develop a nail fungus under artificial fingernails.

Herbal tea soaks or herb-infused oil treatments of comfrey root, oat straw, and horsetail can help strengthen nails and cuticles. Better yet, try combining herbal and essential oil treatments. Daily drinking oat straw, nettle, and horsetail tea can improve your nails (and hair) from the inside out; these herbs are high in silica and other minerals that are important for nail growth.

ANTIFUNGAL NAIL OIL

For this oil, use tea tree oil by itself if you don't mind the smell, but be careful not to rub it in your eyes.

5 drops tea tree or geranium essential oil

1 drop cinnamon bark essential oil

½ ounce neem oil (or calendula-infused oil)

Apply around and under the nail 2 or 3 times per day.

AROMATIC NAIL-CONDITIONING SOAK

This soak is great for dry or torn cuticles.

2 drops lavender essential oil

2 drops bay laurel essential oil

2 drops sandalwood essential oil

½ ounce jojoba or neem oil

Soak nails in the mixture for 10 minutes. Buff to stimulate circulation and bring out a healthy shine.

Aromatic Hair Care

There is nothing more radiant than beautiful, shiny, vibrant hair. Short or long, straight or curly, dark or light, hair is truly our crowning glory. It reflects our self-image, and when our moods or lifestyles change, we often change our hairstyle accordingly. But no matter what the current fashion, clean, healthy hair is always in style. With the help of nature's healing plants, keeping your hair beautiful is easy and fun. Whether it is dry, normal, or oily, all hair can benefit from applications of essential oils and herbs.

Hormonal fluctuations, diet, lifestyle, and stress play a role in the appearance and health of the hair. The ravages of modern life—including pollution, harsh detergents, chlorine, permanent wave solutions, blow-drying, and excessive sun exposure are just a few of the things that can have an adverse impact on your hair's vitality. The obvious advice is to correct poor dietary and lifestyle habits, treat your hair with gentle, loving care, and use high-quality natural hair-care products.

For hundreds of years, women have used vinegar hair rinses for the softening, pH-balancing effects. Acid-balanced shampoos and vinegar alter the electrical charge of the hair, reducing the tendency for "flyaway" hair, and cut through soap scum, removing any detergent residues and leaving hair shiny and soft.

NORMAL HAIR

If you consider your hair "normal," what you currently use on it is probably fine, but check the label for the pH and for harmful or artificial ingredients. Lavender and rosemary are two good essential oils for normal hair. To apply, gently comb out wet hair with a wide-toothed comb, working from the ends to the scalp. When the hair is completely dry, put 1 drop of rosemary essential oil on your palm, rub it into your natural-bristle brush, and brush your hair again from the ends to the scalp. This helps detangle your hair and makes it smooth, shiny, and silky. Too much essential oil can dry the hair, so be careful not to overdo it.

DRY HAIR

Dry hair and a dry scalp go hand in hand, meaning if you have one, you probably have both. When hair becomes dry, the keratin protein it contains turns brittle. Without adequate sebum production by the scalp to protect hair's moisture, it is vulnerable to split ends and can appear unmanageable as well as produce flakes. Drink plenty of water, and look at your diet to make sure you are getting a sufficient supply of essential fatty acids. A supplement of borage, evening primrose oil, or other oil that contains GLA, such as hemp or flaxseed oil, is often helpful. Protect your hair when exposed to extreme drying conditions, such as sailing, biking, or spending a day at the beach. Dry hair is especially vulnerable to any chemical treatments, from perms and dyes to swimming pool chlorine, which strips away its natural oils.

Avoid daily shampooing, and use mild shampoos containing fatty acids and moisturizers. Unfortunately, protein-rich shampoos cannot directly feed the hair, because the hair shaft is no longer alive. However, a protein film will coat dry hair, allowing it to reflect light and appear shiny. The hair will seem thicker and smoother without a "flyaway" look, at least until the protein coat wears off. High-protein herbs such as comfrey leaf create similar effects. Herbal shampoos smell good but simply do not remain on the hair long enough to do much good.

Herbal hair conditioners hold more promise but are best left on for a few minutes before rinsing. Conditioning herbs for dry hair include calendula, chamomile, lavender, rosemary, sandalwood, and burdock root. Hot oil treatments are specific for dry hair, dry scalp, and dandruff. They are simple to prepare but can be a little messy to apply. Oily hairdressings help give damaged hair some shine, but they do not always restore its flexibility and bounce. A small amount of sandalwood oil rubbed between your palms and applied to the dry ends of your hair is helpful, and it leaves a wonderful fragrance that lasts for hours.

OILY HAIR

Oily hair is caused by the same condition responsible for oily skin: excess sebum production. Oil comes from the scalp, so the hair is much oilier near the roots than at the tips. Too much oil in the hair makes it look dull, heavy, and lifeless. However, the right amount of oil makes the hair look shiny, because it fills in minute abrasions on the surface of the hair shaft. Hormonal changes affect the amount of oil the scalp produces, and diet—as always—may also be a factor.

To remove excess sebum and keep oily hair bright requires frequent washing with a mild shampoo. Harsh detergents can dry the scalp, prompting the sebaceous glands to manufacture more oil. Avoid protein and balsam shampoos because these tend to attract dirt and increase oiliness, make the hair heavy. Conditioners with seaweed may improve matters. Brush oily hair thoroughly before washing.

Essential oils of cedarwood, lemon, lemongrass, or sage in your conditioner all discourage oil production by the scalp, as does diluted lemon juice. Adding one drop of patchouli essential oil to your daily dose of shampoo also may help reduce sebum production. Vinegar hair rinses with a drop of spearmint discourage dandruff and keep oily hair in check. If you are concerned about smelling like pickles afterwards, don't worry—the odor of vinegar dissipates within an hour or so. You may also find an herbal rinse of sage tea helpful for reducing dandruff and excess oil.

SHAMPOO

A good shampoo will clean the hair without stripping away the hair's natural oil, abrading the hair cuticle (resulting in "frizz"), or irritating the eyes. Most shampoos are made with sodium lauryl sulfate, a potentially irritating detergent that dramatically increases the production of suds (something most people expect from a shampoo) in both hard and soft water. Some cosmetic chemists feel that compared to other cleansing agents, shampoos containing ammonium lauryl sulfate are less irritating. Many shampoos use a base derived from coconut and other nut oils, but surprisingly, some coconut-based products tend to irritate sensitive skin. Baby shampoos are usually mild and pH balanced, and they are often made from olive and soy oil. One place to look for mild shampoos is professional hair salons, but check the ingredient labels to avoid harsh detergents.

Many books about natural cosmetics give recipes for making herbal shampoos. Most of these are combinations of herbal tea and castile soap flakes, but we have never been satisfied with the results because castile soap is very alkaline and leaves the hair feeling stiff and looking dull. Now you find a pH-balanced castile soap, although they

Herbs and Essential Oils for Hair Care

HAIR TYPE	HERBS	ESSENTIAL OILS
DRY	calendula, comfrey leaf/root, orange peel	chamomile, ho, palmarosa, rosewood
OILY	burdock, lemongrass, lemon peel, sage	clary sage, cedarwood, cypress, lemon, lemongrass, patchouli, sage
DANDRUFF	burdock, sage, willow bark	cedarwood, geranium, juniper, sage, spearmint, tea tree
HAIR LOSS	nettle, peppermint	basil, cedarwood, peppermint, rosemary, spikenard, ylang-ylang
ALL TYPES	chamomile, lavender, rose, rosemary	carrot seed, lavender, Roman chamomile, rosemary

have merely added vinegar to adjust the pH. Test your brand with nitrazine paper to make sure it has a balanced pH of about 5.

We have seen "European aromatherapy" shampoos that sell for exorbitant prices but contain nothing more than detergents to clean, vinegar to balance the pH, salt to thicken, and essential oils to scent. Easily and inexpensively make your own formula by mixing equal parts strong herbal tea and your chosen shampoo base with a few drops of essential oil. We like to use a gentle, nondetergent, unscented shampoo as a base. Make small batches (no more than 4 ounces) to ensure freshness. Try different combinations of herbs and essential oils to suit your hair type, or simply add two or three drops of essential oil per application to your favorite store-bought shampoo. Your homemade herbal shampoo can also double as a body wash if the shampoo base you use is very mild.

HERBAL SHAMPOO

    2 ounces unscented shampoo base
    2 ounces strong herbal tea
    25 drops essential oil
    ½ ounce vinegar (optional)

Add the strained, cooled tea to the shampoo base. Add the essential oils, and shake well before use. The shampoo will be quite thin in viscosity. Use within 2 weeks.

HERBAL HAIR RINSE

    3 drops essential oil
    1 pint herbal tea
    1 tablespoon vinegar or lemon juice

Shake well and pour over the scalp and hair after shampooing. Leave on for several minutes and rinse. Refrigerate any leftover rinse, and use within 3 days.

AROMATIC HAIR TREATMENTS

These luxurious specialized hair treatments pamper and condition your hair with a variety of soothing and therapeutic botanicals.

SCALP TREATMENT

Use this recipe to treat dandruff and falling hair or stimulate hair growth, depending on the essential oils you choose

    25 drops essential oil
    2 ounces carrier (witch hazel, aloe juice, jojoba oil, or neem oil)

Combine ingredients. Apply to scalp, massage in, and cover. Leave the treatment on for 1 to 2 hours and shampoo out.

LICE TREATMENT

Always do a patch test before using this preparation, especially on children. Some people are sensitive to solutions as strong as this one. Take extra care to keep it out of the eyes, and wash it out of the hair at the first sign of any irritation. To thoroughly eliminate lice and hatching eggs, repeat the treatment every 3 days for a total of 3 times.

    20 drops eucalyptus essential oil
    10 drops rosemary essential oil
    10 drops juniper essential oil
    20 drops lavender essential oil
    10 drops geranium essential oil
    5 drops ylang-ylang essential oil
    4 ounces carrier oil (soy or coconut is best)

Mix ingredients, apply to dry hair, and cover with a plastic bag or shower cap. Wrap the head in a towel to help keep the vapors from irritating the eyes. Leave the oil on for 1 to 2 hours. When you are ready to wash it out, directly apply shampoo to the hair without wetting it first to help cut the oil. Work the shampoo into the hair, rinse with water, and shampoo again. The final rinse water should contain a few drops of lavender essential oil to further discourage critters. If you are missing any ingredient, substitute tea tree.

BALDNESS TREATMENT

Every once in a while, yet another magic formula for reversing baldness is advertised, but so far no one has found a wonder cure. This harmless but distressful problem mostly afflicts men; more than half of North American men lose their locks to some degree. Thinning usually starts at the temples, and eventually the front hairline and the crown of the head begin to thin. Once the hair is gone, there is little chance that it will return.

There are, however, methods of keeping the remaining hair healthy and on the head as long as possible. In most cases, even if these treatments do not increase hair growth, they can help by slowing further hair loss.

Better than any secret formula, the most effective way to keep hair roots healthy is to stimulate circulation with a scalp-massage formula containing jojoba oil, vitamin E, and essential oils that improve circulation, such as rosemary. Aloe vera is said to promote hair growth; some studies back such claims but others report mixed results. Hair conditioners containing balsams don't actually foster hair growth, but they do make the remaining hair seem thicker.

HAIR-GROWTH FORMULA

50 drops (½ teaspoon) rosemary essential oil (or a mix of oils from the previous suggestions)

½ cup aloe vera gel

1 tablespoon apple cider vinegar

1 tablespoon jojoba oil

Use nightly. Shake well and massage into scalp for 10 minutes.

CHAPTER 9

Facial Care

NATURE MUST HAVE designed aromatherapy especially for skin care, because it offers such a complete health and beauty package. Throughout history, aromatherapy has cleared complexions, softened hands, and made silky hair for the world's most beautiful women. These beauties knew the secrets that nature holds in her botanical collection. The formulas they passed down to us reveal that plants—especially those containing essential oils—were the key ingredients in their cosmetics.

Modern skin-care products are sold with slick advertising and dazzling packages. Although the array of products may feel, smell, and look different, they are quite similar. Most products follow a basic formula. Behind fancy labels claiming "new" or "improved" ingredients, many consist of mineral oil and water held together with synthetic waxes and emulsifiers and scented with artificial fragrances. Myriad "new" chemical ingredients are also added to make the products look and feel more appealing.

Appealing, that is, until you begin to read the fine print on the labels. Today's more sophisticated cosmetic labels often include names that require a chemical dictionary to comprehend. Reconstructed lanolin and other "chemically altered" emulsifiers and stabilizers help assure that the ingredients don't separate no matter how much heat, cold, or shaking they endure during the long journey from manufacturing plant to your home. The result is a seminatural or semisynthetic product, depending on which way you look at it.

The word *cosmetic* comes from the Greek word *kosmos* meaning "order" or "harmony." We believe in turning to nature for the most harmonizing ingredients. Many cosmetic firms now add botanical derivatives as "active" ingredients to cash in on the trend toward natural ingredients, but a few companies truly concerned about skin care are making an effort to produce totally natural products. Carefully read labels when choosing skin-care products.

If you have the time, you can make aromatherapy body-care products—for a fraction of what you pay in the store. To inspire your creations, we've included our favorite recipes. Instructions for treating specific skin types are explained below. First, we'll take a close look at skin care to help you make informed decisions about the products you buy and make.

Beauty Techniques

Beauty isn't just skin deep—it also reflects your inner health. To maintain a radiant complexion from the inside out and assist the cells in all their metabolic functions, eat a balanced diet and get plenty of rest and exercise to improve circulation. Encourage production of natural collagen in your skin—the substance that gives skin flexibility—by taking vitamin C, including the entire complex of rutin, bioflavonoids, and hesperidin (two of the most destructive influences on collagen are sun exposure and cigarette smoking). Choose skin products that are in the same pH range as skin. Keep your skin moisturized by drinking plenty of water. Although scientific studies don't correlate water consumption with skin hydration, aestheticians urge their clients to drink six to eight glasses each day to avoid skin dryness.

A good rule of thumb (though maybe a bit purist) concerning product ingredients is to never put anything on your face that you couldn't put in your mouth. Though all of our suggestions for product ingredients are natural, some highly sensitive individuals may have allergies to a few of them. It's a good idea to test any suspected ingredients for sensitivities. See "Safety Precautions" in chapter 5 and test as you would for an essential oil.

One of the very best things you can do to promote a glowing complexion is an aromatherapy facial treatment. The basic techniques are cleansing, steaming, exfoliating, applying a mask, toning, and moisturizing. How you employ these methods, as well as your choice of essential oils and herbs, should be determined by your skin type. First, we describe all the facial techniques, then we give guidelines on how to custom design these methods for your own skin type.

CLEANSERS

Beware of many skin-cleansing products on the market. Like soap, many are alkaline so they can clean and penetrate skin better. This translates to harshness as they strip away the natural protective acid mantle from your skin, leaving it vulnerable to bacteria and encouraging the production of rough callous cells in self-defense. Healthy skin produces lactic acid and eventually regains its acid mantle, but this is not an easy task for all skin types. Dry skin is especially susceptible to problems with alkaline cleansers. The result is extreme dryness with sallow appearance and rough texture.

Most bar soaps are alkaline, and many are made with synthetic or partially synthetic ingredients. Sodium lauryl sulfate is the basis of most of the liquid facial and body soaps, as well as shampoos. Even if they are pH-balanced and filled with natural ingredients, such soaps can still be harsh on sensitive skin. The most critical review of sodium lauryl sulfate comes from chemist and aromatherapist Kurt Schnaubelt, who notes, "Sodium lauryl sulfate (SLS) and related detergents [may] cause eye irritation, skin rashes, hair loss, scalp scurf similar to dandruff and allergic reactions. According to a report released by the FDA in 1978, it can combine with other chemicals [such as emulsifiers, TEA, and DEA] to create the cancer-causing N-nitrosamines." Alternatives do exist, such as potassium coco protein and glycine cleansers, which are fairly easy to find these days (see "Resources," page 234). Ground oatmeal is good for washing the face, and in the section of this chapter on skin cleansers, we present a recipe for a homemade cleanser using aloe vera and essential oils.

Before cleansing, remove makeup with homemade cream or vegetable oil. Gently wash your face with warm water, using the cleanser most appropriate for your complexion type, and pat dry.

LIQUID HAND SOAP

To make this soap, purchase nonscented liquid soap in bulk at most large natural food stores. However, there is some concern also about these synthetic liquid soaps. An even better idea is to get liquid soap made from real soap, such as Dr. Bronner's Soap. Use one essential oil or a blend.

    8 ounces liquid soap

    25 drops (¼ teaspoon) essential oil

Combine the ingredients.

STEAMING

Steaming is an excellent way to moisturize the skin and increase circulation. It helps clean the skin and leaves your face looking youthful and vibrant. Steaming won't remove dirt and grime, but it will help soften sebum and unclog pores. You can steam once a week on most skin types—except for couperose skin (see "Skin Types" later in this chapter), which is extremely delicate or extremely dry skin that may be irritated by heat.

Steam carries volatile oils directly to the face, so add essential oil or fragrant herbs to the steam water. Non-fragrant herbs, such as comfrey or plantain, are healing when applied to the skin, but are less effective in steam because they contain no essential oil. In preparing a "facial sauna," brew a strong infusion (tea) using fragrant herbs with boiling water or by adding a few drops of essential oil to plain steaming water. Set up the pan in a location where you can comfortably sit next to it. Lay a towel over the back of your head, put your face over the steam, and secure the ends of the towel around the pan to capture all the steam, creating a miniature sauna. Keep your eyes closed so that the essential oil–filled steam does not irritate them, and keep your face about 12 inches from the steam source. Enjoy the relaxing warmth for a minute or so, then remove the towel, taking a few breaths of fresh air if needed. Put the towel over your head again, and repeat a few times. We recommend that you steam for no longer than 5 or 10 minutes, depending on your skin type. Save the water or tea from the steam for your final rinse water (just make sure it has cooled sufficiently).

If you are in a hurry or traveling and need a quick steam method, place two herbal tea bags (such as chamomile or mint) in a cup, and pour boiling water over them. Using the towel, steam your face over the cup of fragrant vapors.

EXFOLIANTS

Exfoliation is the removal of dead skin cells from the epidermis, the skin's outer layer. Done properly, this brings young, fresh skin to the surface and stimulates cell growth in the lower layers. Exfoliation also gives the impression of erasing wrinkles, because it removes cell buildup on the skin that makes lines appear deeper. Most skin types benefit from exfoliation, but be especially gentle with acne-prone, sensitive, thin, or couperose skin. If overdone, exfoliation can be irritating as it exposes underlying skin before it is ready to face the world. Do not exfoliate too often, and avoid harsh chemical exfoliants.

Some exfoliants, such as cornmeal, work by gentle abrasion, whereas others, such as papaya, pineapple, and ginger, have an enzymatic action on the skin. Among the most popular cosmetic ingredients are alpha hydroxy acids (AHAs), which encourage exfoliation by loosening the tight bond that holds surface skin together. Fine lines become smoother, skin texture becomes softer, spotty skin pigmentation becomes more even, and because AHAs are antibacterial, acne problems improve. In addition, the naturally high acidity in AHAs restores the acid mantle of the skin (dermatologists use highly concentrated solutions to help reduce scar tissue). Since AHAs are also good moisturizers, they provide a very gentle way to exfoliate sensitive skin. AHAs are common in many cosmetics today, including cleansers, toners, masks, and moisturizers.

For all their benefits, the AHA found in most commercial products is a very strong chemically produced acid that you need to dilute greatly before using. Some facial peels with AHA have resulted in burning the skin. For use as a product ingredient, buy AHAs already diluted in liquid form, such as a prepared toner available at most natural food stores, so you can easily add it to your homemade cosmetics.

Even better, use a natural form of AHAs. The use of alpha hydroxy acids is not really a new idea; women have been using natural forms of them on their faces for centuries. Nature offers a variety: glycolic acid is found in certain fruits and sugar, lactic acid in yogurt and sour milk, acetic acid in vinegar, malic acid in apples, citric acid in citrus fruits, tartaric acid in wine. Cleopatra bathed in milk, eighteenth-century European women splashed wine on their faces, and the practice of applying yogurt, sour milk, or fruit to the face is an ancient beauty secret (try starting your day with a yogurt-and-fruit smoothie for breakfast, then spread some of it on your face!).

Dermatologist Ruey J. Yu of Temple University in Philadelphia has been studying the effects of alpha hydroxy acids on skin since the early 1980s. He feels that one reason physical exercise may be so good for the skin is that sweat contains lactic acid that moisturizes the skin. The problem is that most people shower with soap shortly after exercising, and the soap removes the lactic acid, drying the skin.

AHAs are not without some controversy. Some schools of thought express great concern over their use, claiming that they cause inflammation and skin sensitivity. If you choose to use them, pick a natural form such as those discussed earlier, and use common sense if your skin reacts negatively. Avoid sun exposure when using any type of chemical exfoliating agent.

Choose an exfoliant or scrub appropriate for your skin type, and apply in gentle, circular movements. Some exfoliants double as cleansers, masks, or toners.

MASKS

Masks can absorb, moisturize, feed, or remineralize the skin. Many good masks can easily be made at home for pennies. Choose ingredients suitable for your skin type. You may choose several clays as a base: white and green clays are for any skin type, red or yellow clays are very absorptive for oily skin, and gentle blue clay is for sensitive or couperose skin. The colors are natural and reflect the minerals found in the clay.

Clay is the most drying ingredient of the masks, but adjust that with other ingredients. Honey or foods naturally high in oil (such as avocado or cream) are the least drying. Eggs, fresh fruits and vegetables, oats, cream of wheat, yogurt, and nutritional yeast are just a few of the other possibilities for mask ingredients. Fruits and herbs containing skin-softening enzymes act as exfoliants, and you may incorporate them into masks or combine them with other skin-care products to soften and smooth rough skin. Add essential oils or ground herbs to increase the skin-healing properties of the mask.

To make a mask, mash the ingredients into a thick paste, adding hydrosols, herbal tea, or aloe to moisten the dry ingredients (we suggest oats or clay). Apply to the face in an even layer. Avoid sensitive areas around the eyes and the edges of the mouth. Following this step, lie down and relax. Feel the mask working, and visualize yourself with radiant skin.

Leave facial masks on from 5 to 20 minutes, as long as the mask remains comfortable. This varies with skin type and mask ingredients, but don't allow the mask to dry or pull so much that it becomes irritating. Wash the mask off with warm water, and gently pat the skin dry.

TONERS

Toners made of natural ingredients can do wonders for the complexion. They increase circulation, giving your face a healthful glow, improve skin tone, and reduce wrinkles

Herbs and Essential Oils for Skin Care

Use these herbs as a facial steam, compress, face rinse, or in a bath.

SKIN TYPE	HERBS	ESSENTIAL OILS
ALL SKIN TYPES (BOTH OILY & DRY)	calendula flowers, dandelion root, elder flowers, fennel seeds, lavender flowers, red clover flowers	geranium, jasmine, lavender, neroli, rose
OILY / ACNE-PRONE	burdock root, nettle leaves, red clover flowers, rosemary leaves	basil, citruses, cypress, eucalyptus, juniper, lemongrass, myrtle, palmarosa, rosemary (verbenone type), sage, spike lavender, tea tree (esp. niaouli type)
DRY	chamomile flowers, comfrey leaf/root, horsetail, papaya fruit, rose	atlas cedar, carrot seed, chamomile, patchouli, sandalwood, spikenard, vetiver. ylang-ylang
SENSITIVE	chamomile flowers, elder flowers, horsetail, papaya fruit	chamomile, helichrysum, jasmine, lavender, neroli, rose
MATURE / WRINKLES	comfrey leaf/root, dandelion root, elder flowers, fennel seeds, rose, rosemary leaves	carrot seed, clary sage, cistus, fennel seed, frankincense, geranium, helichrysum, jasmine, lavender, myrrh, neroli, patchouli, rose, rosemary (verbene type), sandalwood, spikenard
COUPEROSE	chamomile flowers, elder flowers, rose, rosemary leaves	carrot seed, chamomile, frankincense, helichrysum, neroli, rose
SUN DAMAGED	chamomile flowers, comfrey leaf/root, elder flowers, rosemary leaves	carrot seed, chamomile, cistus, frankincense, helichrysum, lavender, sandalwood
SCARS AND STRETCH MARKS	lavender flowers	atlas cedar, carrot seed, frankincense, helichrysum, lavender, mandarin, patchouli
PROBLEM SKIN	burdock root, comfrey leaf/root, horsetail, nettle leaves, papaya fruit, rosemary leaves	carrot seed, chamomile, eucalyptus, juniper, lemon, neroli, peppermint, rosemary (chemotype verbenone), sage, sandalwood, spike lavender, tea tree, thyme (chemotype linalol)

and enlarged pores—at least temporarily. Toners are often astringent, which means they draw water from underlying skin levels to the surface. This extra water makes the skin puff up slightly so lines and pores seem smaller. The illusion, unfortunately, has a "Cinderella" effect—in a few hours, the magic wears off as the water is reabsorbed and evaporates. Many commercial toners plump the skin with irritating ingredients that cause a slight inflammation, thus diminishing lines. Some are high in alcohol to help remove the mineral oil used in most cleansers.

Some toners can also serve as anti-inflammatory agents or moisturizers and offer a good alternative to oil-based moisturizers for those with very oily or problem skin. Natural AHAs or aloe vera are excellent for these skin types as well as for normal to dry complexions when combined with a small amount of oil or glycerin. They can help to reduce psoriasis, eczema, blemishes, and infections that result from either acne-prone or dry skin. Some individuals are sensitive to aloe vera (or the additives in commercial brands), so test it first somewhere other than the face.

SKIN-CARE PROPERTIES OF ESSENTIAL OILS

The following are just some of the effects of specific essential oils on the skin:

- penetrate to the dermal layer of skin, where new cells are developing
- stimulate and regenerate; produce healthy skin cells quickly following sun damage, burns, wrinkles, or the healing of wounds
- reduce bacterial and fungal infections, acne, and other related skin problems
- soothe delicate, sensitive, and inflamed skin
- regulate sebaceous secretions, balancing over- or underactive skin
- promote the release and removal of metabolic waste products
- contain plant "hormones" that help balance and alleviate hormone-related skin problems
- exert a positive influence on the mental and emotional state, thus alleviating stress-related skin problems

Because of their acidic nature, AHAs can cause a slight burning, depending on the strength. Diluting them will help alleviate the problem, but they won't be as "active."

Make facial toners with plain apple cider, wine, or other natural vinegars, but avoid white vinegar derived from petroleum. Infuse cosmetic vinegars with herbs to boost their healing properties. Vinegars were the rage for centuries, but they lost their popularity with the arrival of modern cosmetics that don't carry that distinctive odor. However, don't let the smell deter you from using vinegar—it lingers only for a short while. Diluted vinegar softens skin, restores the acid mantle, relieves itching, and keeps fungus and yeast (such as candida) in check. A vinegar-based toner used with a moisturizer is excellent for normal to dry skin; when used alone, it may have a slight drying effect on oily skin. All toners made with vinegar must be diluted in water, aloe, or hydrosol. Use a maximum of 1 tablespoon vinegar per ½ cup of water or less vinegar for sensitive skin.

Witch hazel, bought at any drugstore, can be used as a toner. When you infuse witch hazel with herbs (just as you would when making an herb-infused vinegar—see chapter 5), the 20 percent alcohol content helps extract important plant constituents that are beneficial for the skin. It is also possible to get an aromatic hydrosol of witch hazel without alcohol, but the recipes in this chapter refer to the drugstore variety (in the fifteenth and sixteenth centuries, facial toners made with alcohol doubled as potable cordials, sipped by women in the privacy of their dressing rooms!). Alcohol-based toners are acceptable for problem and oily skin and for dabbing on blemishes, but they are not the best choice for dry, delicate, or mature skin.

Combine toner ingredients; for example, blend aloe vera juice with an herb-infused vinegar and add essential oils, or mix hydrosols with AHAs. Toners can be misted on, splashed on, or applied with cotton pads. Toners applied with cotton remove oil and dirt, making adequate cleansers if you're traveling or camping.

AROMATIC HYDROSOLS

Aromatic hydrosols (also known as *hydrolats*) are so effective as toners—and for skin care in general—that we gave them their own section. An aromatic hydrosol produced during essential oil distillation can be a valuable addition to your beauty regimen. Hydrosols are impregnated with water-soluble (hydrophilic) compounds that are not present in essential oils. For example, soothing, anti-inflammatory carboxylic acids are found almost exclusively in hydrosols. Mildly astringent yet nondrying, they are ideal for severe cases of psoriasis, highly sensitive skin, or for any cases in which essential oils might be too strong. Most hydrosols are good to use on normal and oily complexions (or on acne-prone skin), and many are suitable for dry skin. All of them counteract the drying effects from long airplane flights and air-conditioned rooms and cars. The benefits are especially noticeable when used daily.

Use aromatic hydrosols alone as toners or add them to other toner ingredients, such as aloe vera. They are wonderful in masks and lotions. A wide range of pure aromatic hydrosols are not generally available at retail outlets, but you can purchase them by mail order.

The following are examples of hydrosols with cosmetic applications:

- **German chamomile:** Use for sensitive skin and inflammation.
- **Helichrysum:** Rejuvenates damaged or mature skin; heals and soothes inflamed skin conditions.
- **Lavender:** Balances all skin types. Soothes sunburns, irritation, psoriasis, and eczema.
- **Lemon verbena:** Lemon-scented and mildly astringent for oily skin; the odor is light, clean, and refreshing.
- **Melissa:** Very gentle on sensitive skin.
- **Myrtle:** Soothing and gentle, myrtle is also used as an eye compress for irritations and allergic reactions.
- **Orange blossom:** Good for couperose, dry, or sensitive skin; the delicate fragrance soothes and calms.
- **Rose:** Mildly astringent for couperose skin, but suitable for all skin types; soothing (on cotton pads) for irritated eyes.
- **Rosemary:** For sluggish, sallow, devitalized skin that needs stimulation and regeneration.
- **Witch hazel:** Astringent for oily or couperose skin; good as an aftershave tonic.
- **Yarrow:** Mildly scented antiseptic and astringent for problem or oily skin.

FRAGRANT WATERS

Make fragrant waters by adding essential oil to distilled water. We call them "fragrant waters" to distinguish them from true aromatic hydrosols. They are inexpensive but less effective as moisturizing agents, because they don't contain the same hydrophilic compounds as hydrosols. Adding aloe vera juice to fragrant waters can boost the moisturizing properties if you want to use them as toners or as cosmetic body mists.

Fragrant waters have many uses, depending on the essential oils you choose. Spray or splash on fragrant water after your daily shower to cool down on a hot day or whenever you are in the mood for instant aromatherapy. We use them to freshen our faces—and attitudes—on long car trips. Fragrant waters are easy to make and allow the application of diluted essential oils to your skin without the use of vegetable oil.

MOISTURIZERS

Oil alone is not a solution for dry skin; although it adds a silky texture to skin-care products and reduces water loss, no amount of oil by itself can moisturize the skin. However, oil does provide a protective barrier that prevents water from evaporating from the skin's surface, and it smoothes rough, scaly skin cells. Water on its own evaporates quickly from the surface of the skin, causing further dryness. The perfect solution is a cream or lotion that brings together the best of both worlds—water to keep skin youthful, fresh, and plump and oil to hold back water evaporation.

Facial creams generally consist of 40 to 60 percent oil and are suitable for dry-skin problems. Heavy, rich creams with more oil offer greater protection, but they are greasier and usually reserved for the sensitive skin around the eyes that has no oil glands. Standard lotions made with 50 to 90 percent water are absorbed and spread more easily than creams, making them well suited for normal to oily skin or as body and massage lotions.

Liposomes are a popular addition to many cosmetics, especially moisturizers, which contain phospholipids (oils) similar to those found in the skin. They bond to the keratin protein produced by the epidermis (the skin's outer layer), creating a lipophilic film that reduces water loss in the deeper layers of the skin. They also act as carriers to deliver other beneficial substances to the deepest layers of the skin, where new cells are formed. In fact, both liposomes and essential oils are so efficient at permeating the skin, you need to be careful about what you combine with them. Do not use them with cosmetics containing artificial ingredients, and wait at least 15 minutes after using them before applying foundation or sunscreen.

Liposomes come as a thin emulsion, much like a watery lotion, and are derived from animal or plant sources (we recommend the vegetable source derived from soybeans). You can use them undiluted on the skin, but this is very expensive. A 10 percent solution is sufficient in a lotion or cream recipe—and probably much more than most commercial cosmetics contain. Liposomes can be combined with essential oils and are useful for all skin types.

Facial oils made with essential oil diluted to 1 percent in carrier oil offer a simple, easy-to-prepare alternative to making your own creams and lotions. They do not contain the water that creams and lotions provide, but when applied directly after a toner, they are effective skin treatments. Liposomes can also be added to facial oils, but because the water liposomes separate from the oil, shake the mixture before use.

Apply moisturizers in a thin layer over the entire face and neck while the skin is still damp with toner to help seal in precious moisture. Don't forget to moisturize earlobes and neck, right down to the collarbone.

HERBS AND ESSENTIAL OILS FOR THE SKIN

A number of essential oils can be used for all skin types. Lavender, geranium, rose, neroli, and ylang-ylang are so versatile or balancing that many aromatherapists recommend them for more than one skin type. Essential oils can be incorporated into any step of the facial-care routine.

The diverse actions of some herbs make them appropriate candidates for all skin types, especially those herbs that are soothing, anti-inflammatory, healing, and nutritive for skin, such as calendula. Gotu kola and echinacea help strengthen connective tissue and increase the elasticity of the skin. Use herbs as a steam, or incorporate them into our skin-product recipes in the form of teas, tinctures, and oils. See your skin-type category in the following sections for specific oils.

HOME FACIAL ROUTINE

A facial is a real gift to yourself. Better yet, share the experience with a friend. The routine is simple, and after you do it a couple of times, you will feel comfortable enough to alter it according to your own preferences and create your own recipes. You can easily complete a facial in 20 to 40 minutes. If you don't have that much time, do a mini-facial by steaming clean skin (or applying a mask) and then using a moisturizer.

To begin your facial, put on a blouse with a wide or low neck, and pull your hair away from your face. Gather two soft towels, a facial sponge or wash cloth, a pan for heating water, a small mixing bowl for the mask or scrub, and your facial ingredients. Keep your supplies in a box or basket for convenient access whenever you or a friend wants a facial.

The steps and time required are as follows:

1. Cleanse: 2 minutes
2. Steam: 5 to 10 minutes
3. Exfoliate: 3 minutes (with facial scrub)

4. Wear mask: 5 to 20 minutes
5. Tone: 1 minute
6. Moisturize: 1 minute

The difference in your complexion after a facial will be quite noticeable. We always bring mirrors to facial classes so participants can see for themselves how radiant and youthful they look afterward. We have many good stories, but our favorite is about the woman who left an evening facial class and, having nowhere else to take her new complexion, went out for a drink. A handsome young man asked her out, and although she was very flattered, she declined—and never did tell him that she was almost twenty years his senior! We can't always promise results like that, but we're sure you'll find the facial experience enjoyable and the results rewarding.

Skin Types

The eight skin types we will discuss are normal, dry, oily, combination, problem, couperose, mature, and sun-damaged. Carefully observe your complexion, and read the descriptions to determine your skin type. If you are unsure, help diagnose it by testing the oil production of your skin with the following blotting test. Go to bed without applying any facial products. In the morning, before washing or putting anything on your face, pat a few strips of a clean brown paper bag on different areas of your face, especially in the "T zone" of chin, nose, and forehead. Normal skin areas will show a small amount of oil, oily skin will leave a definite oil stain, and dry skin won't leave any oil on the paper. Even though the cheeks will probably not show any oil stains, feel them for dryness.

Many people experience symptoms that fall into more than one skin-type category. Custom design your skin treatments by reading the appropriate sections and then choosing techniques and ingredients to suit you. Expect your skin type to change with your menstrual cycle, age, diet, the season, and other environmental factors.

Typically, skin is normal for children, becomes oily during adolescence, and gradually becomes drier as we grow older. Women (especially those who have fair skin) tend to have drier skin than men, and dryness increases after age forty. As skin matures, you'll need to gradually adjust the way you care for it.

Poor diet or digestion, a sluggish liver, radical changes in weight, lack of exercise, smoking, alcohol consumption, stress, or a generally poor lifestyle all contribute to skin problems. The remedies for these are obvious. You can only expect so much from essential oils and herbs when these factors have not been alleviated. The basics of daily skin care are cleansing, toning, and moisturizing. The complete facial routine adds steaming, exfoliation, and a mask. If you can incorporate this regimen into your life once a week, your skin will thank you with a radiant glow.

NORMAL SKIN

Ah, to be blessed with normal skin—neither too dry nor too oily, but moist and clear with even texture, color, and pore size. Normal skin can usually withstand less attention than other skin types, so count your blessings—but don't neglect your skin! You have a wider choice of ingredients than people with other skin types.

Cleanser: Cleanse once or twice a day with a pH-balanced cream or homemade cleanser.

Steam: Steaming once or twice a week will suffice for normal skin.

Exfoliation: A gentle oatmeal scrub once a week, or occasional use of AHAs, will help maintain normal skin.

Mask: Almost any type, from clay to yogurt, is suitable.

Toner: Aloe vera or hydrosols are best.

Moisturizer: Use light lotions as needed.

Essential oils: Lavender, rose, geranium, and neroli are all good for normal skin. Feel free to add the oils mentioned for other skin types if your skin condition fluctuates.

Herbs: Calendula flowers, comfrey leaf/root, rose flowers, and lavender flowers.

DRY SKIN

Dry skin typically has a fine texture with no visible pores. It feels tight and dry, especially after washing, which is usually caused by underactive oil glands that do not adequately lubricate the skin. Dehydrated skin, which produces enough oil but does not retain enough moisture, is often mistaken for dry skin. Dry skin tends to be sensitive and is susceptible to premature wrinkling and flaking, which is sometimes due to a lack of keratin. It also tends to be thin due to heredity or a lack of water that would help "plump" it up. Low hormone production can also contribute to dry skin. Dry skin is particularly vulnerable to environmental factors such as wind, the hot conditions of summer, and winter's chapping cold, all of which suppress oil-gland activity. Escaping the heat of summer by jumping into chlorinated swimming pools or living in the low humidity produced by air-conditioning present special problems for people with dry skin.

Cleanser: Dry skin that is not subjected to makeup, poor air quality, or dirt may need cleansing only once a day. Foaming cleansers are too drying for this skin type, so use a water-soluble cleansing cream that does not remove the skin's natural oil or a custom-made cleanser. Gently pat the face dry.

Steam: A facial steam can benefit dry skin, but don't overexpose the face to high heat. Cool it down by letting some steam escape during the treatment. Make the entire session short, five minutes at the most. And do not steam too often—once every week or two is sufficient.

Exfoliation: A gentle herbal scrub is ideal because it can help stimulate oil production and exfoliate flaky, dry surface skin. Commercial scrubs often use abrasives such as almond shells, but we prefer the gentle effect of finely ground oatmeal. Make a paste of the oatmeal, and gently massage the face for one minute.

Mask: An emollient mask with ingredients such as honey, whole milk yogurt, avocado, and egg yolks aids dry skin because these ingredients are humectant or contain oils that moisturize the skin. Masks that are beneficial but potentially drying, such as oatmeal, should be used sparingly or applied briefly to avoid even drier skin. A light application of moisturizing cream before applying the mask may prevent problems. If you do use clay, keep in mind that it is very drying so add only a little to a mask, and remove the mask with warm water before it dries completely. A mask is rarely made from clay and water alone, but the two can be mixed together and applied directly to spots of acne and pimples.

Toner: Avoid products containing alcohol. Instead, use aloe vera or a moisturizing hydrosol such as rose to increase the skin's water content. Well-diluted apple cider vinegar is excellent because it softens skin, restores the acid mantle, and relieves the itchiness and flakiness that often accompany dryness.

Moisturizer: Treat dry skin to rich facial creams, especially those that include liposomes. When you wear foundation makeup, choose one that contains moisturizers. Dry skin also benefits from products that include a small amount of glycerin, which attracts water.

Essential oils: Essential oils for dry skin are atlas cedar, cypress, palmarosa, patchouli, rosemary (chemotype verbenone), carrot seed, spikenard, ylang-ylang, vetiver, and sandalwood. German chamomile reduces inflammation of delicate skin. Both chamomile and lavender soothe irritation that can easily develop as outer layers of dry skin flake off. To balance oil gland production, use lavender and geranium. Neroli oil promotes cell rejuvenation, and the hydrosol is moisturizing. Small amounts of peppermint or rosemary stimulate oil production and increase circulation. Geranium, jasmine, neroli, and rose balance dry (as well as oily) complexions.

Herbs: For dry skin, use herbs that heal irritated and injured skin, such as violet flowers, red clover flowers, and marshmallow root. Rosemary leaves help stimulate underactive skin. Comfrey leaf or root (which is more mucilaginous and potent) soothes and mends damaged skin, and St. John's wort flowers help heal damaged nerves in the underlying tissue. Elder flowers promote tone and texture in healthy skin, and soothe dry, chafed skin. These herbs are best used in emollient skin creams. Supplements of GLA, such as evening primrose oil, can improve dry skin from the inside.

OILY SKIN

Large pores, a thick, coarse texture, and overactive oil glands give this skin type its characteristic shine. Excess oil tends to attract dirt that can breed bacteria and infection, clogging pores with dead cells. On the positive side, oiliness protects and lubricates skin as it matures so fewer wrinkles develop.

In summer, overexposure to the sun stimulates overactive oil glands into even heavier production, and when the oil combines with sweat, the skin feels still oilier. In winter, bundling up in scarves and hats and the tendency to wash your face less often worsens oil buildup. Never use anything on your skin that completely eliminates oil production, but many natural ingredients can reduce excessive oil production and accumulation. Restricting hydrogenated dietary fats and fried foods would also be appropriate.

Cleanser: Cleanse oily skin often—at least twice a day—with neutral-pH soap (or cleansing gel) and water to remove excess oil.

Steam: Steaming can benefit oily skin by unclogging pores and releasing excess oil. This skin type is usually sturdy and can benefit from once- or twice-weekly steam treatments, but monitor your skin and reduce the number of treatments when sebum production decreases.

Exfoliation: Avoid vigorous scrubbing that can stimulate oil production. Instead, use gentle oatmeal with cornmeal or powdered herbs as a mild abrasive.

Mask: Facial masks made with ground oats or clay effectively draw out and absorb surface skin oils. Rinse off clay masks before they begin to feel tight and itchy. Beaten egg whites make a good astringent mask.

Toner: Aloe vera, hydrosols, and witch hazel improve the complexion without adding oil. A slight amount of grain alcohol may be used on very oily skin, but drying the skin with too much alcohol produces even more oil to compensate. Never use rubbing alcohol to wipe away excess oil production. It is far too drying for any complexion and we have concerns about its toxicity. Preferably, make a tincture using witch hazel extract or vinegar instead of alcohol, then add herbs and essential oils specific for oily skin. Soak cotton pads with toner, and wipe away excess oil throughout the day.

Moisturizer: Even oily skin needs some moisturizing. When you provide the skin with a little oil, it often produces less of its own sebum. Make a light lotion or facial oil. If you really object to using oil on the face, use aloe gel with essential oils that balance oil production.

Essential oils: The essential oils basil, eucalyptus, cedarwood, cypress, rosemary, spike lavender, and ylang-ylang help normalize overactive sebaceous glands. Sage and lemongrass specifically slow down oil productions and subdue overactive sudoriferous (sweat) glands. All of the citruses may be used, but keep in mind their photosensitizing effects. Geranium, jasmine, neroli, and rose are suitable for both oily and dry complexions.

Herbs: Herbs with astringent and drying properties include yarrow and witch hazel. They can be used in tea form as a final rinse after cleansing or tinctured into witch hazel extract or vinegar.

COMBINATION SKIN

Combination skin—skin that is oily in the "T zone" and dry around the eyes, cheeks, and mouth—is the most common skin type. Treat combination skin like two separate faces, using a combination of essential oils and herbs. Read the sections on dry and oily skin, and follow the guidelines.

Essential oils: Geranium, lavender, neroli, and rose are considered "normalizers," and play double duty by treating both oily and dry skin conditions. Although ylang-ylang is considered better for dry skin, it is often also appropriate for combination skin.

Herbs: Calendula, lavender, rose, chickweed, plantain, and marshmallow root are wonderfully gentle herbs and work well for combination skin.

PROBLEM SKIN: ACNE

Pimples, cysts, blackheads, and whiteheads can occur in dry, but more often oily, skin. Oily skin with a fine texture and small pore size is the most likely candidate for problem skin. Besides all the contributing lifestyle factors, sluggish liver function is often involved. Acne occurs most often where oil glands predominate—on the face, back, and chest. Many dermatologists do not agree, but when researchers at Boston University asked patients what triggered their acne, most said stress. Although stress stimulates production of adrenal hormones in both men and women, female acne patients seem to overproduce testosterone, the cause of most acne. If your acne is hormone-related, it will generally manifest around the chin and jawline. Acne can also be caused by some pharmaceutical drugs, such as those to treat epilepsy or alter hormone production.

Acne may be temporary, especially since it occurs during puberty when hormones rage and cause excess oil production, affecting 80 percent of North American adolescents. However, acne does follow many people into adulthood, particularly if it is hormone-related. Normally, oil travels to the skin surface through hair follicles, but when dead cells and excess oil build up, pores become clogged and the hair canal narrows. The resulting lack of oxygen in the pores encourages bacterial growth, which causes inflammation, infection, and pustules that can leave scars or pits in the skin. If pores are repeatedly clogged, they enlarge, changing the texture of the skin. Oil trapped in pores can also turn into blackheads, which turn dark

as the oil oxidizes (this darkening is not caused by dirt, as many people mistakenly believe).

Acne usually improves in early summer as increased sun exposure provides vitamin D and lightly exfoliates the skin, but it can worsen if the oil-producing glands are stimulated by too much heat and sun.

Cleanser: Acned skin needs thorough cleansing. If your acne is accompanied by oily skin, follow our advice for that skin type, and cleanse the face as often as three times daily. Many people with acne prefer foaming cleansers; just be sure to choose either a pH-balanced cleanser or end with a toner that restores proper pH, such as a hydrosol. If your problem skin is dry, follow the instructions described in that section.

Steam: Steaming acne-prone skin once or twice a week can be helpful, but if pustules open, you may need to lightly cleanse, or at least rinse, the skin before continuing your facial.

Exfoliation: Scrubbing exfoliants can aggravate acne. Natural AHAs, such as vinegar, will help to lightly exfoliate and can double as a toner, especially if you add the appropriate essential oils to it. A papaya fruit mask gently exfoliates due to papain, the natural enzyme it contains.

Mask: An astringent mask on problem skin promotes mild peeling and helps reduce the look of large pores. Clay is useful, especially when moistened with toner and mixed with antibacterial essential oils.

Toner: Diluted cider vinegar has antiseptic properties and helps maintain the skin's acid balance. Aloe vera, with its skin-healing properties and pH of 4.3, is an excellent toner or cosmetic base for products for oily skin. Hydrosols are good antiseptics, and you can use them for problem skin that is oily or dry.

Moisturizer: Use light lotions containing mostly aloe vera to help heal skin damaged from acne. *Calophyllum* (tamanu) oil is a unique carrier oil specifically for oily skin, so include it in a facial oil or lotion recipe. It is proven effective against the primary bacteria responsible for causing acne, *Propionibacterium acnes*.

Essential oils: When dealing with acne, choose oils that are designated for your skin type. The antiseptic and drying essential oils for oily skin with acne are spike lavender, juniper, lemon, eucalyptus, and sage. Rosemary (chemotype verbenone is best), tea tree, and thyme (chemotype linalol) are suitable for acned skin that is dry. Lavender, neroli, geranium, carrot seed, and rosemary help heal acne sores and stimulate new cell growth and can be used on dry or oily complexions. In a study of 124 acne patients, a 5 percent dilution of tea tree oil in a gel base was effective. This is a potent brew with about 50 to 30 drops of essential oil. Although it acted more slowly than the 5 percent benzyl peroxide lotion typically prescribed, skin tolerated it better. The researchers suggested that a stronger solution of tea tree might be ideal. Peppermint and sage are antibacterial agents. Chamomile and helichrysum reduce inflammation, soften the skin, and, along with frankincense, heal injured skin. These oils can also be used on either skin type. Some other suggestions for dry skin that has acne are patchouli, ylang-ylang, and palmarosa. You can do neat (undiluted) spot applications sparingly of tea tree, lavender, *Eucalyptus dives,* or spike lavender on pimples or aggravating cystic acne that never comes to a head. Although this may eventually result in drying, it can be used for a couple of days before it becomes a problem. Tea tree is generally not irritating, but some research points to a possibility of aged oil as potentially irritating.

Herbs: Many herbs come to the rescue of acned skin. Elder flowers, red clover flowers, and licorice root help unclog pores while refining, softening, and healing the complexion. Strawberry leaves discourage excessive oil production. If you make your own products, add herbal tinctures such as goldenseal and myrrh to fight infection, prevent blemishes, and encourage healing.

Any type of problem skin may benefit greatly by internally taking liver herbs. Milk thistle seed and the roots of burdock, yellow dock, turmeric, and sarsaparilla are especially important to use in conjunction with aromatherapy treatments. They should be taken daily as teas or tinctures.

COUPEROSE SKIN

Couperose describes skin marked with tiny dilated capillaries, which are not very noticeable, unless the case is severe, and which are found mostly around the nose or on the cheeks. This condition can be found in any skin type, but it is most common with dry, thin, delicate, or mature skin. It often afflicts people of Northern European descent, especially blonds, redheads, or those with very fair skin. It can also be caused or aggravated by exposure to extreme temperatures, excess consumption of spicy foods or alcohol, cigarette smoking, high blood pressure, or any harsh treatment of the skin that causes capillaries to break. It is a difficult problem to treat, but improvement will be observed over time if the skin is cared for properly. Helpful measures include moderate exercise to increase circulation, aromatherapy treatments, and vitamins, especially those that increase capillary strength, such as E, B2, and the C complex (bioflavonoids, hesperidin, and rutin).

Cleansing: Take extra care of couperose skin by using tepid water while cleansing daily with a cream cleanser. Never use a cold-water splash.

Steam: Avoid steaming unless you keep the sessions short, and expose your face to only moderate heat by holding it far from the steaming pot.

Exfoliation: Take extra care when exfoliating couperose skin. Use gentle AHAs such as yogurt or apply a papaya mask, but avoid scrubs, which increase surface circulation and encourage broken capillaries in such sensitive skin.

Mask: Fruit, yogurt, or honey masks are the most gentle for this type of skin. Clay can be tolerated only if it is adjusted with soothing ingredients such as hydrosols or oil, and it should be washed off before it dries. Blue clay is ideal but hard to find.

Toner: Hydrosols are the most gentle, but you may also use aloe vera.

Moisturizer: Couperose skin may be present in any skin type, so choose your moisturizer accordingly, and add the appropriate essential oils.

Essential oils: Use gentle chamomile (Roman or German) to reduce inflammation, soothe delicate skin tissue, strengthen weak capillaries, and reduce facial puffiness. The essential oils of helichrysum, *Tanacetum annuum,* rose, orange, neroli, and lavender are very gentle and smell very pleasant.

Herbs: Good herbal treatments to soothe broken capillaries include calendula, St. John's wort, and comfrey as teas or oil infusions used externally. Astringent herbal rinses made from oak bark and witch hazel can help unless your skin is very dry. Internally taking hawthorn and ginkgo can improve capillary strength from the inside. Other beneficial herbs are those high in flavonoids, such as St. John's wort and calendula. Foods high in flavonoids include buckwheat and peppers. Green tea contains an important type of tannin called *catechin.* According to a Russian report, tea catechins strengthen capillaries. Tannin-rich green tea also makes a good last rinse in a facial treatment.

MATURE SKIN

As one matures, the complexion tends to become drier. Lines of character and wisdom become more apparent, although they are not always appreciated. The production of hormones that keep skin supple and radiant decreases with age. Skin produces less oil and fewer natural moisturizing factors, so skin treatments need to be adjusted with maturity. Those with fair complexions or a too-thin layer of fat under the skin, as well as those who smoke cigarettes, have a greater chance of developing wrinkles early.

At what age do we achieve mature skin? Some skin specialists say anyone over twenty-five has mature skin, but it is usually defined when lines start to form around the eyes or mouth. Many women begin noticing fine lines on the face at about thirty years of age, but it is never too early to start taking preventive measures. Antioxidant nutrients and limited sun exposure are the most effective defenses against aging of the skin.

The French beauty Ninon de Lenclos, a seventeenth-century courtesan and patron of the arts, bitterly complained, "If God had to give women wrinkles, He might at least have put them on the soles of her feet." Unfortunately, our youth-oriented society has not encouraged most women to feel comfortable about the aging process. If we can learn to love and accept ourselves and appreciate the wisdom that comes with experience and maturity, this situation will undoubtedly change. To treat mature skin, follow the recommendations for dry skin.

Essential oils: The essential oils of lavender, geranium, neroli, rosemary, and rose are historic "antiaging" ingredients for mature skin. Jasmine, frankincense, myrrh, carrot seed, helichrysum, and cistus also rejuvenate this skin type by encouraging the formation of new cells. Clary sage and fennel seed benefit mature skin, perhaps due to their estrogenic properties. Other essential oils are sandalwood and spikenard. Rose hip seed oil offers additional benefits for dryness that can accompany mature skin.

Herbs: Useful herbs include gotu kola, and emollient herbs such as marshmallow and comfrey.

SUN-DAMAGED SKIN

Sun damage can occur at any age, but the effects on the skin, especially premature wrinkling and pigmentation problems, become the most apparent as we grow older. If you want to see sun damage on your skin before it is noticeable, look at your face through the light of a special purple bulb known as a "black light," or more professionally as a "Woods lamp." Some cosmetic counters have this device available as a service to their customers—and to sell products. If you've spent a lot of time in the sun, you will probably be shocked at what the lamp reveals. Most apparent are pigmentation irregularities that may show up later in life.

ESSENTIAL OILS RESEARCHED FOR ANTICANCER ACTIVITY

angelica	ginger	patchouli
atlas cedar	helichrysum	pine
carrot seed	lemongrass	sandalwood
cistus	neroli	turmeric
frankincense	orange	
geranium	palmarosa	

Cells called melanocytes found in the basal layer of the skin produce a dark pigment called melanin. These cells differ from others because of the long, hollow arms that radiate from them. When stimulated by sunlight, these arms attach to neighboring skin cells and inject melanin into them. The result is that the coloration of the skin deepens into what we call a tan to protect sensitive underlying cells from the destructive effects of the sun. But melanin offers only so much protection, and after a few days of repeated sun exposure, the skin thickens in defense. It is a falsehood to think that a deep tan will protect your skin from serious damage. We've all heard it before: There is no such thing as a healthy tan.

As always, prevention is the key. The most important measure to take is to limit your exposure to the sun, which is thought to be accountable for as much as 90 percent of skin aging. In fact, about 70 percent of sun damage occurs without our even trying: It happens as we walk down the street, ride a bike, or drive a car. The long ultraviolet rays (UVA) that penetrate into the skin's lower layers are particularly destructive and harm collagen and elastin, important elements that give the skin vitality and flexibility, and the DNA of the cell. These "aging rays" are present during all daylight hours, even on cloudy days, and they tend to increase susceptibility to the shorter UVB rays that burn the skin (these are strongest at midday). Both types are associated with premature aging and skin cancer. Some experts believe that UVC rays (very short ultraviolet rays) are those most responsible for the worldwide increase in skin cancer, though others don't think they reach the earth. With the depletion of the earth's protective ozone layer, every skin type needs protection from the sun's harmful rays. Depending on the elevation during sun exposure, as little as forty-five minutes of unprotected sun exposure results in skin damage. While getting a little sun is important for the conversion of vitamin D, only about ten minutes of exposure a day to bare arms or legs accomplishes that.

Margaret Kripke, MD, of the Anderson Cancer Center in Houston, Texas, says that sunscreen users may be spending long hours in the sun with a "false sense of security." Kripke thinks that immune suppression caused by ultraviolet light is not stopped by sunscreen. At this point, we still advise using chemical sunscreens—at least on your face if you spend much time outdoors. Although no natural ingredients have yet been found to fully protect us from the sun's rays, minimal sun protection can be obtained from a few natural products. Commercial sunscreens that rely on derivatives from natural ingredients use PABA, part of the B vitamin complex, and the semisynthetic compounds such as oxycinnimate, cinoxate, and cinnamic acid, which are derived from cinnamon. But questions about the safety of these and other chemical sunscreens raise concern; many reportedly cause allergic reactions. A new sunscreen from amino acids found in sea algae has been tested in Australia.

For times when you need only a minimal amount of sun protection, there are natural ingredients to which you can turn. Olive, coconut, and peanut oils, along with aloe vera, block out about 20 percent of the sun's rays. Research shows that sesame oil decreases the impact of the sun's burning rays by about 30 percent. Sesamin, a lignan compound found in the seeds, may also prevent skin problems caused by ultraviolet (UV) light. According to researchers from Suntory Health Care Science Laboratory and Sugiyama Jogakuen University in Japan, one way it does so is by boosting vitamin E levels, which increases the "tocotrienol" compounds in the skin. The Xienta Institute for Skin Research in Bernville, Pennsylvania reports that vitamin E in a 5 percent dilution not only reduces burning, but it also retards cell damage to underlying skin by decreasing oxidation. Helichrysum essential oil also screens some ultraviolet rays, but don't expect it to provide SPF protection. Use a 2 percent dilution (about 10 to 12 drops per ounce).

Phytotherapist Paul Duraffourd points out the cleansing virtues of carrot seed oil, as well as its "positive effect on abscesses, ulcers, and even on epithelial cancers." Carrot seed oil can be used to treat cellular irregularities, but it is always important to seek the advice of a dermatologist for suspicious lesions. A study done in 1990 shows that caraway is anticarcinogenic when used topically. There is evidence that the same is true for citrus oils (which also have photosensitizing effects, so we are not recommending these oils for this purpose until researchers learn more about them). Sandalwood oil also has research that supports its topical use in cancer. Prevention is the best medicine, so consider using these oils in skin preparations for the body.

For a facial routine, follow the directions for dry skin. Sun-damaged skin also benefits from many of the suggestions for mature skin.

Essential oils: Lavender oil in a 2 percent dilution of aloe vera gel (about 10 to 12 drops per ounce) is the best sunburn remedy. When stored in the refrigerator, this remedy provides cool, soothing relief for any burn. Other oils that help sun-damaged skin recover are chamomile and cistus. Rough skin patches, skin damaged by sun or prone to early wrinkles, and precancerous areas respond well to a 3 percent dilution (about 15 to 18 drops per ounce) of carrot seed, frankincense, helichrysum, and sandalwood essential oils applied at least two times a day. See a doctor if the skin condition remains after a few weeks.

Herbs: Oils infused with St. John's wort, calendula, elder, or comfrey ease sunburn. Some herbalists report that St. John's wort may cause skin photosensitivity, so

be cautious with sun exposure if you are using this herb. When applying herbal oils to burns, wait until the "heat" is gone from the burn; applying vegetable oils to fresh burns can make them feel hotter. Use the aloe-lavender solution first, then apply the oil preparation after a few days.

Creating Your Own Skin-Care Products

It is easy and fun to make facial products in your own kitchen, and you can prepare them with minimal cost and fuss. They make great gifts at holidays, birthdays, or just anytime. After many years of experimenting and teaching herbal cosmetic classes, we are glad to share some of our favorite recipes with you. Remember to label and date your creations so some unfortunate family member does not mistake your calendula face cream for mayonnaise (we speak from experience).

Here are a few recipes for each step of a facial routine. Use these ideas and the appropriate ingredients for your skin type to make your own. If you do not have time to make your own cosmetics, increase the effectiveness of commercial products by adding a drop or two of essential oils. Just be sure to look for good-quality products that contain no mineral oil, synthetic colors and scents, or other potentially harmful ingredients (refer to the skin-care sections for suggestions for specific herbs and essential oil ingredients).

SKIN CLEANSERS

Cleansers gently cleanse skin of dirt and other impurities and makeup. The cleansers that we use in a facial routine are really more like toners than soap. They set the stage for the other steps of the facial. If you are blessed with a normal complexion, then skip this step and go on to the steam. When your face is visibly dirty, use a gentle complexion soap first. You can also give either of these cleansers more powerful cleansing action by adding 5 drops of liquid soap. Use one of the true castile liquid soaps (available in natural food stores) instead of the synthetically-made liquid soap that is commonly used as hand soap and body wash.

DRY-SKIN CLEANSING SOLUTION

For the following solution, aloe vera gel makes a thicker solution than the hydrosol.

- ¼ cup hydrosol or aloe vera gel
- 1 teaspoon vegetable oil
- 1 teaspoon glycerin
- 5 drops rosemary essential oil (use rosemary verbenone, if available)

Shake this solution well before each use—it does not lather on the skin. Apply with fingers or cotton pads and then rinse.

OILY-SKIN CLEANSING SOLUTION

- ¼ cup hydrosol or witch hazel
- 1 teaspoon herb-infused vinegar
- 1 teaspoon glycerin
- 1 teaspoon echinacea tincture (for acne)
- 5 drops eucalyptus or cypress essential oil

Follow the instructions above to make a dry-skin cleansing solution.

FACIAL STEAMS

Steams increase circulation, open pores, moisturize, and stimulate the skin. A steam not only clears your complexion, but inhalation of the steam will also clear your sinuses to relieve any congestion that can cause red and puffy eyes.

THE BASIC FACIAL STEAM RECIPE

- 1 quart boiling water
- 1 large handful of herbs (appropriate for your skin type)
- 5 drops essential oils (appropriate for your skin type)

Steep the herbs for 5 to 10 minutes, covered. Remove the lid and add the essential oils, leaving the herbs in the water at this stage. Use a towel to make a tent over the pot, and steam your face for up to 10 minutes. Strain the herbs and save the tea to use as a final rinse water at the end of the facial.

EXFOLIANTS

Exfoliants cleanse deep within the pores and remove dry, flaky, surface skin. Keep some next to your sink and you can use it instead of soap. We suggest making a small amount at a time so it doesn't spoil. Store it in a covered container so that it won't dry out quickly, and use within 3 days.

FACIAL SCRUB

- 1 part oatmeal
- ⅓ part cornmeal
- ⅓ part herbs lavender and peppermint (or your choice of other herbs)
- sprinkle of clay *(optional)*

Grind the ingredients together in an electric coffee grinder to a fine powder, and store it in a closed container. To use the scrub, make a paste using 1 teaspoon scrub powder and enough water or hydrosol to moisten, and apply to a dampened face. Gently scrub your face, and rinse with warm water. You can also use this mixture as a mask by leaving it on for 10 minutes.

HERBAL SCRUB FOR TEENAGE OR ACNED SKIN

Do not use this scrub if your skin is sensitive or has numerous pustules.

 ¼ cup oatmeal

 1 tablespoon dry lavender flowers

 1 tablespoon dry thyme leaves

 1 tablespoon dry rosemary leaves

 5 drops lemon tea tree essential oil

Grind the oatmeal and herbs into a fine powder in an electric coffee grinder. Add the essential oil and mix well. Store the dry mixture in an airtight jar. To use, moisten 1 teaspoon of the scrub with rosewater or aloe vera juice. Gently scrub and rinse.

FACIAL MASKS

Masks increase circulation and moisturize skin by bringing underlying water to its surface layers. A good facial mask will leave you with a smooth and rosy complexion.

FACIAL MASK FOR DRY SKIN

 1 tablespoon facial scrub

 1 teaspoon vegetable oil

 1 teaspoon honey

 1 tablespoon rosewater or aloe juice

 1 drop rose or neroli essential oil

 1 egg yolk *(optional)*

Mix the ingredients and apply to your face. Leave the mask on for 5 to 10 minutes and rinse.

FACIAL MASK FOR OILY SKIN

 1 tablespoon clay

 1 tablespoon witch hazel

 1 strawberry, mashed

 1 drop spike lavender essential oil

Mix the ingredients together and apply. Leave the mask on for 5 to 10 minutes and rinse.

FACIAL MASK FOR ACNE-PRONE SKIN

 2 tablespoons comfrey leaf tea

 ½ cup water

 1 tablespoon bentonite clay (or other facial clay)

 1 teaspoon ground elder flowers

 1 teaspoon ground strawberry leaves

 1 drop lavender essential oil

Make comfrey leaf tea by steeping 1 tablespoon comfrey leaves in ½ cup water. Let cool and mix with the remaining ingredients into a paste. Apply to your face in a thin layer, avoiding the area around the eyes. Leave on for 10 to 15 minutes, or as long as is comfortable, and rinse. Use the leftover tea as a final compress or rinse. (Please note that any potential danger with using comfrey is due to internal use of the root, not using the leaf externally, as we suggest.)

INTENSIVE TREATMENT FOR ACNE

 ½ teaspoon powdered goldenseal root

 25 drops tea tree essential oil

Combine the ingredients into a paste, adding water or tamanu oil if necessary to obtain the right consistency. Apply directly to acne spots. Leave the mask on the skin for 10 to 20 minutes. Rinse.

FACIAL MASK FOR COMBINATION SKIN

 1 tablespoon yogurt

 1 tablespoon applesauce

 1 tablespoon mashed papaya

 1 drop geranium essential oil

Blend the ingredients together. Apply to your face, and leave on for at least 5 minutes. Rinse.

EXFOLIATING MASK FOR ALL SKIN TYPES

 2 tablespoons mashed papaya

 1 teaspoon honey

 1 drop carrot seed oil

 1 tablespoon powdered peppermint leaf or lavender flowers (or enough to firm mixture)

Mix the ingredients. Apply to your skin, and leave on for at least 10 minutes. Rinse.

FACIAL TONERS

Toners nourish the skin and generally improve its pH. Keep a bottle of toner that is designed for your skin type on hand to apply daily. It will be a treat for your skin even when you don't have time to give yourself a complete facial. A convenient and attractive way to bottle toners is in a spray bottle. Just avoid spraying in eyes. (If you plan on using a spray bottle, be sure to use aloe juice, as we suggest in the recipe, instead of aloe gel, which will clog the sprayer.)

TONER FOR DRY OR MATURE SKIN

2 ounces aloe vera juice

2 ounces orange blossom water

1 teaspoon calendula-infused vinegar

5 drops helichrysum essential oil

800 IU vitamin E oil

Combine the ingredients, and shake well before use.

TONER FOR OILY OR PROBLEM SKIN

½ cup witch hazel

½ cup chopped fresh herbs or ¼ cup crumbled dry herbs

2 tablespoons rosewater or aloe vera juice

5 drops lemon eucalyptus essential oil

5 drops lavender essential oil

Soak the herbs and witch hazel together for 10 days. Strain and add the rosewater or aloe and the essential oils. Shake well before each use.

TONER FOR DELICATE OR COUPEROSE SKIN

¼ cup aloe vera juice

¼ cup rosewater or orange blossom hydrosol

¼ teaspoon glycerin

1 drop neroli essential oil

1 drop rose essential oil

Combine the ingredients, and shake well before using. Apply with cotton swabs, or use a sprayer to mist the skin.

FRAGRANT WATERS

Use this spray for your entire body.

10 drops essential oil

4 ounces distilled water

Combine the ingredients in a glass spray bottle. Shake well before each use.

MOISTURIZERS

Moisturizers hydrate and protect your skin. Use creams and lotions whenever your skin is exposed to drying situations. It is best to complete your facial by applying a cream or lotion to your face.

Although it may seem complicated, it is really quite simple to make creams and lotions in your own kitchen. The process requires a bit of patience and preparation, but with a little experience, the results will inspire you.

Become familiar with the ingredients used in lotions and creams and how they can change your product and benefit your skin. This introduction to the subject addresses some of the questions most commonly put to us by students throughout our years of teaching natural cosmetics. Start out simply, using plain oil, distilled water, and beeswax. After you master the processing technique, experiment with the "extras"—different colors, waters, and oils to give you more variation in your lotion recipes. Refer to other chapters to acquaint yourself with unfamiliar ingredients.

Emulsifiers

Emulsifiers bind water and oil together so they will not separate. Chemical emulsifiers are controversial and may slightly reduce the penetrating power of essential oil. Since all lotions and creams need some emulsification to hold the ingredients in suspension and prevent separation of oil and water, we chose the most natural ones: beeswax, lanolin, glycerin, and lecithin. We've included general guidelines to follow when you feel creative and want to design your own products. We came up with these proportions through trial and error, and we want to save you the error part!

Beeswax: Beeswax is the most common natural emulsifier for homemade cosmetics, the best for holding water and oil in suspension. It can slightly thicken a lotion or harden a lip balm, depending on how much you add. After beekeepers extract the honey, they melt the honeycomb, strain it, and pour it into blocks. Beeswax is sold at craft stores, natural food shops, herb stores, and farmers' markets by beekeepers. Be sure you are not buying paraffin or impure beeswax. If the beeswax is brittle, it is probably old. If it is dark, it may contain propolis, an antibacterial material used by bees to seal their hives. A bit of propolis in your beeswax is fine for cosmetics (although it may leave dark specks), and because it is very antibacterial, it may even extend the shelf life. Propolis is also sold separately but will not work as a substitute for beeswax.

For 1 cup base oil, use up to 1 ounce (by weight) beeswax to make a salve, ¾ ounce to make lip balm, up to ¾ ounce to make cream, and up to ½ ounce to thicken lotion. The minimum amount of beeswax that we have successfully used in a lotion recipe is 12 grams (slightly less than ½ ounce).

Lanolin: This is the oil that is removed from sheep's wool. In structure, it is much like the oil of our own skin glands and thus is easily absorbed. There are three types of lanolin: Thick anhydrous lanolin (without water) is the least desirable, because it does not mix well with water. Hydrous lanolin contains a little water, is much easier to work with, and can be used in making lotions. The third type, liquid lanolin, is designed for use as a lotion on its own, but it can also be used as an ingredient for lotions and creams.

Oil-rich lanolin makes a product more emollient and slightly thicker, but too much of it can make a product sticky. However, this may be just what is needed in a water-resistant diaper-rash cream or salve intended to adhere to the skin. A small amount of lanolin will help emulsify a cream or lotion, but don't rely on it alone to thicken the product. The formula still requires beeswax.

Lanolin is sold at most drugstores, but be sure to smell it before purchasing; some smell so strongly of sheep that no amount of essential oil can cover the odor. Stir it into slightly warmed ingredients in the oil portion of your creams to promote melting of this thick ingredient. Liquid lanolin can be added to the water portion in the blender.

Use no more than ½ teaspoon of hydrous or liquid lanolin to enrich 1 cup of base oil. Some people have a sensitivity to lanolin, so test a small amount on the skin before using it in products, especially in those made for babies.

Glycerin: Glycerin is a clear, sweet, sticky product derived from plants or animals or made synthetically. It is often a by-product of making soap. The more expensive "vegetable" glycerin comes from coconut or olive oil soap instead of from the more common tallow and lard soaps.

Glycerin is a *humectant,* meaning that it absorbs water from its surroundings. A little goes a long way, and if you use too much, it makes the product very sticky. Because glycerin draws moisture from the air, it works wonderfully as a moisturizing ingredient.

Glycerin makes a good emulsifier and will mix with either the water or oil phase; but don't rely on it to thicken your creams. Glycerin is also a natural preservative, although at least 20 percent is needed to completely preserve a product. This is more than we use in our recipes; it is so sticky, that few products, except for herbal syrups, contain this much. Glycerin has a long history of use in cosmetic products. Among the most popular glycerin products are Rose Water and Glycerin lotion and Pa's Cornhusker Lotion, both manufactured since the early part of the twentieth century.

Use up to 1 teaspoon of glycerin per cup of cosmetic base.

Lecithin: This emulsifier is derived from soybeans and is found in egg yolk, once commonly used to emulsify bath and hair products. It increases the spreadability of a product and leaves the skin feeling very smooth, although using too much can make it feel tacky. Sold at health food stores for internal use, lecithin comes in granules or liquid form. It can be used in creams or lotions.

Use up to ½ teaspoon granulated or liquid lecithin to 1 cup oil base. It is not water-soluble and is best added when melting oils and beeswax.

Colors

It's fun to color lotions, creams, bath salts, and other products. Experiment with the various possibilities, mixing and matching to develop attractive shades. Green, red, and yellow are easily derived from natural plant pigments; blue and violet shades are trickier. The best way to add color is to use a carrier oil that has been infused with a colorful herb. For example, calendula and turmeric produce rich yellow; comfrey, plantain, nettle, and chickweed provide a nice green; and alkanet is a gorgeous pink to red, depending on how strong you make it. Blue shades are much more difficult to achieve naturally. We have experimented with essential oils such as *Tanacetum annuum* and German chamomile, both of which contain vivid blue chamazulene. Although the smell was incredible, the amount needed to make the lotion blue made it very costly. One more drawback was that although the color was bright to begin with, it soon changed to a gray-blue color that evolved into a muddy green in a few weeks. Still, if money is no object and you plan to use the lotion quickly, you'll love it!

The color of the vegetable oil itself will also influence the color of your final product. Unrefined safflower oil is yellow; extra virgin olive oil is green. Infused vinegar, witch hazel, or tincture used as part of the water base in creams and lotions can lend some color, but the change is less dramatic. A colorless oil and plain water result in a very nice white cream or lotion.

Extras

The addition of special ingredients—such as bee pollen, royal jelly, herbal extracts, flower essences, honey, or glycerin—will set your lotions apart. These ingredients contain vitamins, minerals, and enzymes beneficial to the skin. Add herbal tinctures in the water part of your recipes. Small amounts of these boosters, 1 teaspoon or less, will be sufficient to benefit creams or lotions.

Water and Oil

The basis of creams and lotions is water and oil, which you can mix and match to meet the needs of any skin type. The water portion of your recipe can be any one, or a combination, of the ingredients in the water list below; the same holds true for the oil list. Just be sure to maintain the proper proportion of water to oil in a recipe. All lotions and creams will become firmer as they cool, so it is easier to pour them into wide-mouth jars as soon as they are done. If you use a saturated oil, such as cocoa butter or coconut, the product will be even firmer when cold but will melt readily when applied to the skin.

WATER
distilled water
spring water
aloe vera juice
rosewater or other hydrosols

OIL
any vegetable oil
herb-infused oil
cocoa, mango, or shea butter
coconut oil

Tools to Make Creams and Lotions

You probably already have all of these items in your own kitchen. Make sure everything is squeaky-clean before you begin; optimally, use boiling water to sterilize the instruments.

- blender
- rubber spatula
- chopstick
- Pyrex measuring cup (1 cup)
- small saucepan
- jars
- wide-mouth funnel (optional)

CREAMS AND LOTIONS

For the other cream or lotion recipes below, follow the directions for "Basic Cream." Do not try to cut these recipes in half, because there will not be enough liquid for the blender blades to work and the mixture will not always thicken sufficiently, unless you have one of the smaller new versions to create single-serving drinks.

BASIC CREAM

1 cup oil

3/4 cup (22 grams) shaved (not packed) beeswax

1 cup lukewarm water (distilled is best)

30 to 50 drops essential oils

Add the shaved beeswax to the oil in a Pyrex measuring cup. Set the Pyrex cup in a small saucepan of simmering water that reaches halfway up the side of the measuring cup. Heat just until the beeswax melts, and remove the measuring cup from the pan. Cool for a few minutes, but not long enough for the beeswax to harden. You should be able to put your finger in the oil without discomfort, and a film of cooling beeswax should form at the edge. Put the lid on your blender, and remove the center ring. The use of a wide-mouth funnel will help reduce splattering. Pour the water into the blender through the funnel, turn the blender on high speed, and slowly add the oil-beeswax mixture. This is just like making mayonnaise; proper emulsion and consistency will depend not only on the temperature of the oil mixture, but also on how steadily you

pour the oil into the water. This is not an exact science, however, and there is a fair amount of compensation for both criteria, so don't panic.

The whole concoction should begin to harden after you add about three-quarters of the oil. A chopstick is a handy tool at this point if you need to stir the ingredients as you pour. Be careful to stir only on the top edges, not deep in the center where the blades are. Slowly add the rest of the oil until the mixture becomes too stiff to take any more oil or until all the water is incorporated—which doesn't always happen. Sometimes there is a little water left in the blender; pour it off or carefully absorb it from the edges with a tissue.

You should now have a thick, beautiful cream. Add the essential oils last, turning on the blender just enough to incorporate the oils, being careful not to overblend the mixture. It will usually take 30 to 50 drops of essential oil to scent this quantity of cream, but personal preference will dictate the amount. Adding too much essential oil may thin the viscosity of your cream. Using the rubber spatula, scoop or pour the cream, depending on its thickness, into wide-mouth (1- to 2-ounce) jars. It is best to store extra cream in the refrigerator to prolong shelf life. Use within 6 months.

BASIC LOTION

3/4 cup oil

1 cup water

1/2 ounce (about 2 tablespoons) shaved beeswax

30 drops essential oils

Follow the directions above.

EXOTIC ROSE CREAM

This cream is a luxury for all skin types!

1 cup rosewater

1 tablespoon tincture of rose petals

2 ounces rose hip seed oil

2 ounces macadamia nut oil

1 ounce squalene or jojoba oil

1 ounce alkanet oil

1/2 ounce (15 grams; about 2 tablespoons) beeswax

800 IU vitamin E

20 drops rose essential oil

Follow the directions above.

PRESERVATIVES CONTROVERSY: GRAPEFRUIT SEED SCAM

With all the bad publicity surrounding chemical preservatives, people in the cosmetics trade, even mainstream department store brands, are looking for more environmentally friendly ways to keep cosmetic products safe. A controversy has been brewing for some time over the use of grapefruit seed extract (GSE), which many "natural" cosmetics companies use in place of synthetic and commercial preservatives, claiming it is a natural preservative. However, it has been common knowledge for years that GSE has no preservative qualities on its own and contains chemical preservatives. Grapefruit seed (Citrus paradisi) extract—not the essential oil—is also popular for use as an antimicrobial in many commercial aromatherapy products and to treat skin infection when applied topically. People making their own aromatherapy products at home often rely on it, and many people ingest it at home or on vacations to destroy digestive tract parasites. Its effectiveness as a natural cosmetic preservative is backed by several studies conducted by the primary manufacturer of the product. When the Institute of Pharmacy at Ernst Moritz Arndt University in Germany tested six commercial types of grapefruit seed extract products for their antimicrobial preservative action, five of them did greatly inhibit growth of many infections, including staph, E. coli, Candida maltosa, Bacillus subtilis, Serratia marcescens, Micrococcus flavus, and Proteus mirabilis. However, the researchers also discovered that all five products contained the mainstream chemical preservative benzethonium chloride and three contained the preservatives triclosan and methylparaben as well. The only one without any preservatives had no antimicrobial activity at all. The researchers then prepared their own extract from grapefruit seed and pulp without the added preservatives, but it also proved ineffective. They decided that grapefruit seeds' supposed antimicrobial activity is due solely to its synthetic preservatives! Also, these products were never tested or approved for internal use.

While the grapefruit scam does not seem to have had much affect on the U.S. market, probably because these facts are not widely publicized in the United States, in 2007, France began searching the cosmetic industry to find which products contained the extract because they were imposing fines for the mislabeling. The French Fraud Organization—the Direction Générale de la Concurrence, de la Consommation et de la Repression des Fraudes (DGCCRF)—found benzethonium chloride (0.1 percent) in a U.S. product that claimed it was made from all natural ingredients and did not list the preservative on its label. Other "natural preservatives" are also under question; one is made with honeysuckle (Lonicera japonica), which also showed no effectiveness when tested. A third type of natural preservative contains "a combination of aromatic materials." This is undoubtedly essential oils, which would work since they are naturally antiseptic and thus preservatives.

In fact, the best preservative we can suggest for your aromatherapy products is the essential oils that are already in them. Other things you can do are to prepare your products under very hygienic conditions and use clean containers. You can always run them through a dishwasher or wipe them clean with alcohol before filling them. Also, make small batches, and refrigerate anything that you will not use in a month. Squeeze or pump bottles are preferred over jars since dipping fingers contaminates the products. Formulations that do not contain water—the medium for bacterial growth—such as massage oils, need no preservatives, but extend their long-term shelf life by refrigeration to slow the oxidation of the carrier oils.

NATURAL SUN OIL

Remember, this will not provide sun protection, but it makes a good skin oil after moderate sun exposure.

2 ounces sesame oil

2 ounces calendula oil

2 ounces aloe vera gel

1 teaspoon vitamin E oil

8 drops lavender essential oil

8 drops carrot essential oil

Combine the ingredients. Shake well before using.

LIP CARE

Nothing is more sensuous than full, moist lips. Protect them from drying in windy and cold conditions by using soothing lip balm, and keep them moist by drinking plenty of water. This recipe helps heal chapped lips and keeps them kissable.

LIP BALM

¼ cup herb-infused oil (calendula, chamomile, lavender for healing, or alkanet for red color)

¼ ounce shaved beeswax

10 to 20 drops essential oil

Follow the directions for making salves in chapter 5. You can alter this formula by choosing different vegetable oils and essential oils. Some suggestions for flavoring lip balms are tangerine, anise, peppermint, neroli, and rose essential oils.

Preservatives

Preservation in personal care products is a very contentious subject these days. Products sold in stores must withstand shipping in all sorts of temperatures and months of storage, so many body-care products resort to adding synthetic preservatives. Having a product mold may not be life threatening, but companies are nervous about lawsuits, and any discoloration or change in a product certainly discourages sales.

There is no need for preservatives in homemade products using dry ingredients, such as facial scrubs, bath salts, or powders; however, liquid products, such as creams, lotions, or anything containing water carry a personal invitation for bacterial growth. Even dipping clean fingers into homemade cosmetics contributes to such growth, so it's best to use a small cosmetic spatula or clean chopstick to scoop cream from a jar. Squeeze bottles work well for thin lotions, but creams may be too thick to pass through the narrow necks.

Natural preservatives include beeswax and glycerin, but the best preservatives for your homemade products are the essential oils themselves. Some of the more effective ones are lavender, benzoin, and eucalyptus, but all essential oils are antibacterial or antifungal to some degree. Consider their individual properties and aromas to choose the most suitable oils for your creations. Under most conditions, adding essential oils can provide a three-month shelf life for lotions and creams as long as you keep them uncontaminated with fingers. With refrigeration, most products keep six months. To help extend the life of the fixed oils in your lotions and creams, add 400 IU of vitamin E to the oil portion, or dissolve ¼ teaspoon of vitamin C crystals in the water portion to slow oxidation. We have never encountered detectable spoilage with a lotion containing at least 2 percent essential oil after it was stored for a year at room temperature, but it is best to take every precaution. Start your production with clean tools, including the blender, bowls, and measuring cups, and be fastidious about wiping jar lids after every use of your products. Keep in mind, the less water you have in a product, the less possibility there is of bacterial growth, and lotions have more water than creams. In any case, our suggestion is that you make smaller batches or refrigerate the majority and keep out only as much as you will use in a month.

CHAPTER 10

Essential Oils in the Kitchen

THERE IS NO REASON to confine yourself to the cosmetic and therapeutic applications of essential oils and aromatic hydrosols. Aromatics are wonderful in the kitchen, and with a bit of experience, a few guidelines, and a creative mind, the culinary possibilities are endless.

Culinary herbs have always been a mainstay of creative cooking, adding flavor, color, and nutritional value to recipes. But have you ever considered topping a geranium sponge pudding with a dollop of neroli whipped cream, dreamed of scented sorbet, or imagined real rose ice cream? Iced herbal tea with a splash of aromatic hydrosol is heavenly on a hot summer day! Or how about flavoring your favorite jar of black tea or your sugar bowl with a few drops of essential oil? Try oil of dill in potato salad or caraway oil in cream cheese. Trying a few of the recipes in this chapter should elevate your cooking creations to new heights of inspiration.

Safety is an important consideration in the kitchen, as it is with any aspect of aromatherapy. These are strong flavorings, so diluting them is very important. Be sure to use pure oils from reliable sources, not synthetic scents or flavorings. Essential oils extracted with carbon dioxide are ideal for culinary use because their flavor is true to the plant. Absolutes are never used in the kitchen because of the solvent residues that may be left as a by-product of the extraction process. In general, it is wise to use only those oils that you would normally think of as foods—for example, citrus oils or seed oils such as anise, dill, celery, cumin, and coriander. Also suitable are essential oils from flowers and medicinal herbs such as rose, neroli, geranium, lemon verbena, mint, and melissa. All of these taste great in bubbly water, but adding one drop of ylang-ylang to a bottle of champagne (shake gently!) is an aphrodisiac that must be experienced. Then there are the essential oils from common spices—ginger, cinnamon, clove, nutmeg, cardamom, and black pepper, to name just a few. Oils from commonly used culinary herbs—thyme, rosemary, oregano, savory, marjoram, and sage—are great for savory dishes, but their bitter or overpowering flavors are a bit tricky to work with.

Essential oils, which evaporate as food is heated, yield their best flavor and aroma uncooked. It is best to use the oils in fresh food dishes such as salad dressings, cold soups, blender drinks, and uncooked desserts. In cooked dishes such as soups and sauces, add the oils at the last minute; you only need a drop or two. With casseroles, cakes, and other baked dishes, you may need to add a bit more essential oil to compensate for evaporation. Nothing is more important than dosage—except quality, which we're assuming is good. Experiment, but be conservative until you get the feel of how essential oils flavor food. Start with one drop, and go from there (a little bit really does go a long way; consider that it takes thirty to sixty roses to make one precious drop of rose oil).

Extracts

When you purchase lemon or peppermint extract from the grocery store, you are buying diluted essential oils. Making your own flavoring extracts from good quality food-grade essential oils is easy and economical, and it is a good way to reduce the amount when one drop of essential oil is too much. You can make any essential oil derived from a culinary herb or edible flower into a dilute extract, but the technique is especially appropriate for strongly flavored or very expensive oils.

The usual carrier for commercial extracts is alcohol, but vegetable glycerin or vegetable oil is perfectly suitable and may mix better with some essential oils. Glycerin is sweet and soluble in most mediums. Glycerin is a good carrier for rose essential oil, while alcohol works well with citrus oils and peppermint. Use olive oil for savory extracts such as rosemary or marjoram. Shake all extracts well before using.

To make your extract, use 3 to 5 drops of essential oil per ounce of carrier. Start with ½ teaspoon per recipe, and adjust to suit your serving size.

Aromatic Honeys

This is a delightful way to introduce even the staunchest skeptic to the pleasures of essential oils. Essential oils from herbs, spices, seeds, and flowers make excellent honeys. Favorites include angelica, ginger, cardamom, rose, peppermint, and bergamot. Use the oils individually or in combination: peppermint and ginger, rosemary and lemon, cinnamon and orange are compatible flavors. Aromatic honeys are perfect for flavoring coffee or tea, and are effective digestive aids taken after a meal. They are also very handy for making instant tea when traveling; just add 1 teaspoon honey to a cup of hot water and enjoy. Honeys will keep forever, but may crystallize. To reliquefy, loosen the lid and place the jar in hot water until the honey melts. Never heat honeys in the microwave.

AROMATIC HONEY

¼ cup honey

1 to 2 drops essential oil

Begin with 1 drop; it is usually enough. Stir well.

Aromatic Hydrosols

Aromatic hydrosols add flair in the kitchen. Many gourmet or traditional ethnic cookbooks call for rosewater or orange blossom water in exotic dishes, but imagine using lemon verbena, lavender, or rosemary hydrosol in some of your own recipes. Hydrosols are much milder in flavor than essential oils and are safer (as long as the plant they are derived from is nontoxic). There is little information on the medicinal uses of hydrosols, but we know that the Romans drank rosewater for a hangover. Hydrosols are best kept refrigerated and used within six months.

Because hydrosols are easily added to many recipes, you are limited only by what is available. It is safe to ingest an ounce or two of an aromatic hydrosol at one sitting, but you will find that you do not need nearly that much for flavoring. Rose and orange blossom, frequently called for in Middle Eastern recipes, are the most readily available hydrosols and can often be found in your supermarket or gourmet deli. Be sure not to use an artificially scented water or a product loaded with preservatives or emulsifiers. Hydrosols, like essential oils, are best used in recipes that require no cooking. Always taste a hydrosol before adding it to a recipe; some hydrosols taste burned or overcooked (a hydrosol suitable for flavoring should be fragrant and fresh). One tablespoon of hydrosol is plenty to flavor a cup or two of water, but you will notice the fragrance and flavor with just a sprinkle. Try hydrosols in bubbly water or champagne; you haven't lived until you've tried a neroli hydrosol Cosmopolitan martini.

The following recipes should help get you started and spark your own ideas for creating exotic culinary delights. With a little inspiration, you can dramatically dress up and add excitement to almost any recipe.

LAVENDER LEMONADE

For a special touch, freeze fresh lavender flowers into ice cubes, and serve with the lemonade.

    2 cups prepared lemonade
    1 to 2 tablespoons lavender hydrosol

Combine the ingredients. If you don't have lavender hydrosol, add 1 tablespoon fresh or dried lavender blossoms.

REFRESHING MINT JULEP

Serve with ice cubes that have fresh borage flowers frozen inside.

    ½ cup fresh peppermint leaves
    2 cups cold water
    2 tablespoons lemon verbena hydrosol

Rub the peppermint leaves to release the essential oils; soak them in cold water overnight and strain. Add the hydrosol and serve.

ORANGE-ROSEMARY SORBET

    ¼ cup water
    2 tablespoons honey
    2 cups fresh-squeezed orange juice
    ½ teaspoon finely chopped fresh rosemary leaves
    2 tablespoons rosemary hydrosol

Gently warm the water and honey together until the honey melts. Add the orange juice, hydrosol, and rosemary leaves. Churn in an ice cream maker, and serve in chilled bowls for a refreshing fat-free dessert.

PEACH BLUSH

    3 ripe peaches
    1 cup plain yogurt
    2 tablespoons honey
    4 ice cubes
    1 to 2 drops mandarin essential oil
    1 tablespoon neroli hydrosol

Mix everything together in a blender. Start with 1 drop essential oil and taste before adding a second.

JITTERBUG PERFUME SPRITZER

This recipe was inspired by Tom Robbins's novel *Jitterbug Perfume*.

    ½ cup strawberries
    2 tablespoons honey
    ½ tablespoon beet juice
    1 teaspoon bee pollen
    4 fresh melissa (or peppermint) leaves
    1 tablespoon peppermint hydrosol
    2 cups mineral water
    1 drop melissa essential oil
    fresh jasmine blossoms to garnish

Blend all the ingredients, and serve with a fresh jasmine blossom in each glass. If you don't have beet juice, soak ¼ cup grated beets in the mineral water for 10 minutes and strain.

STRAWBERRY-ROSE ICE CREAM

When my children tasted this, they thought it was "too perfumey" (we absolutely love rose, so we thought it was "to die for"). Try just 1 drop of rose oil the first time you make this.

    1 cup fresh strawberries

    3 tablespoons nonfat dry milk powder

    ¼ to ⅓ cup honey

    ¾ cup plain yogurt

    1 cup heavy cream

    1 to 2 drops rose essential oil

Mix all the ingredients in a blender until smooth. Churn in an ice cream maker until frozen.

AROMATIC WHIPPED CREAM

If you really want to impress and delight your dinner guests, try this recipe from herbalist and aromatherapy enthusiast Diana Deluca, who serves a neroli whipped cream that is out of this world and goes great with chocolate desserts. Experimentation with other essential oils has led to many pleasant results. Cardamom whipped cream on gingerbread, or as an exotic topping for cappuccino or hot chocolate, is fabulous. How about black currant whipped cream atop apple cobbler? Mandarin cream on angel food cake?

For a low-fat topping, add essential oils to yogurt. In either case, for single servings use a diluted extract instead of the full drop that is used for larger quantities of cream or yogurt.

    ½ pint whipping cream

    1 to 2 drops essential oil

Whip the cream to desired consistency, add essential oil, and mix well (start with 1 drop only). Add sweetener if desired.

PEPPERMINT TAPIOCA

Peppermint tapioca is quick, easy, and pleasing to children of all ages. The digestive attributes of peppermint are so good, you could call this a digestive dessert.

    3 tablespoons quick-cooking tapioca

    2¾ cups milk

    ⅓ cup honey

    1 to 2 drops peppermint oil

    1 egg *(optional)*

    1 square (1 ounce) grated semisweet chocolate *(optional)*

Mix together everything except the peppermint oil, and let the tapioca soak for 10 minutes. Cook over medium heat, stirring until the chocolate melts. Bring to a boil, lower the heat, and add a beaten egg to a small amount of pudding; slowly mix it in so it doesn't curdle. Cook for 5 more minutes, and let cool for 15 minutes. Add peppermint oil to taste, and pour into dessert cups. Serve warm or cold.

MIDNIGHT AT THE OASIS BALLS

Present the following aphrodisiac delights to your lover on a warm, sultry night!

    1 cup hulled sesame seeds

    2 tablespoons tahini or almond butter

    2 to 3 tablespoons honey

    1 tablespoon finely chopped dates

    1 teaspoon cardamom powder

    1 teaspoon bee pollen

    ½ teaspoon vanilla extract

    ½ teaspoon rose extract or one tablespoon rosewater

    ½ teaspoon ginseng or maca powder *(optional)*

    shredded coconut, cocoa powder, or whole sesame seeds to garnish

Grind the sesame seeds in an electric grinder. Add the rose extract or rosewater to the vanilla extract to help with the dispersal. Thoroughly mix all the ingredients, and form into balls. Roll in shredded coconut, cocoa powder, or whole sesame seeds. Refrigerate and serve at just the right moment!

LEMON-GERANIUM SPONGE CAKE

Adding geranium essential oil to this low-fat dessert adds a delightful floral hint.

   ⅓ cup honey

   3 tablespoons flour

   ¼ cup fresh lemon juice

   1 teaspoon grated lemon peel

   2 eggs, separated

   1 cup milk

   3 drops geranium essential oil

Preheat the oven to 325°F. Beat together honey, lemon juice, lemon peel, and flour. After adding yolks, milk, and geranium essential oil, mix again. In a separate bowl, beat the egg whites until stiff, and then fold into the lemon mixture. Pour into a buttered 8-inch-square baking pan or into individual custard cups. If available, place fresh rose geranium leaves on top of the pudding. Bake in a hot water bath for 45 to 50 minutes until the cake is set and a knife comes out clean. Serve warm or cold.

FRENCH TOAST WITH FLAIR

Bergamot, anise, or cardamom are nice substitutes for the cinnamon extract.

   2 eggs

   ½ cup milk

   1 tablespoon pure maple syrup

   ½ teaspoon cinnamon bark extract

Mix all the wet ingredients well, and soak the bread thoroughly before frying.

Other Savory Recipes

Using flavored vegetable oils is a great way to tone down the strong flavor of essential oils such as thyme, oregano, basil, savory, rosemary, and sage. Sometimes just one drop of these oils is too much, especially for light flavoring or when making small portions, so having a prepared dilution is handy. Flavored oils are nice for making croutons, as a base for salad dressings, and for basting grilled vegetables and fish. Lemon essential oil in olive oil makes a delicious marinade or dip for French bread.

Vegetable oils make a better carrier for savory extracts than glycerin or alcohol because they tone down the harshness of these oils better than any other carrier. Olive oil serves very nicely as a carrier for good flavoring, but feel free to use sesame, sunflower, flax, or other vegetable oils instead. Combine 4 drops of an essential oil (or combination of oils) to 1 ounce of vegetable oil. Use ½ teaspoon or more (to taste) of the prepared oil in any recipe. For a lighter flavoring, use less essential oil or make infused oil from dried herbs. Whenever possible, add these flavorings just before serving. It is best to store these oil extracts in the refrigerator.

HERBAL VINAIGRETTE DRESSING

This dressing is especially good on organic baby greens, with lightly toasted hazelnuts, dried cranberries, and Gorgonzola cheese.

   ¼ cup balsamic vinegar

   ½ cup olive oil

   2 tablespoons water

   1 teaspoon honey

   1 teaspoon prepared Dijon mustard

   1 clove garlic

   ¼ teaspoon salt

   1 drop black pepper essential oil

   1 drop basil essential oil

   1 drop thyme essential oil

Mix everything together in a blender. Pour onto the salad and toss well.

WILD MISO SOUP

The addition of wild garden greens and herbs makes the following soup a real immunity booster. If you are not familiar with the wild greens in your area, use chard or kale. Purchase astragalus and ginseng roots from an herb or natural foods store.

- 1 onion
- 1 carrot
- 3 shiitake mushrooms (if dried, soak in water for 30 minutes)
- 1 tablespoon fresh ginger
- 1 cup leafy wild greens (dandelion, dock, mustard, lamb's quarters, mallow) or kale
- ¼ cup lovage leaves (optional)
- 1 slice astragalus root
- 1 tablespoon ginseng rootlets
- 1 quart water
- 3 tablespoons dark miso
- 1 drop rosemary essential oil diluted in 1 teaspoon vegetable oil (or 1 teaspoon flavored oil)

Sauté chopped onion, carrot, mushrooms, and ginger in a bit of olive oil for 5 minutes. Add chopped wild greens, lovage, astragalus, ginseng, and water. Bring to a boil, cover, and simmer for about 20 minutes. Remove from heat. In a cup, thin the miso with a little soup stock, and add it to the pot. Add the diluted rosemary oil, stir well, and serve. If you reheat this soup, use low heat and watch it carefully; boiling destroys important enzymes in miso.

ESSENTIAL CREAMY GAZPACHO

This is a cool treat on a hot summer day.

- 3 large fresh tomatoes, peeled and seeded
- ½ avocado
- 1 cucumber, peeled and seeded
- 2 tablespoons fresh cilantro
- 1 clove garlic
- 1 green onion
- 1 tablespoon fresh mint leaves
- 1 cup plain yogurt
- 2 tablespoons white wine
- juice of ½ lemon
- ½ teaspoon salt
- freshly ground pepper to taste
- 1 to 2 drops dill essential oil

Start by chopping the tomatoes in the blender. Add the other vegetables, wine, lemon juice, and salt and pepper, and pulse just until everything is chunky. Add the yogurt and briefly pulse (not so much that it loses its chunky texture). Add 1 drop of the essential oil, mix well, and taste. Add another, if needed. Chill for at least 1 hour before serving.

SAVORY CHEESE TORTA

Stunning creations suitable for a centerpiece, tortas are as elegant as they are versatile. Create a variety of tortas by using different cheeses and layering with chopped olives, pesto, marinated mushrooms, or artichoke hearts, different nuts and herbs, and various essential oils. Go wild!

- ⅓ cup sun-dried tomatoes
- whole basil leaves
- 8 ounces cream cheese, softened
- 1 to 2 drops sweet basil essential oil
- 1 teaspoon paprika
- 2 garlic cloves, pressed
- 3 tablespoons chopped chives
- ⅓ cup lightly toasted pine nuts
- 8 ounces grated sharp cheddar

Soak the dried tomatoes in hot water to soften, if needed; drain and chop. Line a 2-cup bowl or other mold with two layers of cheesecloth. Arrange small basil leaves in a circular pattern in the bottom of the bowl. Stir the cream cheese to a smooth consistency, adding the basil essential oil, paprika, garlic, and chives. Press half the cream cheese mixture into the mold, being careful not to disturb the basil leaves. Add a layer of dried tomatoes and then the pine nuts. Layer in the grated cheddar and press lightly. Finish with the rest of the cream cheese. Fold the cheesecloth over the mixture, cover, and refrigerate overnight. Before serving, unfold the cheesecloth from the top of the mold and invert the bowl onto a bed of lettuce, lift off the bowl, and carefully unwrap the cheesecloth.

PART III

alchemy

And so he would now study perfumes and the secrets of their manufacture. . . .
He saw that there was no mood of the mind that had not its counterpart in the
sensuous life, and set himself to discover their true relations . . . seeking often to
elaborate the several influences of sweet-smelling roots, and scented pollen-laden
flowers, or aromatic balms, and of dark and fragrant woods . . .

—Oscar Wilde, from *The Picture of Dorian Gray*

CHAPTER 11

Blending:
The Perfumer's Art

BLENDING—the art of combining a number of oils to create an appealing and interesting fragrance—can be a challenging, if not overwhelming, prospect for the beginning aromatherapist. However, anyone can learn to create wonderful combinations that are both effective and pleasant. All it takes is a basic understanding of a few elementary principles, a bit of imagination, and an adventurous spirit.

Imagine that you are sniffing a single essential oil, such as lemon. The familiar smell is pleasant enough by itself, but it is very one-dimensional. Your brain responds, "Yes, this is lemon." But add the woodsy smell of cedarwood and the slightest hint of spearmint, and suddenly your nose is experiencing a whole bouquet of fragrances. Your one-dimensional fragrance has been expanded into a collage that will pique interest and continue to intrigue.

This is the effect that perfumers strive for in creating their products: a blend of fragrances, too elusive to pin down, that keeps one coming back for more.

You will use the same blending techniques to create therapeutic formulas. Perfume-blending rules enhance the appeal of any aromatherapy product, whatever its intended use. As the Chinese say, "Every perfume is a medicine."

Develop your sense of smell through practice. One of the best forms of practice we can recommend is to dive into this book and make a lot of aromatherapy products. Your brain will begin to record the different scents and how they combine with each other. Studies show that most people can pick out only three distinct scents in a blend of numerous essential oils. However, we want to train you to pick out the many overlays of scents to aid your ability to blend and to create blends in your imagination.

Blending for Fragrance

Perfume has been used throughout the ages to influence mood or create an image. Inspiration can come from a variety of sources. The four seasons, certain times of day, favorite music or colors, or simple pleasant emotions can all lend themselves to the creation of a characteristic fragrance.

Representational perfumes have fragrances that remind one of a familiar substance such as a flower, leather, or a fine tea blend.

Abstract perfumes embody the feel, or rather the smell, of an experience. They suggest a time or an occasion: a hot summer day, the calm before a thunderstorm, a picnic celebration, or Christmas morning.

Resinous and aromatic gums and roots give us earthy or winterlike scents. These heavier perfumes are deep and sensuous. If you are more of a spring person, you may find yourself attracted to light, fresh scents such as geranium and lavender, whereas summer people go for fruity, rich scents such as the citruses and the sweet smell of ylang-ylang. Autumn types often are drawn to the herblike and pungent scents of clary sage or spicy black pepper.

The object of perfumery has always been to create a sense of intrigue and excitement around the wearer. Keep the mood light, fresh, or fruity for the office, a party, or a sports event. For a romantic evening, choose a heavy, warm, sensuous blend (you will probably want to avoid wearing too much scent for any occasion, however; subtlety, after all, is much more mysterious).

CLASSIFYING ODORS

Perfumers have developed a simple system of classification related to four kinds of odor sensations: fragrant (sweet), acid (sour), burnt (empyreumatic), and caprylic (oenanthic, which is generally perceived as unpleasant in itself but interesting when used to add dimension to another class of scents). Other perfumers use the names commonly associated with the scent, such as minty, balsamic, fruity, rosaceous, and spicy. In *The Art of Perfumery*, Charles Piesse relates the odors to the octaves of a musical scale, theorizing that scents influence the olfactory nerves in much the same way that sounds influence the auditory nerves. As a musician harmonizes sound into a musical chord, the perfumer harmonizes scent into a fragrant bouquet.

The array of synthetic fragrances available to the professional perfumer is somewhat overwhelming and far from our goal as true aromatherapists in using plant-derived ingredients. Blending with pure plant oils simplifies the process of creating perfumes, in part because there are fewer materials to choose from. The following system categorizes natural fragrance ingredients in a practical way that will help you get started in creating harmonious essential oil perfumes.

PERFUME CATEGORIES

In this system, fragrances are divided into six main categories. Familiarity with these categories will enhance your ability to create your own unique blends. The denotations "F" and "M" refer to scents that have been traditionally designated "female" or "male," but don't let such preconceptions limit your choices.

Floral (F): Individual or in combinations (bouquets). Examples include rose, jasmine, ylang-ylang, and neroli (orange blossom). Popular, but synthetic, perfumes in this group are White Shoulders, Arpège, Zen, and L'Air du Temps.

Subgroups: fruity, fresh, sweet, green

Oriental (F/M): Heavy, with a dominant "animal," spicy, or vanilla note. Examples include cinnamon, frankincense, and patchouli. Many popular perfumes are Oriental types, such as Tabu, Opium, Youth-Dew, and Shalimar.

Subgroups: sweet, spicy, and resinous

The following list of oils is by no means complete and categorizing them is subject to opinion, but it provides you with guidelines to begin.

TOP NOTES	MIDDLE NOTES		BASE NOTES
basil	black pepper	marjoram	benzoin
bergamot	chamomile	neroli*	cedarwood
eucalyptus**	clary sage	petitgrain	frankincense
grapefruit	coriander	pine	jasmine
lemon	cypress*	rose*	myrrh
lemongrass	fennel	rosemary	patchouli
lime	geranium	thyme	rose absolute
mandarin	hyssop	ylang-ylang*	sandalwood
peppermint**	juniper		spikenard
tangerine	lavender		vetiver

* middle-to-base
** top-to-middle

Chypre (F/M): Sweet, warm, soft notes. These are combinations of resins, citruses, and woods. The name is French for the island of Cyprus, birthplace of Venus. Examples include oakmoss, bergamot, labdanum, and sandalwood. Miss Dior, Crepe de Chine, and Femme are classic chypre-type perfumes.

Subgroups: fruity, floral, animal, fresh, green, woody, leathery, coniferous.

Green (M/F): Fresh and simple, this group includes lavender, pine, and mint. Perfumes of this group include Acqua de Selva, English Lavender, and Pino Silvestre.

Subgroups: fresh, spicy

Fougère (M): Named after the French word for "fern," this group includes lavender, oakmoss, and coumarin (tonka bean). Fougère fragrance concepts include Skin Bracer, Kouros, Brut, and Boss Sport.

Subgroups: fresh, woody, sweet, floral

Citrus (M): One of the oldest fragrance concepts, this group includes all of the citrus fruit peels, petitgrain, neroli,

bergamot, lemon eucalyptus, and lemon thyme. Examples include English Leather, Drakkar, and Hermès.

Subgroups: floral, fantasy, fresh, green

PERFUME NOTES

Fragrance blending is so analogous to music, we even borrow the terminology. The terms *top, middle,* and *base notes* are used to define essential oils based on their evaporation rates, which also influence and reflect their fragrance or odor tenacity. Fragrances often described as "light and airy," such as citruses, are considered top notes. Base notes are oils we think of as heavy with a tendency to linger, such as patchouli and vetiver. Some essential oils are so complex that they fit into more than one category. Rose, for instance, is sometimes categorized as a middle or base note, while peppermint can be described as either a top note or a middle note. The way an essential oil is extracted may also influence its category—absolutes tend to be heavier than distilled oils.

The most carefully developed perfumes represent varying proportions of all three notes. If you like a light, invigorating perfume, choose a predominance of top notes. If you prefer spicy, sensuous blends, go heavy on the base notes. Suggestions for proportions are given in each of the following categories. Your perfume blend should have a full-bodied character; it should not smell thin or harsh or have "sharp corners." These are guidelines only—feel free to rely on instinct and inspiration, following every spark of creative whimsy.

Top notes: Sometimes called *head notes* or *peaks,* top notes are essential oils that evaporate quickly. In a blend, they are the very first scents that you smell, and they quickly dissipate. They tend to be light, fresh, sharp, or penetrating. The first impression they create lasts about thirty minutes. In perfumery, top notes generally constitute 5 to 20 percent of the blend.

Therapeutically, many top notes are fast acting, stimulating, and uplifting to the spirit, making them useful in the treatment of depression. Examples include all the citruses, melissa, and eucalyptus.

Middle notes: Also called *bouquets, heart notes,* or *modifiers,* middle notes create the main body of the blend, rounding it out with soothing, soft tones. The scent of a middle note unfolds after application anywhere from a few moments to three hours. They usually account for 50 to 80 percent of the blend.

In therapy, many middle notes are harmonizing and balancing to both body and mind. Some affect digestion. Middle notes include chamomile, cypress, marjoram, lavender, and geranium, as well as seed oils such as dill, celery, fennel, anise, and coriander.

Base notes: Also known as *soul, fond,* or *dry* notes, these deep, warm, and sensuous base notes help make blends last longer and add a fixative quality. Their staying power predominates even several hours after application, and they linger long after the top and middle notes have evaporated.

It takes the proper proportion of a base note to give a blend depth and intensity. When used sparingly and mixed with middle and top notes, most base notes are quite pleasant, but when used alone or allowed to predominate in a formula, they can be overpowering. Some base notes are so strong, they may make up only 5 percent of a total blend. Some of the more pleasant base notes, such as sandalwood, cedarwood, frankincense, and jasmine, can be used in larger amounts. Base notes include most of the woods, resins, and gums, including spikenard, vetiver, myrrh, and patchouli.

In therapy, base notes are sedating and are used to promote relaxation and treat anxiety, stress, impatience, and insomnia.

PERFUME FIXATIVES

Most fixative oils—including benzoin, balsam of Peru, balsam of tolu, orris root, patchouli, sandalwood, vetiver, angelica, frankincense, storax, oakmoss, and most balsams, gums, and oleoresins—are base notes. They have the ability to carry lighter scents and keep them from evaporating too quickly, so the entire blend lingers longer. One nice aspect of fixative oils is that although some are quite expensive, your investment will increase with time as the fragrance improves. Unlike most oils, which must be carefully stored away from heat and oxygen, fixative oils generally improve with age. We recommend storing fixatives in bottles with lots of air and shaking them often to distribute the oxygen. Fixatives, particularly orris root as a dried herb, are also used to keep the scent of potpourri alive.

Raw patchouli oil, for example, is clear yellow when it is first extracted from the plant. You can almost see through it. Like most fixatives, it turns amber as it ages, finally becoming a deep brown and thickening to a syrupy consistency. The smell also changes, from a harsh scent to a softer, vanilla-like aroma. People often have an aversion to "young" patchouli, but these same people don't even recognize it—and actually often enjoy it—after it has aged for several years.

Many traditional base notes were once derived from the glands of various animals. Musk (from deer), civet (cat), and castoreum (beavers) were used as fixatives by perfumers. Another animal fixative, ambergris, comes from the intestinal lining of the sperm whale. Although such products once played an important role in the perfume industry, they are for the most part produced synthetically today and are only of interest to the historical-minded aromatherapist. However, ambrette seed is used sparingly as a vegetable replacement for musk.

Aspects of Blending

The principles of blending are as varied as the perfumers who create formulas. Some begin with base notes and build up; others begin with top notes and work down. Here are some basics to help you find your own creative perspective toward blending.

ODOR INTENSITY

Because essential oils vary in odor intensity, we add much smaller amounts of some oils to our blends than others. For example, to obtain equal smell representation in a simple blend of German chamomile and lavender, it takes about five drops of lavender to only one drop of chamomile. Other examples of essential oils with high odor intensities are peppermint, patchouli, spikenard, cinnamon, ylang-ylang, clary sage, and jasmine. Keep in mind that all blends change with time and that different notes become prominent at different times, depending on how long the perfume has aged and whether you are smelling it in the bottle or on the skin. Perfumes also smell different on different people. Biophysiologist Charles Wysocki, PhD, olfactory researcher at Monell, says that "smell is our most intimate, individualistic sense." He discovered that body chemistry and skin type play a great role in determining how long a fragrance will last. Molecules in the oils are more easily absorbed and retained by oily skin and act on a time-release principle. Climate also affects the evaporation of perfumes; dry climates cause natural oils to evaporate more quickly than humid climates.

BEGINNING BLENDING

The middle notes are the easiest to dive in to. If you want to be very safe, choose a middle note that can also be regarded as a base note (see the chart on page 130), or add only a tiny amount of base oil. Finish the blend with at least one top note.

One trick for beginning blenders is to start with oil that has a fairly complex chemistry, which tends to already smell like a blend. Geranium, for example, contains the herblike fragrance (geranyl) common to most scented geraniums, a definite rose scent, a pinelike fragrance (isomenthone), and the fragrance of lemon (citronella), among other constituents. By using geranium, you begin with a premixed "blend" of rose, herb, pine, and citrus. Now expand your formula by adding small amounts of other oils one at a time.

Again, the safest route is to add a second oil that blends well with the complex one. When in doubt, choose a type of fragrance already contained in the complex oil. In the case of geranium, that might be a wood, such as cedarwood or sandalwood, a floral, such as rose, or a citrus—or perhaps bergamot or petitgrain for a more sophisticated fragrance. Finally, add a very small amount of an accent oil to top off the blend. Clary sage, for example, makes a headier fragrance, and spearmint livens things up.

One interesting way to expand upon fragrances in a blend is to choose oils that are similar to each other, such as a combination of peppermint and spearmint, one of lemon and bergamot, or perhaps neroli and another from the citrus group. These are examples of blending together botanically related oils that are different species (or subspecies) but in the same genus to make intriguing combinations. In this case, you would use two oils from the mint family or two from the citrus family. You can also try a mix of spices that have similar scents, such as combining cinnamon and clove or ginger and cardamom. Two similar scents mixed together play a confusing and delightful trick on the nose because they play off one another. You can't pinpoint the aroma, which makes it seem complicated and mysterious.

In his standard essential oil text *Perfumes, Cosmetics and Soaps,* William A. Poucher gives examples of how trace amounts of one oil can change an entire blend. For example, adding a very small quantity of patchouli to a rose base alters the odor very slightly, but makes it smell like a bouquet of white roses instead of red roses (and since patchouli is a fixative, the fragrance is retained much longer).

To sharpen your nose, try methods similar to those used by perfumery students. The table with contrasting and similar odors in this chapter was prepared by the famous French perfumer, Jean Carles of Gasse, known as "Mr. Nose." He was responsible for famous creations such as Tabu, Aqua Brava, and Emir. Dissatisfied with the way he had been taught perfume-making—a trial-and-error approach he termed "happy-go-lucky"—Carles developed a systematic study of blending. Each day, the olfactory student compares a series of essential oils to others that are either similar or contrasting. The apprenticeship period takes many years to complete.

According to Carles,

Anyone may acquire a highly developed sense of smell, as this is merely a matter of practice. A good nose—that is, an excellent olfactory memory—is not enough to produce a good perfumer. By the term "a nose" . . . is meant a perfumer who is able to distinguish a pure product from an adulterated product, who can tell lavender 50 percent from lavender 40 percent. In spite of my many years of experience in smelling essential oils, I am myself only a beginner in comparison to the old "noses" I met in Grasse

who are able to detect olfactorily the geographical area [from which] a given oil of neroli or lavender came.

Perfumer Marcel Carles, son of Jean, describes how he learned blending:

When you smell lemon it contrasts with sandalwood, contrasts with cloves, cloves with orange—you are smelling very contrasting odors. It is much easier to memorize the smell of each of these products individually. . . . When you have finished the study of odor by contrasts, you start over again with the study of odor by family. But here it is difficult to distinguish lemon from bergamot [or] from tangerine. . . . The student whose olfactory memory has been trained in elementary things can go on to the more difficult exercises of studying the odors both by contrast and by family.

Fragrance blends usually improve with age. It takes at least several weeks for a blend to develop its full aroma. During this time, the single essential oils in the blend merge into a cohesive unit. The resulting perfume displays an individual character that is far greater than the sum of its parts as the fragrances marry together.

THERAPEUTIC BLENDING

Blending for therapeutic application allows you to think beyond the classical rules of blending for perfumery. For instance, if you want to create a blend that is deeply relaxing, promotes sleep, and alleviates stress, your formula would contain mostly base notes. In contrast, an uplifting and antidepressing blend could contain mostly top notes.

Safety: Safety is the most important consideration when choosing ingredients for a blend. It is important to use only high-quality oils, especially for therapeutic applications. Be sure to research the oils you choose and familiarize yourself with any properties or actions that may not be desirable in a given situation. Review "Safety Precautions" in chapter 5.

OLFACTORY STUDY OF ESSENTIAL OILS

This chart, prepared by perfumer Jean Carles for his students, has been simplified for your use. Read across the line for oils with similar scents. Read down the column for contrasting oils. Combining both similar and contrasting oils is used in blending techniques. Carles had his students spend at least a day studying just one line or column to become more familiar with the art of scent blending.

NOTES	1	2	3	4	5	6	7	8
citrus	lemon	bergamot	tangerine	orange	orange	bitter orange	petitgrain	lime
woodsy	sandalwood	cedar	vetiver	patchouli	oakmoss	oakmoss	pine	cypress
spicy	cloves	cinnamon	pimento	nutmeg	pepper	pimento	juniper	coriander
anise	anise	—	fennel	fennel	basil	tarragon	cumin	caraway
rose	absolute	—	—	Bulgarian	geranium	geranium	geranium	palmarosa
rustic (camphorlike)	lavender	lavendin	Spanish lavender	rosemary	thyme	eucalyptus	bay	myrtle/sage
balsam	balsam of Peru	balsam of tolu	vanillat	tonka	storax	labdanum	clary sage	balsam copaiba
floral (absolutes)	jasmine	tuberose	jonquil	hyacinth	narcissus	violet	cassie	orris root
resin	frankincense	benzoin	opopanax	myrrh	elemi	galbanum	—	—
orange/ citronella	citronella	lemongrass	verbena	melissa	neroli	petitgrain	—	—
mint & misc.	peppermint	spearmint	pennyroyal	marjoram	rosewood	—	wintergreen	cajeput

Purpose: The intended use will help you decide on the most appropriate ingredients for your creation. Consider the physical and emotional conditions and symptoms the blend needs to address. If you are making a blend that is destined for use as a cosmetic it will be more effective if you know the skin type of the person who will be using it to customize your formula for that individual (see chapter 9).

Application: Decide on the most appropriate method for applying the essential oil blend. Is it best applied by massage, inhalation, footbath, or some other method? Will your blend be most suitable in a vegetable oil, in alcohol, in water, or in some other type of carrier? All of these factors will help you determine the final ingredients, dilution, and instructional use of the blend.

STEP-BY-STEP BLENDING

Before you begin, take a minute to focus: Take a few deep breaths, relax, and center yourself. Think about the purpose of your blend and your intention.

It is important to keep detailed notes of your experiments, including your failures. You might lose a successful blend forever if you don't write it down. Be sure to label each blend with the date, ingredients, dilution, name of the blend, and any other useful information.

To begin creating a blend, make a list of all the oils that are appropriate or desirable for your particular purposes. If you are a beginner, restrict the list to five oils or less. Smell the oils one by one, and try to imagine how they will blend with one another. Remember that many oils are overpowering when smelled directly in the bottle. Briefly wave the cap under your nose for a better appreciation of the true fragrance.

After you sample each oil individually, determine how well they combine. Hold the bottle caps to your nose in different combinations, or better yet, use strips of blotter paper labeled with the names of different oils. Place a dab of oil on each strip and hold different combinations together under your nose. Make notes on paper of the desired possibilities.

REQUIRED SUPPLIES

blotter paper
clean empty bottles
carriers: oils, glycerin, distilled water, hydrosol, alcohol
funnel (optional)
eyedropper(s)
cleanup supplies: paper towels, tissues, alcohol
labels, pencil, notebook

Now you are ready to mix. Start with small proportions, blending drop by drop. Sniff as you go, and continue to make notes on how the blend progresses. It is best to mix the oils together before adding them to a carrier.

When you are satisfied with your blend, add it to a carrier or base such as oil, alcohol, hydrosol, water, or even vinegar. If you prefer, leave your blends in concentrated form for more versatility, lending themselves to a variety of applications such as bath blends or massage oils.

Sample Recipes

Here are a few ideas to get you started. You may dilute the following recipes in 1 ounce of carrier oil (a 2 percent solution) to make a massage or body oil or in an equal amount of jojoba to make a perfume. As an exercise, start by adding 1 drop of each oil. Sniff as you add each drop, and observe how it changes the blend. If you feel adventurous, alter the proportions to suit yourself.

To avoid contaminating each essential oil with the previous oil you used, use separate droppers. Or rinse the dropper in vodka or pure grain alcohol and dry it before dipping it in another scent so you won't need different droppers. Ideally, though, each oil would have a designated dropper or pipette.

AFTERNOON DELIGHT
4 drops orange essential oil
2 drops geranium essential oil
3 drops lavender essential oil
4 drops sandalwood essential oil

EARTH DEW
4 drops juniper essential oil
3 drops cedarwood essential oil
2 drops frankincense essential oil
3 drops jasmine essential oil

KISS ME QUICK
2 drops rose essential oil
3 drops jasmine essential oil
6 drops grapefruit essential oil
2 drops ylang-ylang essential oil

ADOLESCENT AIRS
5 drops lavender essential oil
4 drops mandarin essential oil
2 drops neroli essential oil
2 drops vanilla essential oil

FLORAL SPICE

2 drops ylang-ylang essential oil

2 drops vetiver essential oil

6 drops bergamot essential oil

3 crops cardamom essential oil

REVITALIZE

2 drops black pepper essential oil

6 drops lemon essential oil

3 drops rosemary essential oil

1 drop peppermint essential oil

PERFUME/COLOGNE

Perfumes contain more essential oils and a lower percentage of alcohol and water than colognes, which were originally designed for splashing rather than dabbing. Because natural perfumes are much more concentrated, they command a higher price. As a carrier for either perfume or cologne, use vodka or pure grain alcohol diluted with distilled water. Nevada, Oregon, and Alaska sell Everclear (a 94 percent alcohol) to the public. If you prefer an oil base, consider the application and refer to "Carrier Oils" in chapter 5, "Guidelines." Jojoba oil is best for perfumery due to its long shelf life; this carrier never goes rancid.

ANCIENT PERFUME FORMULATIONS

Chemist Giuseppe Conato, former director of the Laboratory of Experimental Archaeology at Italy's National Research Council, studies ancient perfumes. In the 1970s, he journeyed to the Black Sea to investigate Cleopatra's ancient perfume factory near the En-Gedi oasis. The factory, now partially reconstructed, has two drying kilns, revolving grinding mills for herbs, two large tubs to macerate herbs with oil, a stove to prepare ointments, and a waiting room complete with stone seats. A tower once stood there, possibly to view the plantations of fragrant plants that surrounded the factory.

It might be more accurate if we call this a *cosmetic factory*. Perfumes of that era were vegetable-based body oils made by grinding dried herbs and soaking them in hot oil; the oil was pressed, either through a bag (Egyptian style) or with a screw press (Greek method). The oil base was often *onphacium*, pressed from unripe olives, had only a faint herblike scent, and contained so little fat that it spread easily over skin without being greasy. Perhaps that was part of their beauty secret. We now know that this watery emulsion has great benefits to the skin.

Another ingredient employed in the factory was Dead Sea salt, which contains an unusually high concentration of mineral salts (magnesium, potassium, and sodium chloride)—ten times more than open sea salt. Another component was the famous Black Sea mud, called *asphaltite* by Pliny. Extracted from mud that was rich in petroleum deposits (composted plants), this "pitch of Judea" was used in a popular beauty treatment for the skin.

BLENDING WITH IMAGINATION

Edmond Roudnitska, perfumer for Christian Dior, Elizabeth Arden, Hermès, and Rochas, carried forty years of recipes in one small spiral notebook. He created not with his nose but with imagination. To explain his olfactory genius, Roudnitska said:

A thought comes to mind. I foresee, I visualize a certain form for a perfume. . . . I try first to outline or sketch out the form with products that are most familiar to me, and then I try to modify it, and, step by step, this study goes along, because a study of this nature can last several years, and as it does, I might have my hand on some new raw material, and I say to myself, "Well, now, this might be just the thing I need to complete the form." To create a perfume, you have to live entirely in the universe of odor, think in that universe and, being in it, visualize forms— it is very abstract.

Just as the chef starts in the kitchen, the perfumer starts in a perfumery laboratory by studying the odors, smelling one after the other. After practicing this a great deal, she begins to make small experiments and learns to combine the odors, as a chef de cuisine makes different combinations of tastes or as a painter makes different combinations of colors. It's never done the same way twice.

WEARING YOUR BLEND

Natural scents normally need to be applied more often than synthetics, but take a hint from nature. Plants utilize their aromatic properties either to repel or attract. When too much fragrance is applied, it can repel, but a subtle hint of aroma can draw one closer (attracting pollinators). This is the true art of sensualists—to intrigue, attract, and draw near to find the source of the essence. In other words, use your aroma often but sparingly.

Alcohol Concentrations

PERCENT ALCOHOL	PRODUCT
5–30%	extract or perfume
8–15%	parfum de toilette or eau de parfum
4–8%	eau de toilette
3–5%	eau de cologne
1–3%	splash cologne

PERFUME FORMULAS THROUGHOUT HISTORY

1800 BC: BABYLON

cedar, myrrh, cypress

labdanum, myrrh, storax

1300 BC: EGYPT

kyphi (Tutankhamen): calamus, mastic, henna, juniper, spikenard

1200 BC: EGYPT

"Anointing Oil" (Moses): myrrh (4 parts), cinnamon (2 parts), calamus (2 parts) in olive oil

frankincense, myrrh, cinnamon, cassia, cyperus, saffron, terebinth (pistachio, probably mastic)

storax, labdanum, galbanum, frankincense, myrrh, cinnamon, cassia, honey, raisins

onycha, galbanum, myrrh, frankincense, other spices

600 BC: GREECE

"Megaleion": burnt resin, cassia, myrrh, balanos oil (*Balanites aegyptica*)

(some versions include cinnamon, calamus, spikenard, costus, and balsam)

200 BC: EGYPT

calamus, storax, mastic, "rhodum root," incense, carob

"Cyprinum": henna, cyperus, cardamom, calamus, myrrh, honey, *onphacium*

"Metopion": cardamom, calamus, myrrh, galbanum, bitter almond, honey, wine, *onphacium*

100 BC: ROME

"Telinum" (Caesar): fenugreek, cyperus, calamus, melilot, marjoram, honey, maro, *onphacium*

"Rhodinun": rose, crocus, cinnamon, calamus, rush, alkanet, wine, honey, salt, *onphacium*

"Myrtum Lurum" (Oil of Persia): marjoram, lily, fenugreek, myrrh, cassia, spikenard, rush, cinnamon, myrtle, bay, *onphacium*

"Regale Unguentum" (aphrodisiac for kings of Parthia): costus, cinnamon, cardamom, lavender, myrrh, spikenard, germander, cassia, storax, labdanum, balsam, calamus, rush, Malabar or Indian bay, cyperus, saffron, henna, marjoram, lotus, Indian terminalia, honey, wine, *onphacium*

"Telinum": cyperus, calamus, melilot, fenugreek, marjoram, honey, *onphacium*

AD 100: ROME

"Amarakinon": marjoram, spikenard, myrrh, cinnamon, costus, cardamom, calamus, balsam, honey, wine

"Susinon": lily, balsam, cinnamon, saffron, myrrh, calamus, honey, *onphacium* (some versions include cardamom, orris root, and crocus)

"Irinum": orris root, palm tops, wine

AD 400: EGYPT

"Mendesium": myrrh, cassia, resins, balanos oil (*Balanites aegyptica*)

AD 1100: INDIA

jasmine, cardamom, pine, cloves, coriander, basil, sesame oil

costus, pandanus, agarwood, champac

AD 1100: CHINA

rose, camphor, cassia, citrus, other herbs, alcohol

AD 1200: EUROPE

"Carmelite Water": melissa, angelica, other herbs

AD 1300: EUROPE

"Queen of Hungary waters": rosemary, lavender

AD 1500: ENGLAND (QUEEN ELIZABETH)

musk, rosewater, sugar

marjoram, benzoin in rosewater

PERFUME FORMULAS THROUGHOUT HISTORY

AD 1600: EUROPE

"Honey Water": coriander, cloves, nutmeg, benzoin, storax, vanilla, rose & orange water in honey

"Casting Water": herbs, rosewater

AD 1700: FRANCE

"Brown Windsor Soap": bergamot, cloves, lavender

"Eau de Cologne" (Farina): bergamot, citron, rosemary, neroli, lavender, melissa, rectified grape water

Louis XIV's favorite: aloeswood, nutmeg, cloves, storax, benzoin, rosewater

"Poudre à la Maréchale": ambrette, cloves, calamus, iris, dill, lemon peel, neroli, ambergris

AD 1800

"Jicky" (Guerlain): bergamot, orris root, lavender, synthetics

"Florida Water Cologne": bergamot, lavender, lime, neroli, cloves, cinnamon, rose

AD 1900

"La Rose Jacqueminot" (Coty): rose, violet

"Chypre" (Coty): citrus, bergamot, sandalwood, gum resins

AD 1920

"Emeraude" (Coty): spices, resins

"L'Origan" (Coty): marjoram

"L'Heure Bleue": resin, labdanum, balsam of Peru, synthetics

"Numéro Cinq" (Chanel), Chanel No. 5: ylang-ylang, jasmine, rose, animal scents, aldehyde

"Shalimar" (Guerlain): bergamot, neroli, rosewood, vanilla, geranium, patchouli, sandalwood, vetiver, civet

"My Sin" (Lanvin): jasmine, neroli, patchouli, synthetics

"Arpège" (Lanvin): jasmine, floral scents

AD 1930

"Tabu" (Dana): patchouli, oakmoss, musk, bergamot, neroli, ylang-ylang

"Joy" (Patou): Bulgarian rose, jasmine, synthetics

"Shocking" (Schiaparelli): patchouli, synthetic hyacinth

"Blue Grass" (Elizabeth Arden): jasmine and rose, violet

AD 1940

"Miss Dior" (Dior): neroli, lavender, pepper, coriander, sandalwood, galbanum, patchouli

"Vent Vert" (Balmain/Germaine Cellier): geranium, neroli, lemon, lime, galbanum, with lily of the valley, sage, amber

AD 1950

"Youth-Dew" (Estée Lauder): frankincense, patchouli, vetiver, clove, musk

"Cabochard" (Grès): spices

"Ambush" (Coty): jasmine, oakmoss, sandalwood, patchouli, lavender, with citrus, fruit

AD 1970

"Aramis 700": patchouli

"Bill Blass" (Bill Blass): patchouli

"Charlie" (Revlon): synthetics

"Opium" (St. Laurent): incense resins, spices, florals

"Chloé" (Karl Lagerfeld): citrus, jasmine, tuberose, honeysuckle, oakmoss, patchouli, vetiver musk

"Diorella" (Christian Dior): bergamot, patchouli, vetiver, honeysuckle, fern

"Jontue" (Revlon): jasmine, tuberose, neroli, violet, mimosa, gardenia, jonquil with sandalwood, vetiver, honeysuckle, musk

"Masumi" (Coty): jasmine, rose, sandalwood, patchouli, vetiver, mimosa, violet, hyacinth

AD 1980

"Andron" (Jovan): androsterone

NATURAL INGREDIENTS IN COMMERCIAL PERFUMES

The following are a few examples of natural ingredients in modern popular commercial perfumes and colognes. This is by no means a complete list of ingredients; synthetics are also used in each blend. In additon, many fragrance companies use synthetic versions of natural essential oils.

FOR MEN

Calvin
Top notes: lavender, anise, bergamot, petitgrain, lemon
Middle notes: geranium, marjoram, clary sage, rose, juniper
Base notes: patchouli, vetiver, sandalwood, oakmoss

Obsession
Top notes: bergamot, lemon, clary sage
Middle notes: rosewood, cinnamon
Base notes: cedarwood, patchouli, sandalwood, benzoin, vanilla

Brut
Top notes: lavender, anise, lemon, basil, bergamot
Middle notes: geranium, ylang-ylang, jasmine
Base notes: sandalwood, vetiver, patchouli, oakmoss, vanilla, tonka

Boss
Top notes: bergamot, lemon, mandarin, artemisia
Middle notes: juniper, clary sage, mace, geranium, jasmine, rose
Base notes: patchouli, cedar, sandalwood, tonka

Old Spice
Top notes: orange, lemon, anise, clary sage
Middle notes: cinnamon, geranium, jasmine, pimento berry
Base notes: vanilla, cedarwood, frankincense, benzoin

FOR WOMEN

Tabu
Top notes: orange, neroli, bergamot, coriander
Middle notes: ylang-ylang, jasmine, clove, rose
Base notes: vetiver, cedarwood, patchouli, benzoin, sandalwood, musk

Shalimar
Top notes: lemon, bergamot, mandarin, rosewood, neroli
Middle notes: geranium, rose, jasmine, orris root, sandalwood
Base notes: vanilla, benzoin, patchouli, vetiver

Chanel No. 5
Top notes: bergamot, lemon, neroli
Middle notes: jasmine, rose, violet orris root, ylang-ylang
Base notes: vetiver, sandalwood, cedar, vanilla

Chanel No. 19
Top notes: iris
Middle notes: jasmine, rose, orris root, ylang-ylang
Base notes: moss, sandalwood, musk

White Shoulders
Top notes: neroli, bergamot
Middle notes: jasmine, rose, tuberose, clove, violet (orris root)
Base notes: sandalwood, benzoin

Anaïs Anaïs
Top notes: neroli, galbanum
Middle notes: jasmine, rose, tuberose, orris root, ylang-ylang
Base notes: sandalwood, cedar, vetiver

Extracting Essential Oils

EVER SINCE it was discovered that fragrance could be isolated from plants, human beings have experimented with the best ways to accomplish this. We have learned much since plants were first added to animal fats or steeped in water to extract their fragrances, and refinements in techniques are still being sought today. The goal for the alchemists of the second and third centuries AD was to capture the "quintessence" of the plant—hence "essential" oils, describing the "soul" or "spirit" of the plant.

Distillation

The distillation process of extracting essential oils utilizes steam, heat, and condensation. About 80 percent of all natural oils produced are extracted by distillation. For hundreds of years it has been the best method of extracting pure essential oils, and even with the myriad techniques available today, it still provides a very pure product.

During distillation, fragrant plants exposed to boiling water or steam release their essential oils through evaporation. The oil-laden steam rises and enters narrow tubing that is cooled by an outside source: A larger vessel surrounding the tubing contains cold water that circulates constantly to keep it cold. The tubing is designed (often in a lengthy spiral) to provide a lot of surface area so that the steam, which contains both essential oil gases and water vapor, cools as quickly as possible, thus creating condensation (little droplets of water). As the steam turns back into water and essential oil, both are collected in a vessel traditionally called the *Florentine flask* (named for a city known for essential oil distillation during the Renaissance). Because oil and water don't mix, the essential oil floats on top of the water and can be separated easily (some exceptions are clove, birch, wintergreen, and anise essential oils, which sink to the bottom of water). The still separates the essential oil into one vial and the water (called *hydrosol*) into another.

Examples of commonly distilled plants are lavender, geranium, rosemary, and eucalyptus. Plants are distilled most commonly from fresh material, but in some cases the plant is dried. Dense or thick plant material, especially roots and seeds, are crushed or chipped before distillation to extract the essential oil more efficiently. The technical term for this process is *comminution,* but it is not necessary with very delicate plant parts, such as leaves and flowers, because the steam penetrates them easily.

The amount of essential oil produced depends on four main criteria: the distillation time, the temperature, the operating pressure, and most important, the type and quality of the plant material. Other details that affect yield are harvest time (time of day and year), climatic conditions, and the amount of volatile oil each plant produces. Typically, the yield of essential oils in plants is between 0.005 and 10 percent. For example, plants that produce a relatively high percentage of essential oil, such as sage, thyme, and rosemary, use approximately 500 pounds of plant material to produce 32 ounces of essential oil. These factors all affect the price of the oil.

Historically, there are three types of distillation: water distillation, water-steam distillation, and steam distillation. Water distillation is sometimes referred to as *indirect* steam distillation. Plant material is soaked and heated in water until it boils. The resulting steam carries the volatile oils, and cooling and condensation subsequently separate the oil from the water. This method requires very little equipment and can be done on the spot immediately after harvesting, making it quite inexpensive. Apart from its slowness, the disadvantage of this technique is that the scent deteriorates from constant heat exposure.

The second more sophisticated method utilizes steam. The leafy plant material is placed on a grill above the hot water, carefully distributed for even steaming and thorough extraction, and the steam passes through the plant material. The rest of the process is the same as water distillation.

The third technique, sometimes referred to as *direct* steam distillation, is the most common. No water is placed inside the distillation tank itself, but instead, steam is directed into the tank from an outside source. The essential oils are released from the plant material when the steam bursts the sacs that contain the tiny molecules of oil. Again, the process of condensation and separation at this stage is standard. Direct steam distillation is quick, causing minimal deterioration of delicate essential oil components, and produces a higher quality essential oil than the water and water-steam distillation methods.

As popular and well established as distillation is, there still are several drawbacks. One is that steam does not always disperse evenly, especially when it enters plant material from the bottom. As a result, distillation takes a longer time, and extraction can be inefficient. The heating and cooling needed for distillation also require a lot of energy. Steam must be created with fire, which burns a lot of wood, or with gas or electricity, which can be expensive. Refrigeration to cool down the steam is also costly. In addition, as many as forty-eight hours may be required to thoroughly distill a plant. Over such a long time, oxidation, which chemically alters the original makeup of the essential oil, may occur, often with undesirable results. Some of the problems of steam distillation have been remedied by the invention of other extraction methods that we discuss later.

IMPROVED DISTILLATION TECHNIQUES

Many flowers are so fragile that exposure to the high heat of steam distillation destroys their delicate scents. The new extraction methods still utilize steam, but the techniques have improved and a superior product results thanks to a shorter processing time and lower temperatures. New energy-efficient methods also help to cut costs.

Turbo Distillation
Hard plant materials such as roots, seeds, and barks are processed by turbo distillation. Steaming is combined with cohobation—a process in which the water, known as the *hydrolat,* is recycled back into the still to further obtain volatile molecules and create more steam. The plant material is soaked, softened, and then continuously agitated as it is exposed to the recycled steam. This can reduce the processing time by half.

HISTORY OF DISTILLATION TIMELINE

3000 BC: Terra-cotta perfume containers and a still-like container are made in the Indus Valley in Pakistan.

2000 BC: A still-like container is made in Afghanistan.

Thirteenth to twelfth centuries BC: Egg-shaped vessels with coils are described on Mesopotamian cuneiform tablets.

First century BC: Greek philosopher Aristotle writes about the evaporation and condensation of alcohol, leading some historians to wonder if he experimented with distillation.

First century AD: The invention of a still attributed to Maria Prophetissima the Jewess is described with diagrams in the Alexandrian text, *The Gold-Making of Cleopatra,* the first Western description of a still.

Greek Dioscorides, author of *The Herbal,* which includes a chapter on aromatic herbs, produces "quintessence" of herbs from pine and camphor using a simple process that involves capturing the steam in wool cloth and squeezing it out.

Third century AD: Hieroglyphics on an Egyptian temple wall in Memphis resemble a still, according to the ancient chemist Zozime.

Fifth to sixth centuries AD: Taoist chemists use cold water to cool the steam in the still more quickly and improve the distillation process.

Ninth century AD: Arabian Al-Razi describes a simple method to distill rosewater.

Twelfth century AD: The European still is improved by cooling the tubing with water. Chinese develop a cooling cap for the still that came to be known as the "Moor's head," which resembles the onion-shaped top of a minaret.

Thirteenth century AD: Damascan rose is distilled for export to Europe, India, and China.

Catalan physician Arnaud de Villanova, writes perhaps the first description of the distillation of alcohol.

Fourteenth century AD: Creation of distilled lavender water, Hungary water containing rosemary (1370), and Carmelite Water or *eau de Carmes* by Carmelite nuns, supposedly for Charles V of France, containing melissa, angelica, and other herbs.

Large plantations of lavender, roses, sage, and rosemary are planted in Burgundy, France.

Libellus de Distilla Philosophica, or "Book on Intelligent Distilling," advises avoiding lead and using tight seals on stills.

Fifteenth century AD: Europeans cool distillers more efficiently by coiling the tubing inside a bucket of cold water (called the *serpentine* or *worm*) and add insulation around the distiller..

Sixteenth century AD: Hieronymous Bruschwig (Jerome of Brunswick) writes volumes on distillation, including *Liber de Arte Distillandi de Simplicibus* (a distiller's handbook), and recommends essential oil remedies.

Paracelsus (1493–1541) works extensively with distillation.

Pier Andrea Mattioli (1500–1572) writes *Commentary* on Dioscorides's first century *Herbal* and adds an appendix on distillation.

Giovanni Battista della Porta (1537–1615) writes *Magia Naturalis,* or "Natural Magic" (1558–1569), with sections on distillation and creating perfume, advocates distilling in nonreactive glassware, and describes yields produced by different herbs for the first time.

Lavender is cultivated for distillation in Hertfordshire, En-gland, and rose, in Bulgaria.

Seventeenth century AD: England introduces the stronger flint glass produced with coal instead of wood, due to deforestation there.

Eighteenth century AD: Every European herbalist has access to distilled essential oils and distilled aromatic waters, now often called *hydrosols.*

Hydrodiffusion

In hydrodiffusion, a more energy-efficient variation of direct steam distillation, the steam is forced through the plant material from the top, rather than the bottom, of the still. This method is much gentler than those described earlier, and because less time is required, the resulting essential oil comes closer to the true scent of the plant. Hydrodiffusion is used only with fresh leafy herbs; roots and seeds are left to other, more efficient forms of distillation.

Vacuum Distillation

Unlike many other methods, vacuum distillation provides "dry" distillation, a sophisticated technique in which the steam does not enter the still or come into contact with the plant material. Instead, the steam is contained in a heating jacket outside the still, somewhat like a double boiler. A vacuum effect within the still releases the essential oil from the plant material at a lower temperature. The oil can be collected whole for use in aromatherapy, or portions of the distillate can be collected as they emerge from the condenser.

Continuous Distillation

Continuous distillation, a new process recently introduced in France, utilizes discarded tree branches such as juniper, eucalyptus, and pine, which are cut into small pieces for distillation and exposed to repeated steaming. One method, described by Marcel Lavabre, a former distiller, involves the continuous feeding of plant material through a tube that is exposed to steam. As fresh plant material enters the tube, exhausted plant material is pushed out the other end. The plant material receives extensive exposure to the steam, greatly reducing distillation time. This method also allows for fractionation of different constituents.

Molecular Distillation

Also known as *rectifying,* this process involves redistilling an oil two and sometimes three times. This eliminates the heavier parts of an essential oil, making it smell more the way it does in nature. Some situations, however, require the use of the raw oil produced from the first distillation. In the case of peppermint, the heavier parts in the oil from the initial distillation are "hotter," so this oil is a good choice for use as a liniment. The lighter, redistilled oil is usually preferred for flavoring or for its emotional impact. A number of oils can be redistilled with more favorable aromatic results, including camphor and eucalyptus. The extraction process is rarely indicated on the label, so it may be difficult to tell if you are getting a redistilled oil—unless you have a trained nose or a whole oil with which to compare it.

Fractionation

Fractioning is a technique used to separate specific chemical components from the whole oil. Because each aromatic component in a plant has its own boiling point, each evaporates at a different rate. It is therefore possible to separate the components as they emerge from the condenser, isolating and eliminating individual components as desired. This option is more useful to a perfumer who wants to boost or eliminate a distinctive scent or a chemist who wants to adulterate an oil by increasing a specific aromatic component; aromatherapists are usually concerned with obtaining a whole, natural product.

Other Methods of Extraction

Plants are also extracted by methods other than distillation, including cold expression, enfleurage, solvent extraction, and carbon dioxide extraction.

COLD EXPRESSION

Cold expression is sometimes referred to as *scarification.* This method of extraction is used for citrus fruits, which contain essential oil–bearing pouches in their peel. The peel is shredded and then mechanically pressed. The resulting emulsion, consisting of essential oil, juice, water, and fruit particles, is either filtered or passed through a clarifying centrifuge. The essential oil, which floats on top, is then separated out.

Natural plant waxes resulting from cold expression may contribute to a slight cloudiness or create some sediment in the final oil. This usually does not present a problem unless it is important for the oil to be clear visually or if it will be used in a diffuser that may be clogged by the sediment. Remove the sediment by straining the oil through a fine cloth or a paper filter.

Citrus skins are not always pressed. For instance, lemon and lime peels are also distilled. The smell of the resulting oil is more reminiscent of candy than the fresh-peel smell of cold-pressed citrus oils. Distilled oil of lime is used in many soft drinks, including Coca-Cola, 7-Up, and Pepsi. Oils produced in this way are considered inferior apart from one advantage: They may not be as photosensitive as most expressed citrus oils. Unfortunately, the citrus industry often sprays chemicals and pesticides directly on the peel; these carry over to the essential oil when the peel is pressed. Distilled citrus oils may contain fewer of these pesticide residues. We recommend buying pressed citrus essential oil extracted from organically grown fruit whenever possible.

ENFLEURAGE

Virtually obsolete today, enfleurage is perhaps the oldest method of extracting fragrance from plants. It is used for delicate plants that cannot withstand the high heat of distillation or that continue to exude fragrance after they are picked, such as tuberose and jasmine. Refined lard and tallow were used in small-production enfleurage for centuries. With their excellent ability to pick up fragrance molecules from flowers, animal fats are the preferred medium for this type of extraction.

In the traditional enfleurage process, fat is spread thickly on plates of glass and covered with freshly picked flowers. The layers of glass are sealed to retain the scent. The flowers are left undisturbed for twenty-four to forty-eight hours, then removed and replaced with fresh ones. This time-consuming, labor-intensive process is repeated for several weeks until the fat is saturated with the fragrance of the flowers. The fat is gently warmed and filtered, resulting in a product called a *pomade.* In ages past, pomade was used directly on the skin and hair. Today, it is usually "washed" with alcohol to remove the fat. The alcohol carries the essential oil and is separated from the fat by chilling. At this stage, the product is called an *extrait.*

An *absolute d'enfleurage* is created in the next stage of processing. This semisolid product results after distilling off the alcohol. The final product is coded with a number that represents the number of times fresh flowers were placed on the fat. If you find a "jasmine #42," for example, it means the flowers were replaced forty-two times. The higher the number, the finer (and generally more expensive) the absolute. Technically, absolutes—used mainly by the perfume industry—are not essential oils, though they contain volatile compounds.

An inferior by-product called *absolute de chassis* is made from the flowers after removing them from the fat. Whatever essential oils are left in the blossoms are extracted with solvents. The perfume industry uses the resulting extract to add fullness to synthetic jasmine compounds.

To make your own jasmine-infused oil at home, use almond or coconut oil as a substitute for animal fat. See chapter 5 for directions.

SOLVENT EXTRACTION

Solvent extraction makes it possible to create a whole range of oils that could never be produced before because their structures are too delicate to withstand other methods, especially heat exposure. This is because solvents do not require high heat and water for extraction. However, the method is not without drawbacks and controversy.

Solvents used for extraction include petroleum ether, hexane, toluene, butane, methane, and propane, as well as the more toxic—even carcinogenic—solvents benzene and acetone. Today new nontoxic solvents are being explored. The plant material is submerged in and agitated with the solvent, which dissolves the volatile oils—as well as the waxes and pigments—from the plant. The solvent is removed through evaporation under pressure. The result is a sticky, soft wax called a *concrete*. Because of the waxes and pigments it contains, the product may have cosmetic applications in the concrete stage (as long as the solvent is not toxic). To continue the extraction process, the concrete is mixed with ethyl alcohol and chilled to filter out the solidified waxes, leaving volatile compounds diluted in alcohol. The last step is to remove the alcohol by vacuum distilling the mixture. The final product is called an *absolute*.

Absolutes are said to be relatively free of the solvents and alcohol used during extraction, but solvent-extracted oils may retain a slight residue in the final product. The least harmful solvents are butane, propane, and methane, but one can never be sure what was used. Since solvents are sometimes odorless, it may be difficult to detect them. Solvent-extracted oils should never be taken orally or used to flavor food. Because solvent residues may be present, absolutes are not generally recommended for use in aromatherapy, but are suitable for creating natural perfumes. However, new methods of extracting essential oils are being developed that are said to remove all of the solvents, and some manufacturers recover certain solvents and reuse them.

A *resinoid* is another product derived through solvent or alcohol extraction. The main distinction between resinoids and concretes is that resinoids are produced from tree saps and exudates (frankincense, mastic, labdanum, tolu, and the lichen oakmoss), whereas concretes are extracted from fresh plant materials.

CARBON DIOXIDE EXTRACTION

Supercritical carbon dioxide (CO_2) extraction is a relatively new process used to obtain essential oils through high pressure and low heat and has several advantages. The extraction takes place in a closed chamber and is completed in a relatively short time, so even the most volatile and heat-sensitive fragrance compounds can be collected undamaged and without solvent residues, retaining both fragrance quality and physiological activity. Because the solvent CO_2 is a gas, it is easily—and totally—removed when the pressure is released.

CO_2 extracts come close to the flavor and aroma of the plant, making them excellent candidates for food flavorings, and today the process is used extensively for this purpose (although distillation results in a pure product, it does not always provide an exact representation of a plant's smell or taste).

Of the two types of CO_2 extraction, the first produces *selective extracts,* obtained at a relatively low pressure of 100 pounds per square inch. They are similar (but some say superior) to distilled products in that they consist almost completely of volatile compounds and usually have a liquid consistency. They are suitable for all aromatherapy applications and perfumery. Examples are ambrette seed, frankincense, myrrh, orris root, black currant, and chamomile. The second type of CO_2 extraction produces *total extracts,* which are obtained at considerably higher pressure (350 pounds per square inch). These extracts not only contain essential oils (volatile compounds), but also fats, waxes, and plant pigments. This method of extraction is especially useful for plants specific to skin care. In the case of calendula, it thoroughly extracts all the healing constituents (carotenoids, flavonoids, and essential oils), producing a thick orange tar. The application of this technique to extract lipids such as GLA for the cosmetic and health industries holds a great deal of promise. Some examples of total extracts available today are carrot (root), chamomile, ginger, sea buckthorn, coriander, juniper, lovage, rosemary,

A HOMEMADE ESSENTIAL OIL STILL

Make your own essential oil still with a few things from your kitchen and the hardware store. This homemade still won't produce much oil, but you can use it to make hydrosol and distilled water for aromatherapy projects or for drinking water.

Supplies:

- pressure cooker
- hose clamp
- glass jar
- 10 feet of ¼-inch diameter copper or food-grade vinyl plastic tubing
- 5 gallon bucket

Put the pressure cooker on a stove burner. Fill it up about halfway with water, and place a vegetable steamer inside the cooker (prop up the steamer, if necessary, so the bottom is above the water line). Place the dried or fresh herbs you wish to distill on top of the steamer. Put the lid on the pressure cooker, but instead of placing the regulator vent on top of the cooker, put a 10-foot length of food-grade tubing over the outlet (using a hose clamp to make sure it fits tightly). Tubing with an outside diameter of ¼ inch works well.

About the tubing: Copper tubing is best, although high-grade plastic tubing will also work (and plastic is easy to wind inside the bucket). If you use copper tubing, tape off one end and fill the tube with fine sand (to prevent it from kinking). Slowly wrap it around a small bucket or something else with a cylindrical shape so that the tubing spirals. You want a spiral of tubing that fits into the bucket as described below. You can also use plastic for the section of tubing that spans from the pressure cooker to the pail so the still is easier to make and set up.

Drop the other end of the tubing over the edge of the counter. Place a 5-gallon pail on a chair, and coil the suspended end of the tube inside the pail so that it wraps around at least four times. Put enough cold water and ice into the pail to cover the coiled tubing. Drop the end of the tube that is in the pail over the edge toward the floor. Place a very clean small-mouth jar (at least 1 quart) on the floor, and insert the end of the tube into it, positioning the tubing so it falls straight into the jar. Turn the burner on medium-high.

The water will start to boil, creating steam inside the pressure cooker. As the steam rises through the herbs, it captures and removes the herb's essential oil, carrying it out of the cooker through the tubing. When the steam inside the tubing reaches the cold water in the pail, the steam condenses and converts back to water, literally dropping the essential oil. Now that the essential oils and steam are separated, some oil will float on the surface of the water as it goes into the jar. However, the product will mostly be scented water, or hydrosol, which can be used as you would any hydrosol. Both the pressure cooker and steamer should be made out of stainless steel since aluminum may react with the essential oils.

and vanilla. Like selective extracts, totals are used in the food and cosmetics industries and are suitable for all aromatherapy applications. Some CO_2 total extracts, such as rosemary, ginger, hops, and saw palmetto, are also used in the dietary supplement industry, and nearly every culinary herb is available as a CO_2 extract today.

Until recently, CO_2 extracts were rarely available to the consumer. Today they are generally more expensive than distilled oils because the equipment investment is high; prices should decrease as demand increases.

Quality and Purity

Quality and purity are often regarded as the same thing, but there are subtle differences. *Purity* refers to authenticity, the promise that a product is unadulterated. *Quality* relates to the "grade" of oil, which can be influenced by the growing, processing, or extraction methods. These are important concerns for consumers of pure essential oils, and rightly so. Everyone would like to obtain the highest quality product for the best price. Because most essential oils are produced outside the United States, however, it is sometimes hard to confirm both quality and purity, especially as the growing interest in herb products and essential oils creates levels of demand that are increasingly difficult to meet. This is one reason that many perfume and cosmetics manufacturers have switched to synthetics. Other factors include consistency of aroma and lower cost.

Quality and purity should be especially important to companies or stores that claim to carry "aromatherapy-grade" products. Often store clerks will tell you a line of essential oils is "natural," even when it is synthetic, mostly because they are uninformed. Like many people, they assume that anything labeled *essential oil* is natural and pure, but this is not always so. Most fragrances used in skin-care products are synthetic, even those found in natural food stores. It is no secret that rose is a very popular fragrance, but few companies can afford to use the pure oil and still manage to offer their products at a price most consumers can afford.

Because the aromatherapy industry is unregulated by government, self-regulation is vital—although some standards do exist for essential oils sold in pharmacies or those that carry a Food Chemical Codex (FCC) rating, a standard by the Food and Drug Administration (FDA). Essential oils that carry an FCC rating are food-grade essential oils approved for use as food flavorings or additives; essential oils labeled "USP grade," often available at pharmacies, meet the guidelines of the official *United States Pharmacopoeia*. Still, even though such labels may verify the percentage of constituents or which extraction process produced it, neither FCC coding nor USP grading guarantee quality.

So how can you be sure you have a good quality essential oil product? Although labeling does not ensure purity, it can be an indicator. Ideally, the label should say, "pure plant essential oil"; terms such as "fragrance oil" or "perfume oil" typically refer to synthetics, which should not

A NEW FLAME

The candle market began to boom in 1999 when it hit about $2.3 billion in annual sales in the United States, and it continues to grow 10 to 15 percent per year, according to the National Candle Association. All is not bright, however. Most candles are scented with coal-based, synthetic essential oils that produce intense fragrances that encourage consumers to buy them. These synthetics enter the body through inhalation, even while customers shop in stores that are heady with their scents. There is also concern about petrochemicals entering the air from the evaporating petroleum-based waxes that are most commonly used. These and other candle ingredients can produce toxic chemicals such as acetone and benzene, but candle makers are not required to list ingredients or provide any warnings. Research at the University of Michigan in Ann Arbor suggests another problem: Lead is released into the air by the lead cores that many candlewicks use to increase stability and burning time. A national consumer class action suit was filed against a popular clothing store chain for damages from toxic soot from candles sold at their stores. There are a lot of unknowns concerning the specific dangers, but the safest alternative is to choose candles made of pure vegetable wax, such as soy, or beeswax, that are scented with natural essential oils, and that have a clean-burning cotton or hemp wick.

be used for therapeutic aromatherapy applications. As an informed consumer, you have tremendous power in the marketplace. Ask your suppliers for all the information they have concerning their products, and insist on purity and integrity in the products you choose. It is helpful if the label and accompanying literature indicate the botanical name of the plant, what part of the plant was used, and the country of origin. Many reputable sellers of pure essential oils do not list this information on their labels, but they are usually willing to answer questions.

ADULTERATING ESSENTIAL OILS

Specific agencies may set guidelines for the levels of chemical constituents that an oil should contain, but nature does not always cooperate by remaining consistent from year to year. Unfortunately, unscrupulous vendors try to meet these standards by adding synthetics to their essential oils. Rare and expensive oils are the most likely candidates for adulteration, usually because a seller wants to increase his profit margin. It is often difficult for an untrained nose to tell the difference between the expensive pure essential oils of lemon verbena or melissa and those mixed with cheaper lemongrass or citronella (in fact, these oils are so often mixed with less expensive oils that you may never have smelled the real thing).

Another common method of adulterating essential oils is by "extending" (in other words, *diluting*) them with vegetable oil, alcohol, or solvent. One way to check for adulteration with vegetable oil is to put a small drop of the essential oil on a piece of paper. Because essential oils are volatile, most should evaporate rather quickly, leaving no residue. If an oily stain remains, suspect the product has been diluted. The only pure essential oils that leave slight color stains are dark oils such as benzoin and patchouli, bright blue oils such as German chamomile, and viscous oils such as sandalwood and vetiver. In oils diluted with alcohol, you might detect a slight odor, but it can be hard to tell if an oil is diluted with a clear, non-oily, odorless solvent. This is a potentially hazardous situation, because such solvents are readily absorbed into the body when rubbed on the skin or inhaled into the lungs.

RECONSTRUCTING ESSENTIAL OILS

Pure essential oils can be "reconstructed" by combining specific chemical constituents to match the composition of the natural oil. The constituents may come from natural sources, such as pine or another easily manipulated oil. Fractioning essential oils allows for reconstruction from natural sources. A reconstructed rosemary oil is often created with twenty to thirty-five natural compounds from other plants that match the main aromatic scents found in real rosemary oil. Rose oil is often extended with geraniol (a natural compound found in geranium and other plants), which has a distinctive rose-like scent.

Such adulterations, even if they do originate from natural sources, are not suitable for aromatherapy. Pure essential oils are thought to contain many aromatic molecules not yet detected—unidentified constituents that are active, integral parts of the whole essential oil. When essential oils are reconstructed, even from natural sources, such trace elements may be missing.

In the future, expensive essential oils such as rose and jasmine may be produced in laboratories. Scientists are experimenting with isolating the cells that produce the oils and then growing them in a soaplike solution. They hope the cultured cells will continue to produce essential oils, just as they do in nature. This process will probably yield oils suitable for the perfume industry, leaving more natural oils for aromatherapy.

SYNTHETIC ESSENTIAL OILS

Synthetic aromas are not extracted but are chemically manufactured from a variety of easily manipulated base ingredients—anything from pine oil to petroleum.

Synthetic oils became popular in the 1930s, gaining dominance in the cosmetics and body-care industry.

Aromatherapists do not use synthetics because, at best, they only duplicate scent, and most cannot do that well. A number of other problems make synthetics unsuitable for aromatherapy. To match a real essential oil as closely as possible, the potent aromatic chemicals used in synthetics must be extended in a solvent base, and these potentially toxic solvents may be absorbed through the skin. Perhaps most important, there is no substitute for the "life force" found in plants grown in the earth and nourished by the sun, rain, and other elements, though this perspective is dismissed by the scientific community and many chemists.

If you have trouble identifying synthetics from the real thing, take an aromatherapy course. We tell our students that they'll be spoiled for life. It's not unusual for a student to go home after class and throw out half the items in the bathroom and kitchen, not to mention the medicine cabinet! Your nose very quickly learns to distinguish the good from the nasty. It's almost automatic once you are exposed to a number of real oils made from plants.

GETTING IT RIGHT: SNIFFING OUT SYNTHETICS

Until your nose develops aromatherapy savvy, remember the following tips:

- Many oils are not produced naturally, so if you see lily of the valley, lotus, magnolia, apricot, coconut, peach, amber, strawberry, hibiscus, or apple (and possibly carnation and violet, unless they are very expensive), they are synthetics. In fact, if these particular oils are all the same brand and are sold with oils that look natural, be suspicious of the entire selection.
- Use the prices of the very expensive natural extracts of jasmine and rose as a yardstick against which to compare questionable oils. If you find jasmine or rose oil priced significantly lower than $250 per $1/4$-ounce bottle (or less than $30 per milliliter retail), the oil is probably synthetic (or at best, highly diluted).
- Because you cannot always trust what a label or a store clerk tells you, your nose is ultimately the best indicator of quality. Becoming a good judge of quality really isn't that difficult. When we bring samples of high-quality oils and synthetics to our aromatherapy classes for students to compare, most are able to pick out the synthetics right away.
- Inexpensive synthetic essential oils have a certain cloying/soapy/fruity/too sweet quality, which is what you will most likely find. It's similar to the smell of a cheap scented candle. We can best define it as "making your nose wrinkle."

ANALYZING ESSENTIAL OILS

Gas chromatography–mass spectrometry (GC-MS) is most frequently used to analyze the composition of essential oil. This method uses a gas chromatograph, coupled with a mass spectrometer, to detect individual components. A small sample of essential oil is heated to vapor and then carried along a column by an inert gas, such as helium. As the vaporized oil passes through the column, it separates into individual molecular constituents as it interacts with the stationary phase of the column. The separated constituents pass into the MS module, where they become charged (or "ionized"). The ionized constituents can then be amplified and detected as current by the MS. Each constituent is represented by the level of its peak and a color on a chromatograph. This signature "fingerprint" is then compared to the peaks and colors created by molecules that have already been identified. A library of molecules is used as a reference. GC-MS can detect the purity and often the source of an oil. For example, it shows when two or more similar oils have been mixed together, when an oil's terpene compounds have been removed or rectified, and if there are any traces of solvents or mineral oils. Some companies supply GC-MS results that identify and qualify the proportions and various constituents of the essential oil. However, few consumers are trained to interpret these. Therefore, knowing your source, trusting your supplier, and training your nose are the best means of monitoring quality.

High performance liquid chromatography (HPLC) is another technique used to analyze essential oils. It can separate an essential oil into its many fractions in preparation for analysis by another technique. A liquid solvent carries the essential oil through a column packed with tiny particles to slow down the process and separate the different components. Each individual component is detected as a peak on the chromatograph reading.

Sustainability

Sustainability and social and corporate responsibility are quite the buzzwords today, both for businesses and consumers, and rightly so. To ensure abundant supplies for generations to come, we should all be concerned with the overharvesting of medicinal plants in the wild, biodiversity, responsible wildcrafting techniques, energy conservation, organic agriculture, recycling, clean water and air, global warming, and the myriad other environmental conditions facing our planet today. As social and environmental activists, we deeply believe in these efforts and work toward them through right livelihood in our occupations and commitments to nonprofit organizations such as United Plant Savers (www.unitedplanetsavers.org).

When it comes to plants, we all play a part in ensuring that these supplies remain abundant through managing resources, organic cultivation, responsible living practices, and consumer spending. We often hear the argument that essential oils use too much plant material compared to herbalism, which uses whole plant matter with relatively little processing, but if essential oils are used in the proper dilutions and with the respect they deserve, they can be both economical and environmentally sustainable. This takes us back to the important adage "More is not better when it comes to aromatherapy." One drop of an essential oil *does* represent a lot of plant material, so use it with respect and an understanding of its potency and power. Don't use 30 drops in a bath when 5 will do just as well and is safer for the skin. Aromatherapy is very nearly a homeopathic practice when it comes to dilutions, and in most cases, it should be considered as such.

We prefer to patronize a number of socially responsible businesses—and not just in the realm of botanicals. See the Business for Social Responsibility website as a starting place (www.bsr.org), though many smaller businesses have corporate policies on fair trade and environmental and social justice issues. Stakeholders are pressing companies to step up and publicly report their policies to the extent that there is a "Dow Jones Sustainability Index" to make these nonfinancial disclosures. For instance, companies such as Aveda and Origins implement strident policies, and even Avon mentions their move in this direction. Aveda is one of the largest purchasers of organic essential oil in the world. Their demand for organic materials, based on the company's sustainability directive, has driven more growers into organic supply. The result is fewer chemicals put on our earth, which is a good thing for everyone.

As consumers, we encourage you to ask your suppliers about their sustainability policies and where they get their oils. A certified organic commodity is best, but many oils derived from plants are responsibly wildcrafted or are unsprayed but not certified. Ask questions and let them know you are concerned about these issues; you may be surprised at how loudly your consumer dollars speak.

THREATENED ESSENTIAL OIL PLANTS

The biggest concern we hear regarding aromatherapy is the sustainability of the oil-producing trees that take so many years to grow, since they are generally harvested by being cut down. The other concern is with oil-bearing plants that are harvested for their roots, since they are also killed during harvest. The primary problem with sustainable harvesting appears to be sandalwood, rosewood, and agarwood trees. We contacted several individuals who do fieldwork and visit the growers and essential oil still, and they are also concerned about the sustainability of these plants.

The International Union for Conservation of Nature, also known as the IUCN, which has a Medicinal Plant Specialist Group, rates plants according to whether they are endangered or vulnerable to joining that status. The group also advises governments and issues permits for the import and export of protected plants and animals. The Convention on International Trade in Endangered Species of Wild Fauna and Flora (CITES) is a related branch of the IUCN with almost one hundred countries as members. CITES regulates the international trade in plants and animals threatened by overexploitation. Permits are issued, with more leniency given to cultivated species. Even stricter controls have been adopted by the members of the European Council (EC), the United States, and Australia.

Sandalwood

Sandalwood has a long history of being overharvested everywhere it grows, and it is difficult to cultivate and grows very slowly, taking twenty to fifty years to reach maturity. This parasitic tree must be planted near a host tree while growing, especially in its early years. It feeds off many species but seems to prefer a host plant that fixes nitrogen, such as ones in the *Acacia* genus.

Seventeen species of sandalwood grow in the Pacific from Hawaii to Indonesia, into Australia, and across the Indian Ocean to India. Approximately seven of these are still harvested commercially. Hawaii was the world's largest supplier of sandalwood from 1830 to 1850, when the trees were nearly harvested to extinction (*S. fernandezianum* has become extinct, while *S. haleakala* is considered

vulnerable). After that, Australia stepped in until 1940, when harvesting stopped due to World War II, and then the demand for sandalwood declined with the communist takeover in China, the world's biggest buyer. Today Australian sandalwood is again being produced, with the government controlling the harvest in an effort to keep it sustainable, although there are still reports of nonsustainable harvesting. At this writing, only one company is designated to process the wood and only a couple companies to distill the oil. Both *S. spicatum* and *S. album* are being replanted on plantations and where wild trees have been harvested. In the Cook Islands and Tonga, where the native sandalwood (*S. yasi*) has been almost depleted, so have the plantations. Essential oil production can be expected to begin around 2030.

Australian sandalwood, mainly *S. spicatum,* grows in the western third of the country in very dry conditions, where there is often less than ten inches of annual rainfall. In upper Queensland, a small wild population of *S. album* seems to be *endemic* (native), and some experts believe that it actually originated in Australia. Native species such as plum bush (*S. lanceolatum*) are listed as endangered or threatened. Sandalwood is protected on some reserves, and the bitter quandong (*S. murrayanum*) and sweet quandong (*S. acuminatum*) sandalwoods are protected throughout the country, although the law is not always respected.

There is much speculation as to whether Indian and Indonesian sandalwood is being harvested sustainably. India's sandalwood trade dropped in half during the 1980s. Replanting efforts and the control of poaching have been difficult. Some landowners actually cut down the trees rather than risk poachers, who often arrive armed and dangerous. The export of Indian sandalwood essential oil has long been controlled by the local state governments of Madras and Mysore. Bottles of sandalwood oil are sealed with paper strips verifying these products. However, there is also an active black market. The IUCN lists Indian sandalwood (*S. album*) as vulnerable, though new initiatives have been undertaken to secure sustainable management of indigenous sandalwood by Aborigines, Vanuatu sandalwood *(S. austrocalidonicum)* as threatened, and New Guinea sandalwood *(S. macgregorii)* as endangered.

Rosewood or *Bois de Rose (Aniba rosaeodora)*

While no other oil is exactly like *bois de rose,* many oils contain a high content of it's main compound, linalol. Manufacturers of perfume that include rosewood, such as the popular Chanel No. 5, cannot exactly duplicate its appealing fragrance so they have been demanding huge amounts of rosewood oil since the early 1900s. It is difficult to know the situation with rosewood, except that it grows in South America's tropical rain forests, where most is cut down without replanting and the IUCN lists it as endangered. Brazil's environmental agency, Brazilian Institute of Environment and Renewable Natural Resources (IBAMA), has labeled it as threatened since 1992 and certifies trees that meet their sustainability requirements, which includes replanting areas after harvest and only transporting cut trees by water during the wet season to eliminate the need to build roads. They also use the global positioning system (GPS) to map areas that will be cut and mark individual trees for harvest. IBAMA's projects try to provide indigenous communities with alternative incomes and protect them from "bio-pirates," who coerce them into extracting Amazon plant remedies for export. In addition, they are working with police to stop illegal trafficking of threatened plants such as *bois de rose.* IBAMA is also creating Brazil's first medicinal herb database. While this is all a vast improvement over previous practices, it still results in cutting down wild trees, so we choose not to use the essential oil until it is available sustainably. Meanwhile, essential oil from rosewood leaf, and even small stems, has a similar chemistry and is being researched as a possible source that could be harvested without cutting down trees (note that this essential oil tree is not the endangered rosewood *(Dalbergia* spp.) that is used in construction). Ho wood and coriander seeds are close substitutes.

Spikenard *(Nardostachys grandiflora* aka *N. jatamansi)*

One of the few rhizomes (roots) that are still wildcrafted for essential oil production is spikenard, called *jatamansi* in Ayurvedic medicine. One concern is that the plants grow in alpine forests at high elevations—at four to ten thousand feet. Most commercial spikenard comes from Nepal, not India, as is often assumed. The small amount of Indian production is mostly in Kashmir. Harvesting wild rhizomes is banned in Uttar Pradesh, India, where they have become very scarce (over a quarter of Indian plants are threatened, with nearly 90 percent of Indian herbs used in registered pharmaceuticals collected from the wild, according to the international management consultants McAlpine, Thorpe & Warrier, Ltd.). There are reports of efforts toward better management, and some villages are working on preserving their local botanical resources. However, since it is illegal to transport spikenard from Nepal to India, it is poached and smuggled to meet demand within that country for Ayurvedic medicinal and fragrant products. It is difficult to know the exact status since the amount of essential oil exported is purposely underreported to avoid taxes and much of it is poorly stored and/or adulterated.

Spikenard is being replanted in Nepal, which seems to be building toward a sustainable harvest. A progressive step in communities already harvesting spikenard is that they are distilling it themselves instead of having traders buy the rhizomes (when they change hands four or more times). The Community Forestry Act in Nepal designates forests as being government managed and protected. The Asia Network for Sustainable Agriculture and Bioresources (ANSAB) biodiversity conservation program works with people living near community forests to manage products they already harvest and trade, providing training and technical assistance with quality control, market information, and access to markets and sustainable harvesting information. This increases income in poor, remote villages while conserving plants. Smaller, localized groups have also been forming since 1996. Management of spikenard generally suggests leaving at least 20 percent of the plants for regeneration. Although this is a good step, it is far less than recommended by conservation groups such as United Plant Savers, which is working to save wild medicinal plants in North America.

Tibetan healers called *amchis* use about 375 herbs, and this includes spikenard. They already practice sustainable harvesting based on their Buddhism and Bonpo (Tibet's ancient religion) concepts of universal compassion for all living things. Refuges, such as Tibet's Shey Phoksundo National Park, are being established to preserve medicinal herbs, along with their heritage, thanks to the World Wildlife Fund and the Northern Mountain Conservation Project collaborating with Nepal's Department of National Parks and Wildlife, United Nations Educational, Scientific, and Cultural Organization (UNESCO), and Kew Gardens in England. Villages are establishing medicinal plant management committees. Multidisciplinary teams composed of *amchis,* Buddhist lamas, botanists, park rangers, and sociologists determine plant population sizes and their vulnerability to harvesting. The *amchis* grow spikenard in experimental plots. Traditional Health Care Center clinics use this and other herbs only when they have been cultivated or sustainably harvested. Tibetan medical texts are distributed.

India is also growing spikenard in display gardens at universities and national parks where there is concern about preserving native plants. The Greener Delhi campaign developed a six-acre site in West Delhi where botanists and Ayurvedic practitioners work together cultivating 150 traditional medicinal and cosmetic herbs and giving plants and cultivation instructions to the public.

Agarwood *(Aquilaria malaccensis and A. agallocha)*
Even though it is very expensive, there is a demand for this fragrant wood in China and especially Japan. Most species of agarwood are listed as endangered by the IUCN in India, Malaysia, and Indonesia. In India, the extensive replanting of agarwood trees resulted in a small amount of production by 2006. A large plantation was started in Vietnam, which should yield oil by 2010. Inferior quality and fake agarwood abound, with light-colored agarwood, or even other types of wood dyed and accented in an attempt to look and smell like the true product.

Other Essential Oil Crops
According to the IUCN, other essential oil–producing trees and plants that are considered threatened include the following:

Atlas cedarwood *(Cedrus atlantica* and *C. deodara)* and **Kenyan juniper** *(Juniperus procera):* Also known as cedarwood. Some species of cinnamon in China and India are also threatened, although not the ones that are typically harvested to produce essential oil.

Wild clove trees: The Spice Islands Archaeology Project in eastern Indonesia is striving to save the remaining spice trees on Banda and eight other small islands. They are working on developing management for small island ecosystems and sustainable development that other islands can adopt. These islands were originally the world's sole source of nutmeg and mace. In the sixteenth century, the native people worked as slaves, along with people from all over Asia, for Portuguese and Dutch spice plantations until the price of spices collapsed in the nineteenth century. Since the 1980s, much of what was left of the native spice forests has been cut down.

Essential oil root crops, such as Indian calamus *(Acorus calamus),* are used in Ayurvedic medicine and becoming rare. **Ginger lily** *(Hedychium coronarium)* is also used in Ayurvedic medicine and is considered endangered in some areas of Hawaii, but not in India.

CHAPTER 13

Chemistry of Essential Oils

A GOOD GRASP of the basics of essential oil chemistry adds a new dimension to aromatherapy skills. Becoming familiar with the actions of chemical constituents will help you use essential oils more effectively because you will better understand why and how they work. Daniel Penoel, MD, and researcher Pierre Franchomme first introduced the following approach to aromatic chemistry to aromatherapy students in France. Chemist and educator Kurt Schnaubelt, PhD, subsequently brought the concept to a wider audience in the United States in the late 1980s.

Before we delve into the chemistry of essential oils, let's take a look at how the plant itself manufactures them. Essential oils are secondary metabolites, created and stored in specialized plant structures such as secretory cells, glands, glandular hairs, and oil or resin ducts, and they are always segregated from other plant tissues in these areas. The secretory cells that produce the volatile oils trap the photoelectromagnetic energy of the sun and, with the help of glucose, convert it into biochemical energy in the form of aromatic molecules. In a process similar to photosynthesis, plants create essential oils by trapping and transmitting light and energy.

Volatile oils are produced in various parts of plants. For instance, they are found in fruit peels (citrus), gums and resins (frankincense and myrrh), flowers (rose and lavender), leaves (sage, lemon balm, geranium, and peppermint), barks (cinnamon and sassafras), needles (pine and fir), roots (vetiver and valerian), grasses (lemongrass and palmarosa), rhizomes (ginger), and seeds (fennel, anise, cumin, celery, dill, and coriander). The citrus species *Citrus aurantium*, commonly known as *bitter orange*, provides three different essential oils: petitgrain from the leaf, neroli from the blossom, and bitter orange from the fruit peel.

Plants that produce essential oils do so for a number of reasons that are critical to their survival. Volatile oils in fragrant flowers attract insects for pollination and reproduction. As some essential oils evaporate from the surface of the leaves, they protect against predators and act as antibacterial agents. And in times of metabolic disruption, such as a drought, essential oils serve as protection for the plant.

Whole Plant vs. Essential Oils

When distilling the essential oil from a plant, the only therapeutic properties obtained are those of the volatile oil. Glycosides and many other plant constituents, such as tannins, saponins, and alkaloids, are too large and heavy to carry over during distillation. When you research essential oils in an herb book, keep in mind that the properties attributed to the herb do not necessarily apply to the essential oil, but may instead pertain only to constituents found in the whole plant.

Many of the four to five hundred thousand known plant species in the world have not yet been tested for essential oils or oil components. Although many plants are thought to produce essential oils or their components to some degree, the amounts may be undetectable or too minute to extract. In addition, although some plants produce essential oils in minute to acceptable amounts, the sheer quantity of plant material required for commercial production prohibits their use.

Echinacea is a good example. This popular immune-modulating and infection-fighting herb produces trace amounts of volatile oils, but not enough to make essential oil extraction commercially viable or ecologically sound. On the other hand, some herbs high in volatile oils are not exploited commercially, while many other plants currently used in herbal form are as yet "undiscovered" or at least unavailable. Still, the herbs themselves are wonderful, and you can enjoy the fragrance of oils as well as their healing properties in a simple cup of tea.

Components of Essential Oils

A plant contains a combination of natural chemical components, or *constituents,* that are responsible for its particular taste, smell, and medicinal properties. Such components include alkaloids, saponins, tannins, glycosides, volatile oils, phytohormones, minerals, and vitamins. The constituents relating to aromatherapy are the *volatile* (essential) oils.

There are more than thirty thousand known aromatic molecules. The number and combination of these molecules vary from plant to plant, making each essential oil unique. An essential oil may contain a hundred different aromatic molecules, but the number may also range between ten and five hundred (some have even more). This means that a given essential oil is not composed of just one type of molecule. Its composition is a complex array of components that gives each plant its characteristic odor and flavor, as well as accounting for its unique effects on individuals.

Chemical Groups

Essential oils are mixtures of aromatic molecules built from three basic elements: carbon, hydrogen, and oxygen. Depending on the type of molecules they contain, the constituents of volatile oils classify them into different chemical or functional groups. These chemical groups characterize the nature of the whole molecule and its properties. The main groups are phenols, terpenes, alcohols, ketones, esters, ethers, oxides, aldehydes, coumarins, and acids, although the acid group is not found in essential oils, but in hydrolats. This section explains the actions of these chemical groups, along with examples of plants and the constituents of each group. Classifying essential oils according to the most prevalent group of molecules can be of great value in understanding an oil's basic properties and actions, and it allows us to understand how different oils can share those basic properties and actions.

If you are unfamiliar with chemistry, envision an essential oil separated into segments, some larger and some smaller, each of which represents a different component. For instance, the essential oil of lemon thyme (a variety of thyme with a distinct lemon scent) smells like thyme because of the component thymol (found in many species of thyme), but also smells like lemon because it contains a component called *citronellal.*

Often the same aromatic molecule is found in different plants. Rose, citronella, palmarosa, and geranium all contain geraniol, while cinnamon leaf and clove both contain eugenol. Similar essential oils can give unrelated plants very similar fragrances. Anise and star anise are good examples—both smell and taste like licorice because both have the constituent anethole. Other examples of unrelated plants with similar fragrances are melissa and lemon verbena, both of which have citrus components (neral and geranial) that give them a lemony smell. On the other hand, rosewood, coriander, French basil, and lavender all contain linalol but smell very different due to the other constituents in their makeup.

Certain essential oils may be dominated by only one or two types of molecules. Wintergreen, for example, can contain up to 99 percent methyl salicylate, mustard up to 95 percent allyl isothiocyanate; both are potentially hazardous. Sandalwood, a relatively safe oil, may contain 65 to 90 percent santalol, and clove bud oil may contain 70 to 80 percent eugenol. Exotic (Reunion) basil can contain up to 80 percent methyl chavicol, but the French (sweet) basil is high in linalol (40 to 45 percent) and has approximately 20 percent methyl chavicol. Both come from the same species, *Ocimum basilicum.*

Interestingly, the compound that predominates in an oil is not always the one responsible for most of its activity. The presence of trace components can significantly change the odor and flavor, and sometimes even the action, of an essential oil. Linalyl acetate and linalol make up about 90 percent of the aromatic molecules found in clary sage. A third molecule, sclareol, makes up only 5 to 7 percent, but it is nonetheless responsible for the mild estrogenic activity of the essential oil. Approximately 3 percent of clary sage oil is made up of some three hundred other molecules. Mandarin is 95 percent terpenes, while about seventy-four other identified components make up the other 5 percent.

Many essential oils contain compounds from different aromatic families. Examples include helichrysum, which has esters and ketones; neroli, which has aldehydes and alcohols; and peppermint, which contains both alcohols and ketones. Rose is an example of a chemically complex plant, containing more than 400 different aromatic molecules, including esters, alcohols, and acids. Rose geranium and lavender each have more than 350 molecules from a variety of biochemical groups, including alcohols, esters, and aldehydes. Essential oils extracted by the carbon dioxide process are generally more complex than those derived by distillation, simply because that process extracts heavier components in addition to the volatile oils.

The name of a chemical compound often comes from the botanical or common name of a plant. *Thymol* comes from *thyme, citronellal* from *citronella, pinene* from *pine, geraniol* from *geranium, bergapten* from *bergamot,* and so on. In some instances, the ending of a compound name can provide a hint as to what group it belongs in. For example, terpenes end in "ene," ketones end in "one," aldehydes end in "al," and both phenols and alcohols end in "ol."

Chemotypes

Chemotypes are a phenomenon of nature whereby plants from the same genus and species produce different proportions of aromatic molecules. The specific molecules produced by each plant are determined by genes and enzymes, both of which are influenced by weather and soil conditions, altitude, and variations in light wave-lengths. Chemotypes are reproduced by cloning rather than pollination.

Thyme oil produced from *Thymus vulgaris* grown at sea level is high in thymol. The plant grown under these hot, dry conditions produces different aromatic molecules than a *Thymus vulgaris* plant grown in the mountains, which would be high in linalol. *Thymus vulgaris* has more than eight chemotypes. The different aromatic molecules in a chemotype define very specific applications for each oil, although they all come from the same species of plant. Chemotypes are specified thus: *Thymus vulgaris* CT linalol, *Thymus vulgaris* CT thymol, and so on.

Most of the different eucalyptus oils *(Eucalyptus globulus, E. citriodora, E. radiata)* are not chemotypes, but are from different species. However, *Eucalyptus polybractea* does produce the chemotypes cryptone and cineol, each of which has different applications. *Eucalyptus dives* also produces two chemotypes, piperitone and cineol. *Rosmarinus officinalis* produces verbenone, cineol, and camphor.

Most of the following chemical groups are made up of oxygenated compounds, which means that their molecules come with an oxygen atom attached. The exception is terpenes, which are hydrocarbon compounds and contain only hydrogen and carbon.

PHENOLS

This group contains the most stimulating, bactericidal, and immune-modulating compounds of all the aromatic groups. Phenols are often irritating to the skin and toxic to the liver; therefore, they should be used with caution, in low dilutions, and only for short periods of time. Essential oils in the phenol group include clove, oregano, savory, and specific chemotypes of thyme. Compounds include carvacrol, thymol, eugenol, guaiacol, chavicol, and australol.

TERPENES

Terpenes are antiseptic and stimulating, but they may irritate the skin in concentrated amounts. Essential oils that contain molecules from this group include citrus, mastic, nutmeg, angelica, pine, fir, spruce, and black pepper. Chemists differentiate subgroups of terpenes by the number of carbon atoms they contain. Monoterpenes contain ten carbon atoms, sesquiterpenes fifteen carbon atoms. Diterpenes are C_{20} molecules, meaning they contain twenty carbon atoms. Some constituents in the monoterpene group include limonene, terpinene, camphene, myrcene, sabinene, p-cymene, phellandrene, a- and b-pinene, and thujene.

An important subgroup, called *sesquiterpenes,* are mainly found in roots and woods or from plants of the Asteraceae family (formerly known as the Compositae family). Sesquiterpene compounds include caryophyllene (clove), whose actions are anti-inflammatory and antiviral; farnesol (rose and chamomile), which is antibacterial; chamazulene and bisabolol (blue tansy, yarrow, and chamomile), which are anti-inflammatory and analgesic; and valeranon (valerian), which is antispasmodic and sedative. Other sesquiterpenes include santalol (sandalwood), zingiberol (ginger), veriteron and vetiverol (vetiver), and carotol (carrot seed). Spikenard is almost 100 percent sesquiterpenes.

Diterpenes (twenty carbon atoms) are rarely found in essential oils, and although terpenoid molecules with thirty to forty carbon chains do occur in plants (plant steroids and hormones), their molecular weight is too heavy to allow evaporation with steam.

ALCOHOLS

Toning, stimulating, antibacterial, and antiviral, alcohols are generally nontoxic. Essential oils containing mono-terpene alcohols include geranium, ravensara, rosewood, rose, and tea tree. Generally nonirritating and safe to use, the beneficial constituents found in these plants include geraniol, menthol, a-terpineol, terpineol-4, sabinol, linalol, and thujanol. Monoterpenols include cinalol, geraniol, nerol, a-terpineol, cuminol, carveol, borneol, pinocarveol, sabinol, and menthol. The object of much research and interest, sesquiterpenol molecules in the alcohol group are anti-inflammatory and stimulate immune responses. They include nerolidol (neroli), bisabolol (chamomile), carotol (carrot seed), a- and b-santalol (sandalwood), vetiverol (vetiver), sclareol (clary sage), zingiberol (ginger), patchoulol (patchouli), and farnesol (rose).

KETONES

The actions of ketones are mucolytic (break up mucus), cicatrizant (heal wounds), and lipolytic (dissolve fats). Potentially toxic ketones are found in sage, hyssop, pennyroyal, and thuja, none of which we recommend using. Their toxic effects vary depending on the plant, but irresponsible use of oils in this group can have abortive, convulsive, stupefying, or epileptic actions. Examples of fragrant molecules in the ketone group include thujone, carvone, menthone, atlantone, vetivone, jasmone, fenchone, and pulegone. Subgroups include diones, such as those found in helichrysum, and cytotoxic lactones, which are contained in *Inula graveolens*. Nontoxic oils in this group include jasmine, fennel, and to some extent, peppermint.

ESTERS

A reaction product of acids and alcohols, esters are the most balancing of all the chemical families of essential oils. They are relaxing and soothing, and many have antispasmodic and antifungal properties. Oils that contain a good proportion of esters tend to smell very pleasant; these include lavender, bergamot, clary sage, ylang-ylang, Roman chamomile, and marjoram. Examples of aromatic molecules in this group are linalyl acetate, neryl acetate, geranyl acetate, bornyl acetate, and other acetates.

ETHERS

Plants in this category include basil, tarragon, and cedar. The aromatic molecules are methyl chavicol, methyl eugenol, and cedryl methyl ether. These tend to have antispasmodic actions. Also included are the constituents apiol, found in parsley; transanethole, found in anise; and myristicin, found in nutmeg. Ethers can have a stupefying effect if overused.

OXIDES

Essential oils containing oxides include camphorous oils such as tea tree, niaouli, rosemary, cajeput, hyssop (variety *decumbens*), bay laurel, and eucalyptus. The most important aromatic molecule in this group is cineol, but it also includes piperitonoxide, bisabolol oxide, bisabolone oxide, and linalol oxide. Within the oxide group, potentially toxic molecules can cause convulsions: asarone (from calamus) and ascaridol (found in wormseed oil), both of which are never recommended for use. Menthofuran, which may be present in peppermint oil if the plant was harvested during flowering, is also toxic.

ALDEHYDES

Aldehydes are anti-inflammatory, calming, antiseptic, and sedating, but they may also somewhat irritate the skin if used undiluted. Many lemon-scented oils fall into this category, including lemongrass, melissa, lemon verbena, citronella, and *Eucalyptus citriodora*. Cinnamon bark is also in the aldehyde group, but it has other irritating constituents. Examples of specific aromatic molecules include citral, geranial, neral, citronellal, myrtenal, phellandral, cinnamic aldehyde, and benzaldehyde.

COUMARINS

Coumarins have potentially toxic properties that can cause or contribute to liver damage or photosensitivity, and they are also blood thinners. Therefore, people who have liver problems, have any level of sun exposure, or who take blood-thinning medications should use them with caution. Examples of coumarins are bergapten, herniarine, angelicine, citronene, and furocoumarin. Oils in this group include bergamot and other citruses, cumin, khella, angelica, and to a small extent, lavender.

ACIDS

Some essential oils contain acids, but the majority of acids (e.g., carboxylic, angelic, and quinic acid) are found primarily in aromatic hydrosols. They are anti-inflammatory and antiseptic as well as moisturizing for the skin.

Chemical Groups

KETONES (mucolytic, neurotoxic)	thuja, sage, wormwood, tansy, hyssop, camphor, rosemary, *Eucalyptus dives*, dill
ALDEHYDES (sedative)	*Eucalyptus citriodora*, citronella, lemon verbena, melissa, *Litsea cubeba*, cumin
ESTERS (balancing, soothing)	lavender, clary sage, Roman chamomile, geranium, ylang-ylang
ETHERS (antispasmodic)	basil, tarragon, anise seed, parsley, nutmeg, sassafras
ALCOHOLS (tonifying, energizing)	rosewood, coriander, petitgrain, rose, palmarosa, *Eucalpytus radiata*, neroli, ravensara, tea tree, marjoram, peppermint, spearmint
PHENOLS (stimulating, antibacterial)	thyme, oregano, savory, clove
OXIDES (expectorant)	*Eucalyptus globulus*, bay, *Hyssop officinalis* var. *decumbens*
TERPENES (drying, antiviral)	orange, lemon, pine, cypress, spruce, Douglas fir
SESQUITERPENES (anti-inflammatory)	german chamomile, ginger, sandalwood, patchouli

PART IV

materia medica

Look in the perfumes of flowers and of nature for peace of mind and joy of life.

—*Wang Wei*

CHAPTER 14

Ayurvedic Aromatherapy

AYURVEDIC MEDICINE has been in India for at least five thousand years. India has a rich history of utilizing essential oils, originally as fragrant plants and now often in the form of essential oils. Ayurvedic massage and treatments include several types of traditional techniques that rely on aromatherapy. Before essential oils were commonly available, the herbs were infused into an oil base, usually sesame oil or mashed sesame seeds, which is native to India, or coconut oil. Ayurvedic medicine today still relies primarily on sesame oil for treatments that call for vegetable oil. An ancient branch of Ayurveda called *Dhoopam* relates to healing by inhaling smoke that is produced from certain combinations of aromatic plants. Tibetan medicine also therapeutically uses smoke, and some places have special rooms for these treatments.

Rather than fighting an individual chronic disorder, Ayurvedic theory emphasizes bringing the physical, emotional, and spiritual health of an individual into balance. The goal is to work with and strengthen the body to establish "forgiveness of disease." Ideally, each person has herbal and aromatherapy formulas designed for their particular body type, or *dosha,* which refers to one of three categories. Practioners use age-old forms of diagnosis that involve reading the variations in the pulse, examining the tongue, fingernails, and eyes, and other clues obtained visually and through touch and smell to define each person's constitutional type and treatment. The practitioner looks at the client's biological rhythms and contrasts them with similar properties, or energetics, of the plant. The plant's properties are determined by examining its taste, smell, and sometimes texture. The essential oils or herbs that a practioner chooses for a remedy have the opposite energetics than those that manifest in an individual's personal dosha, to bring that person into balance.

About Ayurvedic Doshas

We use a common shorthand to describe the doshas. These descriptions may not mean much to some readers, but they will be useful to readers familiar with Ayurvedic medicine.

In brief, the doshas are as follows:

VATA (V)

Vata is associated with the elemental nature of infinity (sometimes called ether) and air, and may have a somewhat ungrounded constitution. It manifests as movement, but it can also lead to nervousness, high blood pressure, headaches, and confusion. People of this type tend to be thin and anxious, with sensitive digestion, dry skin, thin hair, and their fingernails may be brittle. They seldom perspire, sleep lightly, are easily fatigued, and often feel cold. In the Western model of body types, it is on par with the ectomorphic type.

PITTA (P)

Pitta is associated with fire and an energetic constitution, and it represents transformation. It often manifests with good digestion and a quick metabolism, but overstimulation can result in irregular hormonal activity and quick anger. People of this type generally have muscular bodies, are warmer than other doshic types, and are prone to becoming flushed or having inflammatory skin conditions such as rosacea. The comparable Western model is the mesomorphic type.

KAPHA (K)

Kapha is associated with the elements earth and water, and manifests in a slower constitution and heavy or stocky bodies. It is commonly nourishing and calm, but it can also mean congestion of mucous membranes with a tendency to laziness and inflexibility. These folks may suffer from phlegmatic and wet conditions such as bronchitis and have a tendency toward oily, moist skin and thick, soft hair. They sleep well and tend to gain weight easily. The comparable Western model is the endomorph.

Ayurvedic Materia Medica

The following are the most widely available essential oils in Ayurvedic medicine. All essential oils are available as steam distilled, unless otherwise noted. Below the common name and its scientific Latin name, we've indicated whether CO_2, absolute (solvent-extracted), or oleoresin is produced. The capitalized letters in brackets indicated how that essential oil affects the doshas (the Ayurvedic constitutional types). Oils that are described further in chapter 15 are indicated with "(MM)." We've also listed Hindi, Sanskrit, and other important alternative names.

The dosha shorthand consists of V, P, or K, along with one of the following symbols:

+ means that dosha is increased
– means that dosha is decreased
o means that dosha has a neutral or mixed action
= means the dosha has the same or balanced action

For example, "KP+V–" indicates that both Kapha and Pitta are increased and Vata is decreased. Some doshas are indicated as "in excess," meaning that the essential oil may not act on the dosha immediately preceding unless that dosha is very strong. There is some disagreement among Ayurvedic experts, as indicated.

Agarwood (*Aquilaria agallocha; A. mallacensis*)

CO_2 [VPK=]

Agarwood, Oud, Aloeswood, Linaloes; Sanskrit: *Aguru;*
Chinese: *Ch'en hsiang;* Japanese: *Jinko*

Used primarily as religious incense, agarwood is also a bitter digestive tonic that relieves indigestion. Ayurvedic medicine uses it as a skin tonic that restores skin pigmentation, an antiseptic, and even to treat snakebites. As a liniment, its eases rheumatic, muscular, and nerve pain. The ancient Indian physician Charaka suggested agarwood as both an internal and external treatment for poisoning and high fevers. In addition, it sometimes flavors the betel leaf combinations so often chewed in India.

Ajowan (*Trachyspermum ammi; Carum copticum*)

[KV+P–]

Ajwain; Sanskrit: *Ajmoda, Agnivardhana*

This Indian curry ingredient, related to caraway, is used to make *Oman water* for digestion and an antiseptic wash. Since the essential oil is very high in the compound thymol—up to 50 percent, making it a common source of pure thymol—use it carefully. As a result, it is highly antibacterial and antiseptic.

Amber

Although many assume that the solid amber perfume is distilled from the ancient fossil stone formed from tree pitch, that amber lost its fragrance long ago. Modern-day amber is actually any of several secret blends that families have passed down for generations. It is a combination of many essential oils, such as sandalwood and storax, though sometimes contains synthetic fragrances. Occasionally, a small amount of grated amber fossil is added to the mix. The fragrance is regarded as a spiritual enhancement and an aphrodisiac—quite a combination!

Ambrette; Musk Mallow Seed
(*Hibiscus abelmoschus; Abelmoschus moschatus*)

absolute/CO_2 [KV–P+]

Musk Dana; Sanskrit: *Lataksturikam*

A popular Eastern spice, these cooling, tonifying, antispasmodic, and aphrodisiac seeds are chewed in Egypt to relieve stomach problems, soothe the nerves, and sweeten the breath. Arabs flavor their coffee with them. The Middle Eastern Unani system of medicine finds that the seeds allay thirst. In India and Malaysia, powdered seeds perfume hair, are burned as incense, and are placed in clothing to deter insects. The Vietnamese consider it an antivenom agent. The essential oil is a substitute for the more expensive musk (from the sexual glands of musk deer) in perfumes. Aromatherapists treat depression and anxiety and relieve headaches and nervousness with ambrette. Externally, it eases cramped muscles and aching joints and improves poor circulation. This species of hibiscus is different than the popular herbal tea from *Hibiscus sabdariffa*.

Angelica, Indian (*Angelica glauca*)

[VPK=P+ (in excess) (MM)

Bhataur-chora; Sanskrit: *Choraka*

Ayurveda uses this native species of angelica mostly as a digestive aid and flavoring.

Basil, Holy (*Ocimum tenuiflorum; O. sanctum*)

[VK–P+] (MM)

Kala Tulsi; Sanskrit: *Tulssi*

Used in ceremonies as much as in cooking, *tulsi* is a popular tonic and blood-cleansing tea. Pressed juice from the leaves is taken internally for skin diseases, including ringworm and even leprosy, and to treat dysentery, indigestion, hemorrhaging, and chronic fever. Mixed with honey and ginger juice, it makes an expectorant cough syrup that is also used to clear the mind.

Black Pepper (Piper nigrum)

[KP+V– or K–PV+] (MM)

Kalimrich; Sanskrit: *Marichs;* Chinese: *Huchio*

Long pepper *(P. piper longum)* is also used in Ayurveda, although it is not readily available as an essential oil.

Calamus, Indian (Acorus calamus)

[VK–P+]

Bach; Sanskrit: *Vacha;* Chinese: *Shui chang*

The deep but pleasantly sweet scent relieves nervousness, headaches, and dizziness. It is an aphrodisiac and is used as an ingredient in perfumes, especially in India. A traditional formula infuses the charred roots in oil to rub over rheumatic inflammation, paralyzed limbs, or the abdomen to relieve indigestion. However, only use the herb topically, and only sniff the essential oil, which contains 80 percent of the compound b-asarone (banned in 1978 by the U.S. Federal Drug Administration). Western calamus is slightly less toxic, even though it is the same species.

Camphor (Cinnamomum camphora)

[KV–P+]

Kapur; Sanskrit: *Kapoor* and *Karpuram*

Although potentially toxic, camphor is used in Ayurvedic and Traditional Chinese Medicine, mostly as a heating liniment and to relieve itchy skin.

Cardamom (Ellettaria cardamomum)

CO_2 [K –P+ and V+ or V–] (MM)

Chhoti; Sanskrit: *Ela*

Cardamom is used to open the body's energy or *prana.*

Cedarwood, Tibetan (Cedrus deodara)

[VK–P+ or VPK=] (MM)

Deodar; Sanskrit: *Devadaru*

Thanks to the essential oil it contains, a tea made of the bark relieves fever and skin disorders and is a snakebite antidote.

Celery Seed (Apium graveolens)

[KV–P+]

Ajowan; Sanskrit: *Ajmoda*

Celery seed extensively flavors food and drinks (alcoholic and soft drinks) and scents some soaps and cosmetics. Distilled from the flower head, the warm, spicy, and sweet scent opens even chronic sinus congestion. It has hormonal properties, stimulates mother's milk, and relieves liver congestion and genitourinary problems. In Ayurveda, it stimulates poor appetite, digestion, and relieves the pain of arthritis, rheumatism, gout, and sciatica. The absolute is bright blue in color.

Champa (Michelia champaca)

mostly absolute, concrete, CO_2 [PK–V+ (in excess)]

Champaca

This towering tree becomes covered with thousands of fragrant, golden flowers that are often infused into vegetable oil to heal skin irritations. Antiseptic, anti-inflammatory, and cooling, they treat rheumatism and gout and are an aphrodisiac. From Indonesia and India, this heady scent is expensive, so it is sometimes adulterated with ylang-ylang. It is also sold as concrete and absolute and often distilled with sandalwood as an attar.

Cinnamon (Cinnamomum tamala)

[VK–P+] (MM)

Dalchini; Sanskrit: *Twak*

Ayurveda looks to this species of cinnamon for general digestive complaints, as an adjunct to bitter tonics, and a strong laxative. Cinnamon or laurel berry *(C. glaucescens),* also available as an essential oil, is chewed to relieve indigestion and sweeten the breath.

Coriander (Coriandrum sativum)

CO_2 [PKV= or VPK–] (MM)

Dhaniya; Sanskrit: *Dhanyaka*

The seed relieves gas and indigestion and is used for scorpion stings and snakebites.

Costus (Saussurea lappa)

[KV+P–]

Costus; Sanskrit: *Kustha*

The finger-sized roots of this Himalayan thistle are prized as a respiratory tonic, aphrodisiac perfume, Arabic body oil, and incense, especially in Japan. Kashmir merchants used the roots, as rug merchants used patchouli, to protect shawls from moths. We advise caution even for topical application, although the essential oil is made into an antiseptic salve that destroys *Staphylococcus* and strep infections and is a muscle and rheumatic pain-relieving liniment. Tibetan medicine uses the herb to help people with emotional problems.

Cumin (Cuminum cyminum)

CO_2 [KP–V+]

Jeera; Sanskrit: *Jiraka;* Apiaceae (Umbelliferae)

Cumin seed was mentioned in Egypt's *Papyrus Ebers* (1550 BC) and by the first-century AD herbalist Dioscorides. It stimulates saliva and other digestive juices, relieves digestive-related headaches, obesity, and fluid accumulation, and may help stabilize blood sugar. It also increases poor circulation and is slightly sedative. The seeds are historically used to relieve menstrual cramps. Studies find cumin may be slightly estrogenic and inhibit cancer cell growth.

The fragrance counteracts emotional and physical exhaustion and helps instill stability. It may have aphrodisiac qualities but use it sparingly, because it is reminiscent of male underarm odor! It can also irritate skin and be slightly photosensitizing. The seeds flavor lemonade and tamarind juice for their cooling action and are often in formulas for hoarseness, chronic indigestion, or diarrhea. Don't confuse it with the carrier oil black cumin (*Nigella sativa*).

Cyperus (Cyperus rotundus)

[PKV–]

Korehijar; Sanskrit: *Nagar-Mustika*

The tubers of this smoky-scented sedge, called nut grass in English, has a deep, rootlike, stimulating fragrance. They are found in many Indian hair conditioners, colognes, and perfumes and are also used as antiseptics for skin rashes, infections, and slow bleeding. Indian researchers found that their anti-inflammatory action is comparable to the drug cortisone. Cyperus seems to have estrogenic properties. Traditionally, it has been infused into oil that is rubbed over the abdomen for menstruation problems and on the breast to increase milk. *C. scariosus* is more prevalent as essential oil, the scent of which is said to increase creativity and calm the mind. Do not confuse it with the cypress tree (*Cupressus sempervirens*).

Davana (Artemesia pallens)

CO_2 [PVK]

Dhavana

Davana regulates menstruation, increases circulation, soothes skin irritations, and is an aphrodisiac. Ayurvedic panchakarma treatments use it to treat ovarian and other cysts. Aromatherapists find that it balances energy, reduces anger, and releases negative thoughts.

Fennel (Foeniculum vulgare)

CO_2 [VKP=] (MM)

Saunf; Sanskrit: *Shatapushpa*

The appetizer, digestive, and stimulating seeds are chewed.

Fenugreek *(Trigonella graecum)*

CO_2 [VK–P+]

Sanskrit: *Methi;* Chinese: *Huluba*

The seed paste is traditionally placed on boils and slow-healing wounds. It aids the nervous and respiratory systems.

Frankincense, Indian; Boswellia

(Boswellia serrata)

[KV–P+] (MM)

Luban; Sanskrit: *Shallaki*

Mixing it into a paste with lemon juice is a traditional remedy for skin problems such as boils, ulcerations, and ringworm.

Galanga *(Alpinia galanga)*

[VK–P+]

Kulanjan; Sanskrit: *Malayavach*

The rhizome of this Chinese native is similar for use in cooking and medicine. It decreases indigestion, inflammation, pain, and fungal infection. Studies back its use for bronchitis and asthma, showing that the essential oil stimulates and opens the bronchial passages. It also treats Epstein-Barr virus and seems to act on the immune system. The herb flavors Thai soups, Indian and Indonesian curries and digestive bitters (such as Boonekamp and Abtei), and Russian beer. A paste of the powdered rhizome is applied to skin conditions, such as acne. Considered an aphrodisiac, it is in Indian perfumes, deodorant body powders, and breath fresheners. It is often confused with false or Malaysian ginger *(Kaemferia galanga)* oil.

Galbanum *(Ferula galbaniflua)*

[VPK= (V+ in excess)]

Gandhabiroza; carrot (Apiaceae) family

Native to the Middle East and West Asia, the root was burned as a woody and spicy incense and found its way into Europe as the "poor man's angelica." Resembling a

NON-INDIAN ESSENTIAL OIL DOSHAS

bay [P+KV– or VK+]

benzoin [VPK=]

bergamot [VK–P+]

cajeput (Sanskrit: *Katupruhi*)—[VK–P+]

chamomile [VK–P+ or PV–K+]

citronella [PK–V+]

clary sage [VPK–]

clove bud (Sanskrit: *Lavanga*) [KV–P+]

cypress [VK= or VKP+]

eucalyptus [KV–P+]

geranium, rose [PK–V]

lavender [PK–Vo]

lemon [PV–Ko]

lemongrass [PK–Vo]

lime (Sanskrit: *Nimbuka*) [PK–V+]

marjoram [KP–V+]

myrtle [PK=V+]

neroli (orange blossom) [PV–K+]

orange [VK–P+]

palmarosa [VPK–]

peppermint [PK– and V+ or Vo]

petitgrain [PK–Vo]

pine [VK = P+]

rosemary [KV–P+]

sage [KV–P+]

tangerine [VPK=]

thyme [VK–P+]

tuberose [VK–P+]

giant fennel plant, it is cultivated as food flavoring, perfume fixative, and for use in pharmaceuticals, mostly as a bronchial inhalant called Luba. It has been used to dress inflamed, abscessed wounds, tone mature or irritated skin, and is thought to promote cell regeneration. It also treats indigestion, asthma, poor circulation, and soothes emotional tension and aching muscles and joints. The oil is distilled from the oleoresin, which is collected by incising the stem base. Persian oil is solid, the Levant type is liquid, and the Galbanol type has most terpene compounds removed, making it somewhat water soluble. It is related to the Indian garlic substitute asafetida *(Ferula asafoetida).*

Ginger *(Zingiber officinale)*

oleoresin/CO$_2$ [VK–P+] (MM)
Adrak; Sanskrit: *Shunthi*

A paste of the powdered rhizome is applied to the forehead to relieve headaches and on toothaches, and it is rubbed on skin to increase blood circulation.

Ginger Lily *(Hedychium spicatum)*

[P–VK+]
Kapur-kachri

Related to Hawaii's white ginger *(H. coronarium),* these lilies grow in the Himalayan foothills. Used to relieve depression, as a nerve tonic, and as both religious and secular incense, the scent is a cross of ginger, camphor, and violet.

Guggul *(Commiphora mukul)*

[KV–P+]
Gogal; Sanskrit: *Goggulu*

It is antiseptic and anti-inflammatory and has long been used to reduce pain and stiffness and improve movement in arthritics. The resin, as a dietary supplement rather than essential oil, lowers cholesterol. These uses are backed by science. Arabian women use this incense to smudge (smoke) a birthing room after labor. Sometimes called Indian myrrh, it is less expensive and sometimes adulterates myrrh, although it is not often made into essential oil.

Jasmine *(Jasminum officinalis)*

absolute, concrete [KP–V+ (in excess)] (MM)
Chameli ka tel, Mogra; Sanskrit: *Jati*

A poultice of the dried flowers is applied to the breasts of nursing mothers to slow milk production. It is used to cool down anger and even to counter insanity. It is traditionally used for mouth problems.

Jatamansi; Spikenard *(Nardostachys jatamansi)*

CO$_2$ [KV–P+] (MM)
Jatamansi; Sanskrit: *Jatamansi*

The rhizomes are mixed with sesame and rubbed on the head as a sedative, as well as to keep hair dark. It has also been used to heal leprosy sores.

Juniper *(Juniperus communis)*

[P+ and VK+ or KV–] (MM)
Aaraar; Sanskrit: *Hapusa*

Powdered berries are rubbed on painful, swollen, and arthritic joints.

Keawa; Screw Pine (*Pandanus tectoriu; P. odoratissimus*)

[PK–V+]
Kevda; Sanskrit: *Ketaki*

A mature tree produces thirty to forty of the fragrant, 10- to 20-inch-long spathes (leaflike spikes enclosing the flowers) that grow along the central stalk. They yield a pungent, woodsy-scented infused oil said to help rejuvenate and stimulate the mind. Calling it *keora* oil, Ayurvedic physicians use it to treat headaches, earaches, and allergies and rub an antispasmodic liniment on tight muscles and sore joints. The hydrosol is sold in the United States in Indian markets.

Lotus (*Nelumbo nucifera*)

absolute/concrete [PV–K+]
Kaner; Sanskrit: *Karavira*

This expensive oil has only recently become available again after a long time of not being distilled commercially. Regarded as very cooling, a honey tonic made from it, called *padmamadjhu,* is used for eye disorders. The flowers soothe skin eruptions, snakebite, and scorpion stings, and a syrup treats coughs and bronchitis.

Nutmeg (*Myristica fragrans*)

CO_2 [VP–K+]
Jaiphal; Sanskrit: *Jatiphalam*

The scent of nutmeg is used for insomnia. Potentially toxic to the nervous system, the ancient Indian doctor Charaka recommended nutmeg for external use only. However, small amounts are used for skin care, including ringworm and to prevent scars, and are added to massage oils, hair pomades, and some Oriental-type perfumes. A plaster made of the ground nuts is applied over rheumatic pain. Nutmeg is the basis of the Ayurvedic formula *Jatiphaladi,* which is used to treat nausea, dysentery, and smoker's cough. The tea of nutmeg is used for insomnia, but is very drying internally (it is therefore good for Kapha types, although they don't normally have trouble sleeping).

Saffron (*Crocus sativus*)

only as absolute [VPK=]
Kesar, Kumkuma; Sanskrit: *Nagakeshara*

This is one of a handful of *tridoshic* remedies that are good for every constitutional type and very balancing to the mind. It is a sedative, and studies show it is an antidepressant, although it can be stimulating in small amounts. Collected from the flower's stamen, it is quite expensive, so it is commonly infused into sesame oil. It is still popular in India for the golden glow it imparts to dark complexions, and small amounts in powder reduce acne and allergic skin reactions. A paste is applied on bruises or nerve pain, and on the chest to relieve congestion. It also promotes digestion, regulates the menstrual cycle and menopause, and is used for depression.

Sandalwood (*Santalum album*)

CO_2 [PV–Ko] (MM)
Safed Chandan; Sanskrit: *Chandana*

A paste or emulsion made from the wood is used as a cooling dressing to treat swelling, overheated conditions, and hot skin eruptions, such as prickly heat. The essential oil is used neat to eradicate scabies outbreaks. The powdered wood is drunk in coconut milk to alleviate intense thirst or heat or sweetened and mixed with rice water for dysentery.

Turmeric (*Curcuma longa*)

CO_2, oleoresin [K–V– and P+ or P=]
Haldi; Sanskrit: *Harida*

Turmeric rhizomes are often cured in pits before being steam distilled. A strong antioxidant, it is beneficial to the liver, although the herb may be stronger than the essential oil. It is also antibacterial and relieves inflammatory conditions such as arthritis. Studies show turmeric

ESSENTIAL OILS TO BALANCE AYURVEDIC DOSHAS

These essential oils provide the opposite, or balancing, effect on the dosha for which they are listed. For instance, Vata oils are calming, warming, or moisturizing so they soothe and balance a person who has a Vata constitution, which tends to be dry, cold, and excitable. Some oils are in more than one category because they have several balancing qualities, although not all of the doshic qualities are indicated on this list. Use this modified, quick reference to help you choose an appropriate essential oil or to create a blend that is designed for an individual's constitution. Essential oils are often diluted in fixed oils to make cosmetics and medicines.

Vata oils warm, moisten, and ground the cold, dry, and flighty qualities of a Vata constitution.
Pitta oils cool and calm the fiery nature of those with Pitta qualities.
Kapha oils are drying, providing movement and stimulation for this damper, sluggish constitution.

VATA-BALANCING OILS	PITTA-BALANCING OILS	KAPHA-BALANCING OILS	
Grounding, wet, warming, soothing	*Cooling, calming, floral, anti-inflammatory*	*Stimulating, drying, warming, expectorant*	
Atlas cedar	ambrette	anise	lemon tea tree
benzoin	cassie	basil	lemongrass
bergamot	chamomile, blue/Roman	bay laurel	lovage
cardamom	davana	bergamot	marjoram
cinnamon leaf/bark	geranium	birch	myrtle
cistus	ginger lily	black pepper	nutmeg
clary sage	helichrysum	cardamom	orange/bitter orange
clove	jasmine	cinnamon leaf/bark	oregano
fenugreek	lavender	cistus	palmarosa
frankincense	neroli	citronella	peppermint
ginger	peppermint	clary sage	petitgrain
grapefruit	rose	clove	rosemary
helichrysum	sandalwood	coriander	sage
lavender	vetiver	cypress	spearmint
lemon	ylang-ylang	eucalyptus, all types	star anise
mandarin		fennel	tea tree/niaouli/cajeput
nutmeg		fir/pine	wintergreen
orange		frankincense/benzoin	
palmarosa		ginger	
patchouli		grapefruit/mandarin	
petitgrain		hyssop	
rose		juniper	
star anise		lavender/spike lavender	
vanilla		lemon/lime	
vetiver			

decreases inflammatory substances produced by the body. Ayurvedic medicine considers it cooling and applies it in a paste over sprains and inflammatory, heat-producing skin diseases. Chinese medicine also uses it for many complaints, including toothaches and chest pain.

Vetiver; Vetivert (*Andropogon zizanioides; Vetiveria zizanioides*)

CO₂ [KP+V–] (MM)

Khus, Kiryata; Sanskrit: *Kirta, Ushira*

Ayurvedic medicine uses this scent to cool both the physical body and overheated emotions or headaches, heatstroke, and to delay the onset of senility. The related ginger grass *(Andropogon nardus)* is an invigorating scent used mostly in perfume.

Chakras

Chakras are an important aspect of traditional Ayurvedic medicine. The word *chakra* means "wheel" in Sanskrit. These energy centers in the body were acknowledged by the healing practices of many ancient cultures, such as the Egyptians, Chinese, Hindus, Greeks, and Romans. Traditional Chinese Medicine acknowledges chakras through acupuncture meridians and *qi* (chi), while Ayurvedic medicine relates to them as *prana*. According to these ancient philosophies, when chakras are unbalanced, dysfunctional, or blocked, a range of emotional and physiological imbalances manifest. Balance is important in achieving overall health, and chakras are said to play a role in regulating emotional states and physical and spiritual well-being.

Though anatomically undetectable, the location of each chakra is associated with major nerve bundles in the body, reflecting the degree of balance or imbalance in that area. Ancient Hindus recognized seven main energy wheels vertically arranged along the spine, which physically holds the base of nerves that reach out to all the organs and hormonal centers. One theory is that chakras are connected to the hormonal output and endocrine gland and thus affect the entire body. They are visualized as mandalas or flowers with different colors that radiate energy into the body as they spin clockwise.

BALANCING THE CHAKRAS USING ESSENTIAL OILS

According to Ayurvedic principles, the chakras represent "balanced" energy. Essential oils for chakras can be used individually or blended together for direct inhalation, used in a bath or massage oil, or diffused into the air. Incorporating them into meditation practice or ceremony can be effective, as can specific yoga poses, breathing exercises, and affirmations.

First Chakra: *Root/Base*

Purpose: physical transformation

Element: earth

Color: red

Keyword(s): courage/security

Endocrine gland: adrenal

Sensory perception: smell

Location: base of spine (perineum)

Description: The focus of the first chakra is primal, tribal, and survival energy; it denotes vitality, strength, determination, and courage. As the foundation of the other chakras, it provides a solid base to build growth and awareness. When balanced, one feels secure and brave with a healthy body awareness. Deficiencies can manifest as fear, selfishness, lack of ability to care for life's basic necessities, or feeling "ungrounded." The first chakra can be connected to problems in the lower limbs or colon. The oils are the deep, earthy, and grounding roots and resins.

Affirmation: "I am responsible for my life and capable of caring for myself. I nurture my body in healthy ways and can cope with any situation. I have a deep sense of belonging and deserve the best that life offers; my needs are always met."

Myrrh warms and energizes, especially when this chakra is depleted.

Vetiver grounds and balances all chakras.

Frankincense unites body and spirit from root to crown chakras.

Other essential oils: ylang-ylang, spikenard

Second Chakra: *Sacral*

Purpose: creative transformation
Element: water
Color: orange
Keyword: creativity
Endocrine gland: ovaries/testes
Sensory perception: taste
Location: sacrum (lower spine below the navel)
Description: The second chakra is associated with emotion and creativity, whether it manifests in creating life or works of art, music, poetry, and so on. Imbalances result in indiscriminant sexuality or infidelity, addictions, a lack of satisfaction, or creative blocks. It can be connected to reproductive organs and lower back problems. The oils for this area are slightly lighter than root oils; they harmonize the reproductive area and balance emotional and creative flow. Since flowers are the sexual parts of plants and represent creativity, they are included.

Affirmation: "I am worthy of love. I honor my beautiful body and am balanced in my sexuality. My creativity provides a healthy outlet for the expression of my inner self. In balance, I am faithful, satisfied, content, and productive."

Sandalwood is an aphrodisiac and offers further grounding to transition from the first chakra.

Jasmine is the king of flowers; balances yin and yang, transcends physical love into its most spiritual form, favors artistic development, and makes one more responsive to beauty.

Rose is the queen of flowers; represents the best of feminine energy and connects to the higher octave fourth chakra to transform sexual love to a deeper, spiritually connected devotional love.

Other essential oils: balsams, patchouli, vanilla

Third Chakra: *Solar Plexus (Navel)*

Purpose: transformation of individual will
Element: fire
Color: yellow
Keyword: manifest
Endocrine gland: pancreas
Sensory perception: sight
Location: solar plexus (navel)
Description: The third chakra represents one's relationship to the world in the manifestation of will, strength, and expression of identity. It radiates to the other chakras and, more than any other, is affected by stress and shock. Imbalances may be associated with Type A personalities, nervousness; feeling stressed, impatient, lazy, or directionless; or "not finding one's place in the world." Physically, it may be associated with digestive or liver problems. When balanced, this chakra supports spiritual harmony, assertiveness, confidence, patience, and awareness of one's purpose in life.

Affirmation: "I accept myself and know that I have value in the world. I am true unto myself and face each challenge with strength, determination, and serenity."

Vetiver protects and balances.

Juniper counters the effects of having others intrude on your space.

Carrot seed strengthens intent and removes mental obstacles.

Other essential oils: ginger, mandarin, petitgrain, peppermint, spearmint, cinnamon bark, nutmeg

Fourth Chakra: *Heart*

Purpose: emotional transformation

Element: air

Color: green, although pink is a subcolor

Keyword: joy

Endocrine gland: thymus

Sensory perception: touch

Location: near the heart

Description: The theme is love in its most healthy form: love of self or another or devotional and spiritual love. The fourth chakra unifies the three upper centers (which are more spiritually oriented) with the three lower chakras (which are more oriented with the physical world). A balance of body and spirit from the heart chakra links the body (feeling) and mind (thinking) to mediate on how thought processes affect emotions. It reflects the relationship of yin/yang or the masculine/feminine. This chakra may be connected to emotional trauma, depression, abuse, selfishness, or lung or heart problems. In Traditional Chinese Medicine, lung ailments represent the air element and are a manifestation of grief. In balance, we are compassionate, responsible, and nurturing with others and with ourselves. This is the higher octave of the second chakra.

Affirmation: "My heart is open to receiving the love I know I deserve. Every experience deepens my compassion and understanding of the principles of love. Love radiates from me unconditionally, and gratitude fills my heart."

Rose is the essence of love and an excellent reproductive system tonic; helps heal grief, envy, and jealousy.

Bergamot allows love to radiate and permeate, promotes moral courage, and helps people acknowledge their own highest gifts and use them appropriately.

Lavender balances upper and lower chakras.

Other essential oil: geranium

Fifth Chakra: *Throat*

Purpose: expressive transformation

Element: infinity (ether)

Color: blue

Keyword: truth

Endocrine gland: thyroid/parathyroid

Sensory perception: hearing

Location: throat

Description: The fifth chakra deals with expression and speaking your truth. In fact, public speaking or another form of outward expression such as singing is paramount to a balanced throat chakra. An imbalance may be connected to denying an outward expression of who one is, feelings of rejection, and difficulty in voicing feelings or repressing emotions. The fifth chakra may be connected with throat or thyroid problems. A throat chakra in balance allows for creativity, trust, and acceptance of others. This is the higher octave of the third chakra.

Affirmation: "I speak my truth and know that my voice is worthy of being heard. I delight in my special brand of self-expression because it is a manifestation of who I am."

Myrrh helps those who keep quiet out of fear.

Roman chamomile encourages expression of spiritual truths.

German chamomile is blue in color, imparting a calming strength and enabling truth to be spoken without anger.

Other oils: benzoin, lemon, marjoram

Sixth Chakra: *Third Eye*

Purpose: intuitive transformation

Element: none

Color: indigo

Keyword: vision

Endocrine gland: pituitary

Sensory perception: infinity (space)

Location: between and slightly above the brows

Description: The sixth chakra rules intellect, intuition, discrimination, and wisdom. Those who are overly analytical may benefit from more attention to their intuition. Acknowledging spirituality and attention to the lessons of life are useful. When the sixth chakra is out of balance, one may be unaware, absentminded, narrowminded, intellectually egotistical, and may suffer from memory loss. The appropriate essential oils focus on meditation and the "opening" of the third eye (the intuitive center).

Affirmation: "I trust myself to find the right answer. I know that every experience allows me to develop more fully. I am protected."

Rosemary clarifies thought and connects with the mind to provide clarity and the understanding of one's spiritual principles.

Helichrysum stimulates the right brain to enhance intuition and access the unconscious; fosters compassion and creativity.

Juniper assists intuition for altruistic outcomes.

Other essential oils: clary sage, marjoram, benzoin

Seventh Chakra: *Crown*

Purpose: spiritual transformation
Element: none
Color: violet
Keyword: inspiration
Endocrine gland: pineal
Location: top of head

Description: The seventh chakra is depicted as the *thousand-petaled lotus,* representing the unfolding of consciousness. It is the sum of all the chakras and embodies spirituality and self-realization. It is a focal point during some forms of meditation and is often visualized as white, violet, or golden light streaming in from above in a rainbow of all colors. This chakra is blocked when one dwells in the ego, is fearful of spirituality, or becomes consumed by the material aspects of life. When balanced, it represents inner wisdom and the awareness of spiritual connections.

Affirmation: "I lift myself up to higher levels of awareness and transformation. Spirit guides my way."

Frankincense enhances the ability to connect with the Divine and links to the base chakra forming a continuous, energetic circuit.

Elemi means "as above, so below"; further enhances energy from root to crown.

Lavender resonates through its physical manifestation of the color violet, encourages the opening of the crown chakra, and manifests creative potential.

Other essential oils: angelica, cedarwood, sandalwood, resins

Using specific essential oils to balance the chakras can help to encourage positive transformation and influence a greater sense of well-being in body, mind, and spirit.

CHAPTER 15

Materia Medica

THIS CHAPTER lists and describes the most important essential oils used in aromatherapy and thus summarizes the whole book. To help you, we grouped together oils that are related either by genus or by association. The plant names are arranged alphabetically by common name, and the botanical name appears in italics. We present historical or anecdotal information and then details of the aspects described below.

Family: This is the herb's botanical family. Some family names have changed, so we indicate a previous name in parentheses to eliminate confusion.

Extraction: This lists the methods of extracting the essential oil and the parts of the plant used. All of these methods are described in detail in chapter 12. The oil's fragrance is also described in this section.

Medicinal action: This summarizes the therapeutic activity of the essential oil. Refer to chapters 5 and 6 for instructions on their uses and for sample recipes.

Cosmetic/skin use: This categorizes essential oils by skin type and recommends the best oils for the treatment of various types.

Emotional attributes: The commentary on a fragrance's emotional attributes comes from a combination of scientific study, historic folklore, personal experience, and the observations of other aromatherapists. This means that much of the information is unproved territory, but it is presented for your interest and for utilizing the oils for emotional purposes.

Considerations: These warnings apply to the essential oil, but most do not apply to the herb itself, which you may substitute for the oil. Potentially toxic essential oils, which should be avoided altogether, are listed in chapter 5.

When you review the properties of essential oils, remember that although they are a very active component of an herb, they are often not the only active ingredients in that herb. That means that most herb books, and many aromatherapy books, list properties that are not found in the essential oil. We have looked into the scientific research and studied each essential oil's active compounds to help determine the actual properties of each essential oil.

Since essential oils are so potent, also consider that the best way to use them is often by using the whole herb. This is especially true in treating digestive tract complaints. You can always rub on a product containing diluted essential oils, but drinking a tea made from the appropriate herb directly gets to the problem. If the herb has a fragrance, essential oils are present, and the more aromatic the herb, the more essential oils it contains.

ANGELICA

Angelica archangelica

Thought to have originated in Syria, angelica was one of the few aromatics exported to the ancient Orient. This essential oil has long been a flavoring and apothecary drug, and it still flavors Cointreau liqueur.

Family: Apiaceae (Umbelliferae)

Extraction: Distilled from the root or seed; absolute. It offers little fragrance until you bite into a seed or snap a root. The seed oil is spicy/peppery, while the stronger root oil is earthy and slightly more expensive.

Medicinal action: During the plague, people burned roots and chewed seeds to fight infection. Besides being antiseptic, angelica regulates menstruation and is a digestive tonic that stimulates appetite and alleviates belching, gas, stomach cramps, and indigestion. It also aids the respiratory system and reduces coughing.

Emotional attributes: The fragrance relieves depression (especially when nerve-related) and provides a new outlook on problems. Religious significance was once attributed to angelica as the "Root of the Holy Ghost," and thus, it was historically used to increase the feeling of safety and protection. When you see how it hovers over the herb garden as if its large leaves were wings, it's no wonder!

Considerations: Use angelica carefully and in small amounts, since it can overstimulate the nervous system. Like a number of plants in this family, the root oil contains the photosensitizing compound bergapten. A few sensitive people experience skin reactions when products containing the oil are applied on skin that is exposed to the sun.

Associated Oils

Indian Angelica (*A. glauca*): See chapter 14.

Korean Angelica (*A. gigus*): Researchers found that simply inhaling the fragrance of this root may reduce behavioral and neurological sensitizations produced by nicotine, deterring the addiction. It seems to regulate the brain's release of the neurotransmitter dopamine, which is associated with addiction. It is not readily available as essential oil.

Lovage (*Levisticum officinale*): This large European and western Asian plant tastes and smells like spicy celery reminiscent of angelica. It treats digestive spasms, rheumatism, poor circulation, and menstrual irregularity. However, the oil distilled from leaves and stalks, or especially the fresh root, can be photosensitizing and potentially toxic, so it is rarely used.

ANISE

Pimpinella anisum

Originally from Asia Minor and Egypt, anise now grows throughout the Mediterranean. William Turner's 1551 *Herbal* says it "maketh the breth sweeter." The oil flavors pharmaceuticals, confections, toothpaste, mouthwash, and "licorice" candy in the United States, not to mention tobacco and alcoholic beverages. Examples are French anisette and pastis, Turkish raki, Latin American aguardiente, Latvian kummel, Russian allasch, Spanish ojen and pacharan, and Greek ouzo. There is also anise schnapps, reputed to promote appetite and digestion, as well as being an aphrodisiac. In India, anise water is splashed on as cologne; curiously, the scent attracts pigeons.

Family: Apiaceae (Umbelliferae)

Extraction: Distilled from the seed. Anise has a sweet, licorice-like scent. The oil solidifies at room temperature. **Turkish Anise** (*P. anisetum*) is cultivated exclusively to produce a very similar essential oil.

Medicinal action: In addition to being flavorful, anise is a potent antibiotic that quells indigestion, coughing, and muscle spasms, including menstrual cramps. Mildly hormonal, it encourages mother's milk, as was described by Pliny the Elder in the first century AD.

Emotional attributes: Sniffing anise is both stimulating and calming, enhancing emotional balance, and even one's sense of humor. It relieves stress from overwork, forgetfulness, and is said to be an aphrodisiac and help overcome heartache, as well.

Considerations: Large amounts of the oil can be narcotic and slow circulation, so caution is always advised. However, older studies may not be reliable, which may mean it is less toxic than once thought. It is estrogenic so should be avoided during pregnancy and by those who have problems related to high estrogen, such as estrogen-promoted cancers, until more is known about this action. The anethole compound causes skin dermatitis in sensitive individuals.

Associated Oil

Star Anise *(Illicium verum):* The seeds from this Oriental tree sometimes replace anise. It has similar chemistry, flavor, and scent, but differences in minor compounds make it a safer essential oil. Since it is also probably estrogenic, those cautions still apply. It is distilled mostly from seed but occasionally from the star-shaped fruit surrounding the seed. In 2006, star anise provided compounds that the Swiss drug company Roche used to make Tamiflu (oseltamivir), an antiviral to counter avian flu (although the large quantities required to be effective are toxic). The related *I. religiosum* was once combined with rue and pyrethrum for a natural fumigant that kept bugs out of books, especially holy books, thus its name.

BASIL

Ocimum basilicum

Basil comes from India, but it has been cultivated in the Mediterranean for thousands of years and is now grown in North Africa. The genus name *Ocimum* probably comes from the Greek word "to smell." The basils are so diverse in their scent, some botanists want to reclassify them according to their chemistry. You need to grow your own to have a complete collection, since only a few types are distilled. We have fun home-distilling a variety of spicy, citrus, and fruity basils into hydrosols.

Family: Lamiaceae (Labiatae)

Extraction: Distilled from the leaves and flowering tops; CO_2. The fragrance is sweet and spicy. The Reunion type from the Comoro and Réunion Islands (hence its name) is harsher since it contains little linalol, but has 70 to 88 percent methyl chavicol, a skin irritant. It flavors food and dental products, but use it carefully.

Medicinal action: Sniffing basil's scent relieves headaches, sinus congestion, head colds, and the resulting loss of smell. Basil also treats nausea—even from chemotherapy—indigestion, arthritis, and sore muscles. It hormonally stimulates adrenal glands, menstruation, childbirth, and mother's milk. Research shows the essential oil destroys germs, intestinal worms, and a number of detrimental insects. It even wipes out multidrug-resistant strains of *Staphylococcus, Enterococcus,* and *Pseudomonas* infections and urinary tract infections.

Cosmetic/skin use: Basil treats skin and hair that is oily or has bacterial or fungal infections. In studies, it works better than commercial antiseptic products to heal wounds, pimples, and boils and reduce inflammation. Its antiviral action is effective against herpes and shingles, although it has been shown to work differently than the antiviral drug acyclovir, helping cells build up their protective coating rather than directly killing the virus. Once made into cleansing water for the hands and feet, it provides an inexpensive substitute for mignonette (lily of the valley) in perfume and soap.

Emotional attributes: Basil's uplifting effect overcomes a lack of confidence, indecisiveness, negative thoughts, stress, rattled nerves, hysteria, depression, fear, anger, and mental fatigue. It is also said to increase awareness of one's surroundings. John Gerard found the buoyant smell "good for the heart" and said it "taketh away sorrowfulness." Aromatherapists use it to help detoxify the brain of the effects from either pharmaceutical or recreational drug use.

Considerations: Large dosages of the essential oil can be overstimulating and eventually stupefy. It is estrogenic, so it should be avoided during pregnancy and by those with problems related to high estrogen, such as estrogen-promoted cancers, until we know more about its actions.

Associated Oils

Some of basil's species and chemotypes can contain a large amount of essential oil (up to 1.4 percent) that have high percentages of thymol, methyl cinnamate, or eugenol, making them harsh on the skin and the liver.

Hairy or Hoary Basil *(O. canum; O. americanum):* There are several chemotypes of this East African basil, which is commercially grown in Asia. It is usually high in camphor, but is delightfully spicy due to methyl cinnamate compounds. Other types have more linalol or citral and so are less harsh.

Holy Basil *(O. tenuiflorum; O. sanctum):* Known in India as *tulsi,* or sacred basil, it has been shown to aid relaxation and increase sleeping time. A strong antioxidant, preliminary research shows that it may protect the stomach from ulcers by inhibiting pepsin secretion. The essential oil varies considerably, containing either the compounds citral or chavibetol, making it lemon-scented, or a combination of estragole, linalol, and cineole. It is also grown in southern Asia, South America, the Caribbean, and Africa.

BAY

Laurus nobilis

Bay "laurel" leaf crowns were once placed on the heads of headache sufferers and Greek scholars. Today, we still confer a *baccalaureate* degree, which means "noble berry tree" in French. A bay-infused vegetable oil makes fine salad dressing, and one or two leaves are a well-known addition to stews and soups. The essential oil flavors commercial soup, a few liqueurs, and some men's colognes. Placing a leaf in stored grains keeps away grain weevils.

Family: Lauraceae

Extraction: Distilled from the leaf and occasionally the berry. Bay smells pungent and spicy.

Medicinal action: Bay is a stimulant to digestion, lymph, sinuses, lungs, and circulation. According to studies, it counters drug-resistant strains of *Campylobacter jejuni,* the most common bacterial cause of diarrhea. It also makes a good muscle liniment.

Emotional attributes: Smelling bay is stimulating, improves memory, and cures headaches and stress. Apparently, bay has even more curious properties; ancient Greek priestesses at Delphi sat over the burning fumes to increase their prophetic visions!

Considerations: If you crush a leaf, the smell is so intense it can produce a headache as easily as cure one! A few people develop contact dermatitis when their skin is exposed to this oil.

Associated Oils

Allspice *(Pimenta dioica; P. officinalis):* Familiar to cooks, this culinary seed tastes and smells like a combination of cloves, cinnamon, and pepper, thus the name *all*spice. The name comes from the Spanish *pimento* because the seed (actually a berry) looks like black pepper. It is the source of pimento water, an indigestion remedy in its native West Indies. The antibiotic action is effective against *Salmonella* and *Staphylococcus.* It is sometimes sold as "bay" oil, although it is spicier and hotter and more readily irritates skin. The essential oil flavors herbal liqueurs such as Chartreuse, Benedictine, and Aromatique, and it scents perfume, cologne, and soap. *Pimenta dioica* is available as an absolute.

Bay Rum *(Pimenta racemosa):* Cooler and sweeter than true bay, this is the source of most commercial "bay" oil. It scents bay soap, cosmetics, and Bay Rum cologne, which is originally from the Virgin Islands and yes, made with rum. It is sometimes called "oil of pimento."

BENZOIN

Styrax benzoin

The Arabs, who traded benzoin as a frankincense substitute, called this Southeast Asian tree "incense of Java," or *luban jawi.* The Europeans heard this as *benjawi* and called it *Benjamin,* making solid "vanilla" pomades from it.

Family: Styracaceae

Extraction: The solvent-extracted gum resin (absolute) is quite thick, but can be diluted in alcohol. It is often thinned with ethyl glycol to make it liquid. The scent is sweet and vanilla-like. The sweeter Sumatran *S. tonkinese,* especially as thick "almond tears," is considered the best quality.

Medicinal action: The French burned the gum around people who were ill and still refer to it as *baume pulmonaire,* or pulmonary (lung) balsam. Friar's balsam was an inhalant for lung conditions and a wound antiseptic that became the official pharmacist's Compound Benzoin Tincture. Sweet *pastilles* are sucked in Europe to fight flu and colds and soothe sore throats. Benzoin is also used for poor circulation and muscular soreness.

Cosmetic/skin use: Benzoin is antiseptic and antifungal, and it increases skin elasticity, heals wounds, and protects and repairs chapped or irritated skin.

Emotional attributes: This fragrance is for those who feel anxious, emotionally blocked, lonely, or exhausted, especially from a life crisis. It creates a "safe space" that protects one from outside interference.

Considerations: Benzoin sometimes sensitizes skin after extended use.

Associated Oils

Stoyrax *(Liquidambar orientalis):* The vanilla-like resin from this tree is used for indigestion, intestinal worms, poor appetite (especially due to illness), insomnia, menstrual irregularity, and skin disorders, including ringworm. It is in Compound Benzoin Tincture and the solid Indian "amber" perfume.

Balsam of Peru *(Myroxylon balsamum* var. *pereirae):* The gum of this El Salvadoran tree got its name because it was shipped with Peruvian goods. It is slightly hotter than tolu and can be skin sensitizing.

Balsam of Tolu *(Myroxylon balsamum):* This Colombian tree was cultivated by the Incas for its vanilla-like fragrance and medicine. The oil, distilled from the gum resin, treats lung congestion, scabies, eczema, and ringworm. It can be skin sensitizing.

BERGAMOT

Citrus bergamia

These small, green Mediterranean citrus fruits aren't edible, but the rind emits a wonderful scent! First mentioned in the seventeenth-century *Parfumeur François,* it was named after the town of Bergamo, Italy, where the oil was first distilled. It is still grown in Italy, mostly in Calabria. Bergamot scents many colognes and flavors Earl Grey tea and some candies. Don't confuse this citrus with the common herb garden bee balm *(Monarda didyma),* also called bergamot.

Family: Rutaceae

Extraction: Cold-pressed from almost-ripe fruit rind. Bergamot oil has a fresh, clean scent.

Medicinal action: An anti-inflammatory, antifungal, and antiseptic, bergamot also enhances immunity and helps heal wounds and skin growths and prevent scarring. It treats genital, urinary, mouth, throat infections, and flu and eases muscle pain and inflammation. It aids digestion and is a traditional Italian folk medicine for fever and intestinal worms.

Cosmetic/skin use: Bergapten-free bergamot is suitable for most skin conditions and eczema and is a deodorizer. It is an antiviral against the related herpes, shingles, and chicken pox.

Emotional attributes: Sniff bergamot to reduce stress, depression, anxiety, insomnia, or compulsive behavior cycles (including eating disorders). It balances emotions, instilling composure.

Considerations: Bergamot is photosensitizing due to the furanocoumarin compound bergapten, so it occasionally causes a rash when skin is exposed to the sun. Most commercial oil has had the bergapten removed, but search labels to see "bergapten free" or "FCF" (furanocoumarin free).

Associated Oils
See Lemon, Neroli, and Orange.

BIRCH

Betula lenta

This North American tree is the source of most "wintergreen" essential oil, since the two share similar chemistry, properties, and fragrance. The formula for the popular nineteenth-century Russian Leather men's fragrance (so named because it also was used to keep book bindings soft) was closely guarded, but we now know it was mostly birch oil.

Family: Betulaceae

Extraction: Distilled from the inner bark after maceration in warm water. Sweet Birch oil has a sweet, sharp scent, like candy. A smoky scented, thick birch tar is produced through the "destructive" steam distillation of burned bark for skin infestations, such as scabies, but is slightly toxic.

Medicinal action: Birch is a muscular and arthritic pain reliever, a diuretic, and a circulatory stimulant. As a liniment, it warms the area by increasing peripheral blood circulation.

Cosmetic/skin use: A skin softener, it soothes irritation and psoriasis and helps prevent dandruff.

Considerations: Use birch and wintergreen oils carefully, and since they smell like candy, be sure to store them safely away from children.

Associated Oil
Wintergreen *(Gaultheria procumbens):* Native to northeastern North America, wintergreen is a short ground cover. The true oil is rarely available and toxic if taken internally.

BLACK PEPPER

Piper nigrum

India produces most of the world's peppercorns for seasoning and essential oil. Some also comes from Indonesia and the Orient. Pepper has a rich history, with wars fought to gain the ability to have control over growing this climbing, tropical shrub.

Family: Piperaceae

Extraction: Distilled from partially dried, unripe fruit; oleoresin; CO_2. The scent is spicy, sharp, and slightly herbaceous. Oil with a more fruity fragrance is produced from the fresh, green fruit.

Medicinal action: This potent germ-fighter treats food poisoning, indigestion, colds, flu, urinary-tract infections, and congested lungs. In one study, it killed all bacteria tested, including *Salmonella* and *Staphylococcus.* It is an antioxidant and aids digestion. It also lowers fever and improves poor blood circulation.

Cosmetic/skin use: In liniments, the warming sensation of black pepper produces is surprisingly mild. In Ayurvedic and Arabic medicine, a pepper ointment treats skin diseases, including scabies. A paste of the seeds is rubbed on the skin to increase circulation and relieve rheumatic pain, and a poultice soothes sore throat, hemorrhoids, toothache, and problems with paralyzed nerves. It also helps with urinary tract problems and sexual debility.

Emotional attributes: The fragrance is emotionally stimulating and, some say, an aphrodisiac.

Considerations: Although nontoxic, black pepper irritates the skin of some people.

Associated Oils

Cubeb *(P. cubeba; P. officinalis):* The essential oil is distilled from the immature berry of this Malaysian relative of black pepper. It treats urinary tract infections, headaches, and is an expectorant for lung congestion. It sometimes flavors tobacco and soap, and it is a "secret" ingredient in gingerbread. It substitutes for litsea, although it is more peppery and is not known to have the same properties.

Peruvian Pepper Tree *(Schinus molle):* This South American tree is a popular ornamental California pepper tree. Used to replace pepper in cooking during World War II, essential oil now substitutes for it in perfume. South Americans use the berries and gum resin as a light laxative and digestive aid and as a very strong fungicide to prevent food from spoiling. It is considered safe, although eating large amounts can cause vomiting and headaches, especially in children. The gum resin is antibiotic and heals wounds, especially mucous membranes such as vaginal inflammation.

CAMPHOR
C. camphora

See Ravensara.

CARAWAY
Carum carvi

Thirteenth-century Europeans learned about caraway from the Arabs. Today the seeds are more likely to find their way into rye bread than aromatherapy products. The essential oil flavors several liqueurs.

Family: Apiaceae (Umbelliferae)

Extraction: Distilled from the seed. The fragrance is sharp and somewhat bitter.

Medicinal action: Caraway treats colds, poor circulation, dizziness, and nerve pain such as toothaches. Preliminary studies found that it relaxes tight muscles and mild digestive tract spasms, and relieves gas and some intestinal parasites. Nursing mothers can drink caraway tea or use it in food to promote milk. It also increases menstruation.

Cosmetic/skin use: A medieval European love potion, facial water, and cordial called *Huile de Vénus,* it remained popular through the Victorian era. It toned muscles, softened skin, lightened the complexion, and decreased bruising (it was also sipped to quell indigestion).

Emotional attributes: The fragrance helps overcome mental strain and improves energy efficiency.

Considerations: Caraway is a skin irritant for some individuals.

CARDAMOM

Eletteria cardamomum

The seeds of cardamom, a relative of ginger, were a valued export item from the Middle and Far East, finding their way to ancient Greece. They flavor Turkish coffee and East Indian chai tea, as well as Angostura Bitters, Chartreuse liqueur, and Cordial-Médoc.

Family: Zingiberaceae

Extraction: Distilled from the seed; oleoresin; CO_2. The best quality is sweet and spicy, while inferior seeds are harsher, with a hint of eucalyptus.

Medicinal action: The seed stops intestinal spasms. Mixed in honey in a traditional Ayurvedic formula, it is diuretic, or, with honey, ginger, cloves, and caraway, cardamom treats indigestion, poor appetite, diarrhea, and coughs. It also decreases inflammation, pain, and muscle spasms.

Emotional attributes: The scent is emotionally invigorating and overcomes stress and anxiety. Ayurvedic medicine uses the seed to stop dizziness caused by indigestion! It has long been considered an aphrodisiac and is used to counter impotency.

CARROT SEED

Daucus carota

Carrot seed is distilled in France from wild Queen Anne's lace, the ancestor of our common vegetable carrot, for perfume.

Family: Apiaceae (Umbelliferae)

Extraction: Distilled from the seed. The fragrance is fruity, sharp, pungent. In cosmetics, carrot root–infused vegetable oil is usually used, and a fixed oil pressed from the seed is sometimes used.

Medicinal action: Carrot seed stimulates liver and lymphatic function, increases circulation, and eases genital, urinary, and digestion problems. It is rich in beta-carotene, which is the precursor to vitamin A and produces a deep orange color.

Cosmetic/skin use: Carrot oil improves skin tone and elasticity and is specific for mature or dry skin. It deters wrinkles, dermatitis, eczema, rashes, and skin discoloration, and treats precancerous skin conditions, sun damage, and ulcerated skin.

Associated Oil
French Marigold *(Tagetes minuta; T. erecta; T. patula):* Marigold is sometimes used on calluses, bunions, and even scars. In India, *attar genda* is found in perfume. High in beta-carotene, it is occasionally sold as "carrot oil." The essential oil is phototoxic and the tagetone compound it contains is potentially toxic and a skin irritant, making calendula-infused oil a better choice.

CEDARWOOD

Cedrus species

This North American tree has lost popularity since the nineteenth century, when cedarwood matches were commonly burned for their scent. It still scents soap and cologne, and the oil makes the wood resistant to wool moths and other insects.

Family: Cupressaceae

Extraction: Distilled from the wood; resinoid; absolute. It has a soft, powdery, woodsy, earthy, and sweet scent. Many "cedar" essential oils are actually juniper (*Juniperus* sp.).

Medicinal action: Antiseptic cedar treats respiratory and urinary infection.

Cosmetic/skin use: Cedarwood is an astringent for oily hair and skin conditions, acne, and dandruff and is said to encourage hair growth. It relieves dermatitis, insect bites, and itching, and helps prevent scarring. It is among the most recommended oils for cellulite.

Emotional attributes: Cedar increases memory, emotional fortitude, and stabilizes emotions by "grounding" an individual. It enhances meditative relaxation, intuitive work, and helps to relieve depression, tension, aggression, and even emotional dependency.

Considerations: Avoid all cedars during pregnancy.

Associated Oils

Atlas Cedar *(C. atlantica):* This cedar oil comes from the Atlas Mountains of North Africa. It is very similar to **Moroccan Cedar** *(C. libani),* the legendary "Cedars of Lebanon" prized by ancient cultures, who nearly eliminated it (even the word *Lebanon* comes from the Akkadian *lubbunu,* meaning "incense").

Tibetan Cedarwood *(C. deodara):* Also called "Himalayan cedarwood," Tibetan cedarwood comes from India. It has a warm, almost spicy fragrance, and it is the least toxic cedar oil.

Thuja *(Thuja occidentalis):* Known as "cedar leaf" or *arborvitae,* the oil is distilled from leaves, twigs, and bark. It contains the skin irritants thujene and thujone (a neurotoxic ketone), so it should be used externally for short periods of time (or as an herbal tincture) and not at all by anyone prone to seizures. Thuja treats pelvic congestion, enlarged prostate, urinary infections, and warts, including the condyloma virus.

CHAMOMILE, GERMAN

Matricaria recutita; M. chamomilla

The Greeks, inspired by chamomile's distinct applelike scent, named it *kamai* (ground) *melon* (apple). In Spanish, it is still called *manzanilla,* or "little apple."

Family: Asteraceae (Compositae)

Extraction: Distilled from the flowers. The scent is deep, sweet, and herbaceous. German chamomile oil contains blue chamazulene (*azul* means blue), a potent anti-inflammatory constituent produced during distillation. In 1664, when chamomile was first steam-distilled in glass, the distillers were surprised to see it turn blue, which they previously thought was a reaction to the copper stills. Chamomile absolute is not blue since it is not exposed to heat, but does contain other anti-inflammatories, including bisabalol and matricine, a precursor to azulene.

Medicinal action: Ancient Egyptians infused the flowers into oil to rub on sore muscles. This versatile essential oil also eases sprains, tendons, joints, menstrual pain, and headaches. It alleviated pain, in some cases as well as drugs, in clinical studies in which hospital patients were undergoing painful procedures. It also treats indigestion, diarrhea, stomach ulcers, and PMS. It is also used to treat asthma, allergies, and to improve immune system activity.

Cosmetic/skin use: The essential oil inhibits the activity of bacteria, fungi, and various toxins on the skin. Chamomile is ideal for all complexion types, including sensitive, puffy, or inflamed conditions, boils, rashes, broken capillaries, and allergic skin reactions. Research shows it improves the rate of healing for wounds, burns, skin problems, and eczema. It is suitable for all types of hair, and herb tea brings out blond highlights as a rinse.

Emotional attributes: An antidepressant, the scent helps those who experience emotional oversensitivity, stress, anxiety, hysteria, insomnia, or suppressed anger (especially when associated with the past). It decreases hyperactivity in children. In one hospital study, it reduced anxiety and fear in new mothers. In the seventeenth century, *Ram's Little Doeden* recommended that "to comort the braine, smel to camomill . . . ," and herbalist Nicholas Culpeper noted that "bathing with . . . camomile thaketh qawy weariness, easteth pains to what part of the body soever they be applied. It comforteth the sinews that are over-strained, mollieth all swellin . . . by a wonderful, speedy property."

Associated Oils

Several types of chamomile are distilled for essential oils. They act as antidepressants and are anti-inflammatory, and they treat burns, eczema, and skin irritation.

Roman Chamomile *(Chamaemelum nobile,* formerly *Anthemis nobilis):* This short-growing perennial produces very little of German chamomile's blue chamazuline compound, so the resulting oil is pale yellow. In fact, the two have different chemistry, making Roman chamomile a stronger digestive stimulant and antispasmodic, but less anti-inflammatory. This perennial ground cover is still planted in English lawns to emit a wonderfully sweet aroma when walked upon. Medieval monks built raised "healing beds" in their gardens so invalids could lie upon chamomile to relieve emotional depression. In one study, a massage with the oil greatly reduced anxiety in hospital patients. As a sleep aid, it counters insomnia.

Moroccan Chamomile or **Ormenis** *(Chamaemelum mixtum; Anthemis mixta; Ormenis mixta; O. multicaulis):* Native to West Africa and Spain, ormenis is distilled in Morocco. Generally a little less expensive than other chamomiles, it is anti-inflammatory and sedative but lacks the subtle and pleasant fragrance of a true chamomile.

Cape Chamomile *(Eriocephalus punctulatus):* This South African daisy (Asteraceae family) known as *wild rosemary* is neither rosemary nor chamomile. However, the dark blue distilled oil does produce azulene, which gives German chamomile its fruity fragrance. It relieves stress and depression, and it has sedative, anti-inflammatory, pain-relieving, digestive, and antiallergenic properties. Considered a restorative tonic, it seems to benefit the liver and nervous system. Usually less expensive than other chamomiles, the essential oil is starting to appear in high-class perfume. **Cape Snowbush** *(E. africanus),* used in South African cooking, has similar properties.

Blue Tansy *(Tanacetum annuum):* Tansy has erroneously been sold as "blue chamomile" but is a stronger oil that needs to be used with more care and not during pregnancy. It is anti-inflammatory and an antihistamine, so it is used for hay fever, asthma, and hives, as well as other rashes, eczema, and dry skin. A related *Tanacetum vulgare* essential oil is toxic and should not be used, although it is rarely available.

Great Mugwort *(Artemisia arborescens):* This blue oil contains azulene and is occasionally passed off as "blue chamomile." It is actually related to wormwood and common mugwort *(Artemesia vulgaris),* with a sweet fragrance similar to *Tanacetum annuum.* It treats inflammation, bruising, and pain, but contains potentially toxic ketone compounds such as those in wormwood, so it is not recommended for long-term use on skin. Use it carefully at very low dilutions even just for sniffing.

CINNAMON

Cinnamomum verum; C. zeylanicum

Cinnamon was a popular aphrodisiac and antiseptic in India and Europe. Often fought over, it first caused the Portuguese to seize Ceylon in 1505, the Dutch to take the country from them, and the British to grab it from the Dutch. Small amounts of the oil spice Oriental perfume blends. The scent also sends cockroaches running!

Family: Lauraceae

Extraction: Distilled from the leaf or bark; CO_2. Cinnamon essential oil has a sweet, spicy-hot fragrance with bark oil that is much sweeter. Today the bark of this large tree has been commercially harvested in Madagascar, Africa, Indochina, and Sri Lanka twice a year for at least thirty years. The bark comes off the tree in long, slender sticks that curl together into "quills." The chemistry changes as it ages, so newly dried bark has a better, more complicated aroma. The main compound, cinnamaldehyde, increases with age and is responsible for most allergic and irritating reactions to cinnamon. The compound eugenol is isolated from the bark oil to make the synthetic vanilla called vanillin, though this is typically done from cheaper synthetic sources.

Medicinal action: Cinnamon improves appetite and seems to aid digestion by slowing and steadying digestive tract movement, similar to peppermint. Although doctors usually discourage eating spices if you have stomach ulcers because they might irritate the lining, it does inhibit the *Helicobacter pylori* bacteria responsible for ulcers. In the laboratory, it counters food poisoning bacteria, including *E. coli, Salmonella, Staphylococcus aureus,* and *Listeria monocytogenes.* It also treats genital and urinary infections and diarrhea. There is evidence that it improves blood vessel integrity and reduces the resulting accumulation of fluid in cells. In addition, as a potent antioxidant, it destroys free radicals in the body and makes a natural preservative for aromatherapy products. Cinnamon is a common pain-relieving liniment ingredient to warm skin and underlying muscles by increasing the surface blood circulation. The leaf oil destroys head lice, but keep in mind that this is hot stuff!

Emotional attributes: The smell of cinnamon relieves tension, steadies nerves, and invigorates the senses. Used in very small amounts, cinnamon has an old reputation as an aphrodisiac (interestingly, cinnamon has been found to increase sperm mobility and count in rodents).

Considerations: Both bark and leaf oils can irritate mucous membranes and burn sensitive skin. Some people are even sensitive to cinnamon chewing gum and toothpaste. The hotter, and more expensive, red-brown bark oil contains 40 to 50 percent cinnamaldehyde and 4 to 10 percent eugenol. The leaf has the opposite proportions of 3 percent cinnamaldehyde and 70 to 90 percent eugenol, making it similar to clove oil, so use it even more carefully.

Associated Oils

Cassia *(C. cassia; C. aromaticum):* This less expensive "Chinese" cinnamon substitute comes from a tree from China and Southeast Asia, where it is used as *kuei pi* for medicine, seasoning, and incense. The thick bark must be removed in small chunks from twisted tree branches, so it doesn't form quills like cinnamon, although it has a similar composition. It flavors cola and lemonade drinks and scents the famous Brown Windsor Soap from England, a favorite of Queen Victoria. Many other species of cinnamon are used as spice but probably don't sneak into cinnamon essential oil. Don't confuse it with the cassie *(Acacia farnesiana)* used in Oriental-style perfume and to overcome stress and nervous tension. Along with its relative **Mimosa** *(A. decurrens* var. *dealbata),* it is available as absolute or concrete.

CISTUS/LABDANUM

Cistus ladaniferus; C. incanus

Native to Spain and Greece, this is the rock rose grown in North American gardens and possibly the bible's *onycha* and "rose of Sharon" (Song of Solomon 2:1). It often replaces ambergris and is an ingredient in the East Indian solid "amber" perfume. Long popular in Spain, it remains the major producer today. Another name is *labdanum,* so don't confuse it with *laudanum,* an old-time pain remedy made of opium or cistus *(Helianthemum canadense),* which is sometimes distilled from the frostwort plant to help skin problems.

Family: Cistaceae

Extraction: Leaves and twigs are boiled, resin skimmed off, then aged and distilled or extracted into an absolute; a fixative. Cistus has a warm, spicy, balsamic scent. Shepherds in ancient Crete drove their herds through the plants so the sticky gum would collect on the animals' coats; after combing it out, they took the gum to market.

Medicinal action: Labdanum is a nervous system sedative, used in the treatment of rheumatism, colds, coughs, menstrual problems, cystitis, and hemorrhoids.

Cosmetic/skin use: Antiseptic to wounds, acne, dermatitis, and boils. It is specific for sun-damaged and mature skin.

Emotional attributes: Labdanum is both emotionally elevating and grounding, improving meditation and intuition. It raises consciousness, calms the nerves, and promotes sleep, yet it is also known as an aphrodisiac.

CLARY SAGE

Salvia sclarea

This relative of sage flavors muscatel wine and tobacco; the largest U.S. grower is the tobacco company R.J. Reynolds. Don't confuse this large, thick-leafed herb with the delicate, tricolored-leaved sage sometimes also known as *clary.*

Family: Lamiaceae (Labiatae)

Extraction: Distilled from the flowering tops and leaves; concrete; absolute. Similar to ambergris, the winelike scent is sweet, herbaceous, green, and heady.

Medicinal action: Clary eases muscle and nervous tension, pain, menstrual cramps, PMS, and menopause problems, such as hot flashes. It also stimulates adrenal glands, and Europeans use it as a sore throat remedy.

Cosmetic/skin use: Clary was mixed with ambergris, cinnamon, brandy, and sugar to make a popular European cordial that improved the complexion (and was also sipped to ease digestive problems). Use clary on any skin or hair type, but especially for mature or acne-prone complexions, inflammation, and dandruff. It rejuvenates cells and is said to encourage hair growth.

Emotional attributes: Clary's fragrance provides a wonderful remedy for depression, especially when related to the hormonal imbalance of postnatal depression, PMS, or menopause. Other stress-related conditions it treats are panic, paranoia, mental fatigue, and general debility. The twelfth-century abbess Saint Hildegard of Bingen recommended curing a headache by placing lightly cooked clary sage leaves on the forehead covered with a cloth before going to sleep. Clary produces relaxation, dramatic dreams, euphoria, and smiles—we pass it around classes to perk up the students and to improve communication (once the giggling dies down). On the other hand, small amounts are excellent to relax children. Sixteenth-century herbalist William Turner said that clary "comforts the vital senses, helps the memory [and] quickens the senses."

Considerations: Large amounts of clary sage can actually stupefy a person. Combined with alcohol, it increases drunkenness and nightmares, and in lab studies, it potentiates hypnotic drugs. It contains a rare ketone compound called sclareol that mimics estrogen, so women who suffer from breast cysts and uterine fibroids or other estrogen-related disorders should avoid long-term use until more is understood about this action.

Associated Oil
See Sage.

CLOVE BUD

Syzygium aromaticum; Eugenia caryophyllata

Europeans and East Indians sweetened their breaths with cloves, as did envoys to the court Chinese Han Dynasty during audiences with the emperor. Pierre Poivre risked his life to steal clove trees from the Dutch colonies. Today's supply comes mostly from trees planted by the British on islands off Africa. To discourage Indonesians from chewing betel nuts, the Dutch introduced clove cigarettes named *kretek* (describing the crackling sound as cloves burn), although smoking them turned out to be even more harmful than tobacco itself. A popular sixteenth-century Italian cologne combined clove with lavender, musk, and ambergris. To keep away the plague, the similar Guard's Bouquet was dabbed on handkerchiefs, and doctors wore leather beaks filled with cloves over their faces. It still scents cologne, aftershave, and soap.

Family: Myrtaceae

Extraction: Distilled or concrete; absolute; oleoresin; CO_2; from immature flower bud. The scent is powerful, spicy, and hot. Oil distilled from clove leaves contains more of the harsh compound eugenol. Sometimes leaves, flower stalks, or very young fruit are distilled with clove buds to produce inferior oil. Once established, the trees bear their woody buds for at least a century.

Medicinal action: Clove oil is a popular tooth pain remedy and is found in a number of dental products. Mouthwashes and some fillings contain the oil or its main component *eugenol.* A strong antiseptic, it kills mouth bacteria, including the *Helicobacter pylori* bacteria that promote stomach ulcers. It also heals the stomach lining, stops nausea, destroys intestinal parasites, and aids digestion, stimulating the flow of digestive juices and bile. It relieves flu, colds, bronchial congestion, and, sometimes, migraine headaches, probably because it opens constricted blood vessels and slows inflammation. Finally, clove is also a powerful antioxidant, destroying free radicals in the body and slowing the spoilage of fatty food dishes. Studies indicate that it protects cells from carcinogenic substances and slows the formation of blood clots. As a liniment, it provides warming relief for sore muscles and arthritic pain. The herbalist abbess Saint Hildegard of Bingen was already aware of the exotic cloves in the twelfth century, prescribing them to ease headaches and ear infections and regulate hot and cold sensations.

Cosmetic/skin use: Antiseptic, antifungal, and antiviral, diluted clove oil can be dabbed on scabies, warts, athlete's foot, and fever blisters. Studies show that it inhibits reproduction of the herpes simplex virus.

Emotional attributes: Small doses are stimulating and help to overcome nervousness, mental fatigue, or poor memory. Sniffing it can even reduce anaphylactic shock reactions.

Considerations: For all its attributes, the clove essential oil is irritating to skin and mucous membranes, so use it in a 1 percent dilution or less. Although it is a folk remedy for teething babies, it can create more pain than the tooth itself unless it is greatly diluted. Before using anything on a baby—or an adult, for that matter—first experiment on yourself, and consider that 1 drop of clove oil for a fifteen-pound baby is equal to about 10 drops for an adult, which would be considered an overdose. We recommend diluted chamomile (1 drop in ½ teaspoon of vegetable oil) as a clove substitute applied to the jaw to ease the teething pain in infants.

CORIANDER

Coriandrum sativum

One of the oldest spices mentioned in literature, coriander was one of the bitter herbs eaten at Passover. It is discussed in the Old Testament, ancient Sanskrit texts, and the *Papyrus Ebers* (1550 BC), and it has been used in China for at least two thousand years. The Romans flavored their wine with it, bringing seeds with them as their troops invaded central Europe. Now coriander scents soap and deodorant, and it is mostly used as flavoring for aperitifs and liqueurs, such as Cordial-Médoc and Danziger Goldwasser. It is a good substitute for endangered rosewood oil, since they share a similar chemistry. It can be brought closer to rosewood by adding rose or the less-expensive geranium or palmarosa.

Family: Apiaceae (Umbelliferae)

Extraction: Distilled from the seed; CO_2. Grown commercially in Russia, it has a spicy, sharp scent. Cilantro oil is also distilled from leaves.

Medicinal action: Coriander soothes inflammation, rheumatic pain, headaches, cystitis, flu, urinary tract inflammation, intestinal gas, and diarrhea. It is also a good antiseptic and antifungal, and a mild antispasmodic that aids digestion and food assimilation. Studies show that it may also regulate cholesterol levels.

Cosmetic/skin use: Regardless of its reputation as a love potion, fourteenth-century nuns included coriander in their Carmelite water. It remained popular for complexion care for the next four centuries and eventually was produced as cologne. It once dominated longtime Paris favorite Eau de Carmes cologne, and is still the base of the modern Coriandre perfume.

Emotional attributes: Uplifting and motivating, the scent relieves stress. This seed, which has been described as smelling similar to bedbugs, may seem a surprising choice for fragrance, let alone an aphrodisiac. However, the secret is to blend it with other oils.

CYPRESS

Cupressus sempervirens

Landscapes of southern France and Greece are graced with this statuesque evergreen. Related to juniper, it appears in many men's colognes and aftershave lotions.

Family: Cupressaceae

Extraction: Distilled from pruned twigs and needles and—sometimes—cones; concrete and absolute. Its scent is sharp, pungent, and spicy.

Medicinal action: Cypress treats low blood pressure, poor circulation, and hemorrhoids. As a good gargle at the first signs of a sore throat, it alleviates laryngitis, spasmodic coughing, and lung congestion. It is antiseptic and deodorant. Smoke from burning the gum was once inhaled in southern Europe to relieve sinus congestion, and the Chinese chewed the small cones to reduce gum

inflammation. This astringent oil also treats excessive fluid and urinary tract problems.

Cosmetic/skin use: Use cypress on oily hair or skin or to reduce excessive sweating, dermatitis, itching, allergic reactions, skin injuries, varicose veins, and even skin growths. This is one of the favored essential oils to reduce cellulite.

Emotional attributes: Cypress eases insomnia, depression, anxiety, nervousness, and grief, and increases stamina, helping people get on with their lives after emotional crises. Cypress has long been used to help people in the process of dying and those dealing with grief. Egyptians used the wood to build their coffins, while French and Americans plant the tree in graveyards.

ELEMI

Canarium luzonicum

See Frankincense.

EUCALYPTUS

Eucalyptus globulus

With more than six hundred species, eucalyptus offers a variety of scents. The blue gum variety is most widely cultivated and produces most of the oil. It was introduced at the Paris Exposition in 1867 after the Melbourne, Australia, botanical garden's director suggested it as an antiseptic replacement for cajeput. The French government planted trees in Algeria to ward off "noxious gases" thought responsible for malaria. It worked because the trees transformed the marsh into dry land, eliminating the mosquito's habitat. Australia's "blue forests" are named for the haze produced by the tree's essential oil, which mutes the surrounding scenery. Today eucalyptus is used liberally in industrial preparations, aftershaves, cologne, and mouthwash.

Family: Myrtaceae

Extraction: Distilled from the leaf and small twigs. The scent is pungent, sharp, and somewhat camphorous.

Medicinal action: A potent antiviral, antibacterial, and decongestant, eucalyptus treats sinus and throat infection, fever, and flu. Its drying activity is especially useful for respiratory conditions that produce excessive mucus.

Cosmetic/skin use: Studies show that eucalyptus is antiseptic on wounds, boils, insect bites, and lice, and antiviral on chicken pox and herpes simplex virus when applied as a 3 percent concentration. It also enhances skin repair and reduces itching and inflammation. Most liniments and vapor rubs contain it or its eucalyptol compound.

Emotional attributes: The scent increases energy, countering physical debility and emotional imbalance. It can reverse headache, shock, and stress.

Associated Oils
Most of the eucalyptus species are referred to by their Latin names.

Australian Eucalyptus *(E. australiana):* This Australian oil is specific for treating lung congestion and sore throats.

Peppermint Eucalyptus *(E. dives):* There are two chemotypes that look identical but have different scents. One is rich in the compound cineol and specific for acne, while the other contains piperitone, a ketone compound that reduces mucous but is somewhat toxic. It is similar to the **Peppermint Eucalyptus** *(E. piperita)* that is used in mouthwashes and veterinary supplies.

Lemon Eucalyptus *(E. citriodora):* A high percentage of the compound citronellal gives this eucalyptus a wonderful lemony scent, making it more relaxing than blue gum eucalyptus and an inoffensive bug repellent. It also decreases inflammation and fungal and bacterial infections, especially *Streptococcus.* This is a good choice for

oily skin, herpes, cystitis, or arthritis, or symptoms that include heat, such as thirst and fever.

Blue Mallee Eucalyptus *(E. polybractea):* There are two chemotypes of this species. Cineol (cuminol) is specific for sinus and bronchial congestion. Cryptone treats genitourinary tract problems, including chlamydia and condyloma virus, cystitis, cervical dysplasia, uterine fibroids, and uterine and prostate infection.

Grey Eucalyptus *(E. radiata):* Commonly referred to by its Latin name, *Eucalyptus radiata* treats overall ear, nose, throat, and upper respiratory conditions, acne, vaginitis, ear infections, and herpes. Its action is cooling and anti-inflammatory.

Gully Gum Eucalyptus *(E. smithii):* An energizer and immune modulator, this species is mild, making it a good choice for children or sensitive people. It is also helpful in treating muscle pain.

FENNEL

Foeniculum vulgare

A tall, feathery Mediterranean herb, fennel loves to grow by the sea. Italian fishermen brought it to California, where it flourishes along the coast. It is called *licorice plant* due to its taste and smell. Pliny the Elder praised it as medicine in his *Natural History* in the first century AD, but fennel traces its written history back to Babylon in 3000 BC.

Family: Apiaceae (Umbelliferae)

Extraction: Distilled from the seed; CO_2. The scent is herbaceous, sweet, and similar to licorice. A bitter fennel oil is distilled from the whole herb.

Medicinal action: Romans ate the seeds as a digestive in after-dinner cakes that also contained anise and cumin seeds. In similar fashion, East Indians often serve the seeds after dinner. The twelfth-century herbalist abbess Saint Hildegard of Bingen agreed, saying the seeds are "beneficial for anybody, whether healthy or ill, when it is eaten after some food." The old formula called gripe water, a syrup of fennel, dill, and baking soda, is still given to colicky babies in Europe. Hildegard also recommended inhaling smoke from fennel seeds for severe sinus infections, although modern aromatherapists suggest using a steam instead. While anise stimulates appetite, fennel (and its cousin dill seed) has traditionally been used to decrease it, as well as water retention and obesity. Fennel also treats urinary tract conditions and bacterial and fungal infections. It has estrogen-like properties, slightly stimulates adrenal glands, increases mother's milk, and helps relieve menstrual cramps.

Cosmetic/skin use: Encouraging cell repair, fennel refines all complexion types, especially mature skin, and heals bruises. It has been used for centuries in antiwrinkle creams and remains a popular facial cream today. Small amounts scent cologne, perfume, and soap.

Emotional attributes: Stimulating and revitalizing, fennel increases self-motivation and enlivens the personality. Hildegard said fennel makes a person happy and that a warm fennel compress on the forehead relieves insomnia.

Considerations: Since it can overexcite the nervous system, use fennel oil carefully. It also has mild estrogenic properties. Individuals with nervous system problems, epilepsy, or estrogen-related disorders should avoid the essential oil and stick to eating the seeds.

Associated Oil

Dill (*Anethum graveolens*): Dill essential oil is distilled from the seed. Early Americans chewed the seeds to inhibit appetite during church services. Like fennel, it treats obesity, water retention, and refines the complexion. It also reduces muscle spasms and increases digestive juices, including saliva to ease indigestion. Babies were put to sleep on fragrant "dilly pillows," which were filled with dill seeds, lavender, and chamomile, to prevent indigestion from returning.

FIR

Abies alba and other species

The fir is native to northern Europe. This is the well-known Christmas tree and the tree that provides the Yule log. The oil is also distilled from Siberian fir (*A. siberica*) and the sweeter Canadian balsam (*A. balsamea*).

Family: Pinaceae

Extraction: Distilled from the twigs or needles of many different species, even from spruces, pines, and other conifers. The scent of fir essential oil is fresh, soft, and forestlike.

Medicinal action: Fir lessens asthma and coughing, and it inhibits bronchial, genital, and urinary infections. As a liniment, it soothes muscle and rheumatism pain, increasing poor circulation. Fir, pine, and spruce oils are all considered tonics for adrenal glands, usually applied as a massage oil rubbed on the lower back.

Cosmetic/skin use: Sometimes used on skin infections, it is drying on oily and acne-prone skin.

Emotional attributes: The scent is used to increase a feeling of family harmony and goodwill. It combines the sensation of being grounded and elevated at the same time, and it increases intuition and releases energy and emotional blocks.

Associated Oils

Pine (*Pinus nigra; P. pinaster;* etc.): Very antiseptic and inexpensive, pine is often used in cleaning solutions. European bath preparations and liniments use it to increase circulation. The fragrance replaces apathy and anxiety with peacefulness and invigoration. According to Daniel Penoel, MD, **Scotch** or **White Pine** (*P. sylvestris*) treats male impotency (pine pollen is used similarly).
Black Spruce (*Picea mariana*): The fresh scent of spruce is stimulating. The oil treats muscle spasms, adrenal gland insufficiency, and fatigue.

Hemlock *(Tsuga canadensis):* Hemlock is often sold as fir or spruce oil (probably so it is not confused with the poison hemlock, *Conium maculatum,* that Socrates was compelled to drink).

FRANKINCENSE

Boswellia carterii

This small tree grows on rocky hillsides in Yemen and Oman. An important incense since ancient times, frankincense is also known as *oleum libanum* or "oil of Lebanon." The ancients so prized it for religious ceremonies that it was largely responsible for establishing the spice routes.

Family: Burseraceae

Extraction: Distilled from oleo gum resin that exudes from incisions in the trunk and hardens into "tears"; absolute; CO_2. The finest quality is North African, with some produced in Somalia. The scent is balsamic, powdery, and similar to incense. *Olibanum (B. papyrifera)* is inferior and less expensive.

Medicinal action: Frankincense is antiseptic and anti-inflammatory for muscles, arthritis, and the lungs. It treats genital and urinary complaints, stomach ulcers, chronic diarrhea, and breast cysts. It can encourage menstruation.

Cosmetic/skin use: Frankincense is excellent to help dry, sensitive, mature, couperose. and sun-damaged skin and acne. It helps counter bacterial and fungal skin infections, boils, hard-to-heal wounds and scars, skin growths, and distended varicose veins.

Emotional attributes: Used throughout the ages to enhance spirituality, mental perception, meditation, prayer, and consciousness, frankincense fortifies and soothes the spirit as it slows and deepens breathing. It improves memory and sleep, and releases anger, anxiety, depression, and stress.

It is considered one of the best oils to heal deep-seated wounds of the soul that may manifest in physical illness.

Associated Oils

Indian Frankincense or **Boswellia** *(B. serrata):* Ayurvedic and Traditional Chinese Medicine practitioners use *Boswellia* to treat pain, inflammation, hemorrhoids, chronic degenerative diseases, and liver and lung conditions, especially asthma. They also use it to provide a sense of well-being and counter sluggishness and pain related to nervous system problems. Drugstores sell Boswellia cream to ease arthritic and other forms of pain. Studies show that it is an excellent NSAID (non-steroid anti-inflammatory pain killers) that relieves inflammatory pain better than pharmaceutical drugs prescribed to treat colitis and Crohn's disease. It also destroys liver and colon cancer cells in the laboratory. This less expensive frankincense finds its way into soap and cosmetics.

Elemi *(Canarium luzonicum):* This tropical Philippine tree is distantly related to frankincense and was a less expensive alternative in ancient trade. Distilled from the gum, it scents soap and cosmetics and sometimes even flavors food. It treats congested lungs, inflammation, infection, and mature complexions. Emotionally, it reduces stress and nervousness. It is also available as an absolute.

GERANIUM

Pelargonium graveolens

Seventeenth-century Europeans took a fancy to this tender African perennial, also known as "rose geranium," and propagated it in their greenhouses. The resulting hybridization increased the species number to more than six hundred including many rose types. The French planted it in Algeria and Réunion, or "Bourbon," the name for geranium from this area. It is also grown in Morocco, South Africa, and China. Although the leaves resemble common geranium (hence its name), the two are only distantly related.

Family: Geraniaceae

Extraction: Distilled from the leaves; absolute; concrete. The fragrance is a rose-citrus-herb combination. The oil varies considerably, depending on growing conditions and species. Chinese oil is slightly less sweet but produces a good yield, making it less expensive. The pharmaceutical industry widely isolates the geraniol compound, which is used as a starting point to make synthetic rose and to extend real rose. This is the only type of "scented" geranium distilled commercially, except for a small amount of cape rose geranium *(Pelargonium capitatum* x *radens)* and lemon geranium *(P. odoratissimum).*

Medicinal action: A light adrenal gland stimulant and hormonal normalizer, geranium is a balancing agent for many conditions. Just sniffing the fragrance can regulate blood pressure by at last a few points. Geranium treats PMS, menopause, menstrual cycle irregularities, fluid retention, breast engorgement, and sterility. In one study, it killed all bacteria tested, including *Salmonella* and *Staphylococcus* and in another, it inhibited all fungi being tested.

Cosmetic/skin use: A popular skin treatment, geranium reduces inflammation and infection of wounds, insect bites, eczema, acne, and burns, and enhances skin repair. It is used to stop bleeding, scarring, stretch marks, enlarged veins, lice, shingles, and herpes. It balances all hair and complexion types, including couperose and mature skin, and is said to delay wrinkling.

Emotional attributes: The fragrance relieves anxiety, depression, discontent, irrational behavior, and stress and associated headaches. It is used to balance passive-aggressive natures, heal poor relationships, and enhance one's perception of time and space. It is often described as a sedative, although some aromatherapists consider it stimulating to the point of inducing insomnia. This discrepancy may be due to its balancing action.

Associated Oil

Zdravets *(Geranium macrorrhizum):* Don't confuse this oil from the *Geranium* genus with scented geranium *(Pelargonium).* It doesn't have the same amazing scent but it does scent perfume. Studies show that it strongly inhibits *Staphylococcus, E. coli,* and *Candida* infections. The herb is used medicinally in Bulgaria.

GINGER

Zingiber officinale

Native to the tropics, ginger's thin, broad leaves are attached to a succulent, spicy rhizome. The herb originated near the Indian Ocean, but it is now grown throughout the tropics. Its aromatic properties were described by Pliny the Elder in the first century AD and in ancient Indian Sanskrit texts.

Family: Zingiberaceae

Extraction: Distilled from unpeeled, ground rhizome; absolute; concrete; CO_2 extraction. The fragrance is spicy, warm, and sharp.

Medicinal action: Ginger essential oil treats fevers, migraine headaches, inflammation, and genital, urinary, and lung infections, reducing inflammatory compounds called *prostaglandins* in the body. It stimulates saliva, bile, and digestive enzymes to improve digestion, food assimilation, appetite loss, nausea, and intestinal movement. It helps prevent stomach ulcers. It destroys many types of intestinal parasites, bacterial infections, including *Salmonella* and *Staphylococcus,* and viral infections, including Epstein-Barr and the common cold. A warming liniment or a hot ginger compress is an excellent remedy for menstrual and other muscle cramps. Studies show that ginger rhizome increases drug and herb absorption, normalizes blood pressure, and helps protect the liver, although these actions may be stronger in the herb form than essential oil.

Cosmetic/skin use: Researchers found ginger destroys the herpes virus in a different manner than the drug acyclovir. They assume that it helps cells build a protective envelope rather than directly killing the infection.

Emotional attributes: Ginger is a stimulant and an aphrodisiac.

Associated Oils

Plai *(Z. cassumunar):* This relative of ginger is common in Thailand, where it is used extensively in massage to treat inflammatory conditions and skin ailments.

Galanga or **Galangal** *(Alpina officinalis):* See chapter 14.

GRAPEFRUIT

C. x paradisi

See Orange.

HELICHRYSUM

Helichrysum angustifolium; H. italicum

Known also as *everlast* or *immortelle* since the flowers last so long, the herb is native to the Mediterranean and North Africa, and it is cultivated in Spain, Italy, and Yugoslavia. The plant is also called "poor man's curry" because it was used in cooking in place of expensive Oriental curry.

Family: Asteraceae (Compositae)

Extraction: Distilled from the flowering tops. The pleasant fragrance is spicy, sweet, and almost fruity.

Medicinal action: Helichrysum treats infection and the inflammation of chronic cough, bronchitis, fever, muscle pain, arthritis, phlebitis, and liver conditions. It helps counter allergic reactions such as asthma.

Cosmetic/skin use: Helichrysum stimulates production of new cells, so it is used on acne, dermatitis, scar tissue, bruises, burns, boils, insect bites, and couperose, mature,

and sun-damaged skin. The extract is included in some commercial sunscreens to protect skin from ultraviolet ray damage. It also counters irregular skin growth and is valuable in treating precancerous skin conditions. In addition, it is antifungal and antibacterial. It is a fixative to retain the fragrances of cosmetics and perfume.

Emotional attributes: The scent helps lift one from depression, lethargy, nervous exhaustion, and stress. Some aromatherapists find it helps with detoxification from drugs, including nicotine.

Associated Oil

French Helichrysum *(H. stoechas):* The distilled oil has an orange hue, while the absolute and concrete are both brown-red. Essential oil from several other species are sometimes available.

HYSSOP

Hyssopus officinalis

Hyssop comes from the Mediterranean. Most of the essential oil now goes into expensive perfumes and Benedictine, Chartreuse, and Kartäuser liqueurs.

Family: Lamiaceae (Labiatae)

Extraction: Distilled from the flowering tops. The scent is spicy, strong, and herbaceous.

Medicinal action: Hyssop treats the respiratory system, stimulates blood circulation, and somewhat reduces muscle cramps. The essential oil improves digestion, although the bitterness of the herbal tea makes it a better remedy.

Emotional attributes: Hyssop eases grief, fear, oversensitivity, and hysteria while increasing mental clarity.

Considerations: A nervous system stimulant due to ketone compounds, use hyssop oil with caution since it can trigger asthma or epilepsy and large doses may raise blood pressure. An alternative is to use the herbal form, although even drinking hyssop tea daily isn't recommended.

Associated Oil

Hyssop *Decumbens* (H. *officinalis* var. *decumbens*): This variety contains none of the hazardous ketones, so it is preferred in aromatherapy. High in the compound linalol, it is a sinus and lung decongestant that can safely be used with allergies, asthma, and nervous conditions. It is a good antimicrobial, even acting against strong strains of tuberculosis and *Candida albicans* yeast infections.

INULA, SWEET

Inula graveolens; I. odorata

This native to Asia is now cultivated in many locales. It produces an essential oil that very effectively breaks up congestion. It can be dispensed from a diffuser for respiratory problems.

Family: Asteraceae (Compositae)

Extraction: Distilled from the root, resulting in a rich blue-green oil. The scent is strong and pungent, somewhat resembling eucalyptus.

Medicinal action: Inula is especially helpful for chronic lung inflammation, sinus congestion, bronchitis, and related muscle tension.

Cosmetic/skin use: Inula relieves skin rashes, herpes, and itching.

Considerations: Sweet inula is regarded as quite safe, but it hasn't been tested for toxicity, so don't use it on children, pregnant women, or anyone who is frail. On the other hand, elecampane (*I. helenium*) essential oil is an irritant that is high in potentially toxic ketones, so it is not used except as tea or tincture. In one study, it caused skin allergies in twenty-three out of twenty-five test subjects.

JASMINE

Jasminium officinale and *J. grandiflorum*

Probably an Iranian native, jasmine has captured the imagination for centuries. Forty-three different species are grown in East India, where it is poetically called "moonlight of the grove" and the "king of fragrance." The complex scent is a part of most great perfumes. Try as chemists do to reproduce it, synthetic jasmine is so harsh that it demands a touch of the true oil to soften it.

Family: Oleaceae

Extraction: Absolute; produced through enfleurage at one time. The fragrance is fruity, floral, and sweetly exotic. The most prized oil comes from France and Italy, although about 80 percent on the market is Egyptian.

Medicinal action: Jasmine is a nervous system sedative that reduces menstrual and other muscle cramps. The seventeenth-century herbalist Nicholas Culpeper suggested rubbing it into "hard, contracted limbs." It is occasionally suggested to alleviate prostate problems.

Cosmetic/skin use: It is used for dry, sensitive, or mature skin.

Emotional attributes: Jasmine's fragrance soothes headaches, insomnia, depression, anger, fear, grief, and worry, dissolving apathy and lack of confidence. At the same time, it reverses fatigue. This is the supreme aphrodisiac, for which it has been used for centuries.

Associated Oil

Sambac Jasmine (*J. sambac*): This is also called Chinese jasmine, although it comes from India. Rather than having jasmine's heavier base notes, this rich scent is fruitier, with a touch of neroli.

JUNIPER

Juniperus communis

Named after *genièvre* (which is French for "juniper berry"), the berries of this North American and European shrub have long flavored gin and other alcoholic drinks, including Juniper schnapps and Genever.

Family: Cupressaceae

Extraction: Distilled from the ripe berries; resinoid; absolute. The pungent, peppery, camphorous scent is similar to pine. Berries offer the highest quality oil, but needles, branches, and berries that have already been distilled into gin are sometimes used. The proportions of compounds in the oil vary depending on the country it comes from, the altitude where the trees grow, and when it was harvested. Cade oil is a thick, smoky tar produced through the "destructive" distillation of burned roots for use on skin parasites. It gives food a smoked flavor but is best avoided in aromatherapy.

Medicinal action: Traditionally the fragrance was thought to ward off contagious disease. Until World War II, the French burned the branches in their hospitals as an antiseptic. Native Americans living in the high deserts of the West still burn them during purification and healing ceremonies. It does help with respiratory infections, but its reputation is mostly for relieving genital and urinary tract infections, inflammation, fluid retention, and cystitis. It also promotes digestion. Juniper is used in the treatment of arteriosclerosis and hemorrhoids. As a liniment, it warms an area by increasing peripheral blood circulation. In one study, the essential oil decreased joint pain in people with rheumatoid arthritis.

Cosmetic/skin use: Juniper is suitable for acne, eczema, and greasy hair or dandruff. It is used on dermatitis, boils, insect bites, bacterial infections, and inflamed, itchy skin. As a circulatory stimulant, it helps with congestion-related conditions such as varicose veins and cellulite.

Emotional attributes: Juniper is good for those who suffer from general debility, mental fatigue, insomnia, anxiety, or feel emotionally drained. It provides a feeling of protection when the demands of others pull too strongly.

Considerations: Juniper is usually considered harsh on kidneys, although modern studies have not supported this earlier observation. It is still suggested that it not be used for more than a week at a time if kidney problems exist or to choose gentler oils until science has more data. Pregnant women should still avoid it.

Associated Oils

Virginia Cedarwood *(J. virginiana):* This juniper is the real source of most "cedar oil"—and most wooden pencils! It provided the "Lebanon cedarwood" that perfumed many Victorian handkerchiefs. Texas cedarwood *(J. mexicana)* oil is also produced, while the low-priced East African cedarwood *(J. procera)* scents soap and sometimes cologne. The most toxic of junipers, *J. sabina,* should be avoided.

LAVENDER

Lavandula angustifolia; L. vera; L. officinale

A well-loved Mediterranean herb, lavender has been associated with cleanliness ever since Romans added it to washing water. In fact, the word comes from the Latin *lavare* (meaning "to wash") as do "lavatory" and "lavage." Lavender remained popular as facial water from the fourteenth through the nineteenth centuries. It was the basis for palsy drops, which were recognized by the *British Pharmacopoeia* for more than two hundred years, until the 1940s, and was used to relieve muscle spasms, nervousness, and headaches. The modern lavender water formula by Yardley adds rose, musk, and neroli. When in doubt, use lavender!

Family: Lamiaceae (Labiatae)

Extraction: Distilled from flowers; absolute; concrete. The scent is sweet floral and herbal with balsamic undertones.

The term "40 percent ester," which is often seen on lavender oil, means that it has a high ester content—boosted, if necessary, with natural esters extracted from lavender or more likely, lavandin. Often called *English lavender,* some of the finest quality actually hails from France.

Medicinal action: Lavender is among the safest and most widely used oils in aromatherapy and is considered a universal first aid oil. Studies show that the essential oil destroys a wide range of fungal and bacterial infections, including *Staphylococcus,* strep throat, and pneumonia, as well as most flu viruses. It treats lung, sinus, and vaginal infections, including *Candida,* and is excellent for laryngitis and asthma. It relieves muscle pain, headaches, and cystitis. It also treats digestive disturbances, including colic, and may help boost immunity.

Cosmetic/skin use: Lavender is suitable for all skin and hair types, including a couperose complexion. A cell regenerator that helps prevent scarring and stretch marks, it has a reputation for slowing wrinkles. It is used on sun-damaged skin, skin growths, wounds, rashes, skin infections, varicose veins, and anything that is swollen. There is no better remedy for burns than lavender. This is one of the few times we recommend using a few drops of the oil neat (undiluted) to stop the itching of insect bites and on small, first-degree burns several times during the first day of treatment. However, dilute the essential oil with aloe gel when treating overall sunburn.

Emotional attributes: Nervousness, exhaustion, insomnia, irritability, depression, and even manic depression are addressed by lavender. Producing balancing effects on the emotions, it both relaxes and stimulates, depending on dosage and, probably, the individual's needs. It is specific for central nervous system conditions. Preliminary Japanese studies indicate that lavender's scent affects the autonomic, sympathetic, and parasympathetic nervous systems as well as adrenal glands. Quite a few studies on lavender show the scent alone helps counter insomnia, depression, mental stress, anger, and anxiety and improves one's mood and memory. It even reduced aggressive behavior of elderly people with Alzheimer's. Lavender-scented rooms also worked as well as drugs to lull hospital patients to sleep. It was shown to work in a manner similar to sedative drugs such as diazepam, but without the drug's intensity or side effects. On the other hand, it also improves concentration levels. For centuries, lavender was brought into birthing rooms and made into baby pillows. Old texts say it "raises the spirit," and it was the main ingredient in Victorian "smelling salts" to revive the all-too-common fainting due to a lack of oxygen from wearing restricting corsets. Victorian women also revived themselves with lavender-filled "swooning pillows." In his sixteenth-century *Herbal,* William Turner wrote that lavender could "comfort the braine."

Associated Oils

Lavandin *(L.* x *intermedia; L.* x *hybrida):* This is English lavender crossed with spike lavender. Strains of this hybrid, such as Abrialis, Grosso (the most productive and common), Standard, Super, and Maime Epis Tête, have a slightly camphorous fragrance that is less refined than their parent lavenders. About twenty times more of the less-expensive lavandin is produced than true lavender, which produces less essential oil with its shorter and fewer flower spikes. Lavandin has similar, but probably less pronounced, healing properties; use it for muscle pain and as disinfectant and deodorant.

Spike Lavender (L. *latifolia; L. spica):* Sometimes called *aspic,* this camphorous species relieves congestion and is good for acne. Its high yield makes it less expensive. It is grown mostly in Spain and is slightly more toxic, so one needs to use it more carefully than English lavender.

Stoechas Lavender *(L. stoechas):* This oil is used mostly to heal wounds and reduce inflammation, but it is slightly more toxic than other lavenders—so use it cautiously and never on babies.

LEMON

Citrus limon

The lemon tree originated in Asia but is now widely cultivated in Italy, Australia, and California. The fragrance is popular in household cleaning products. The flowers have a pleasant aroma, but only the peel oil is produced commercially for body-care products, cologne, and bath salts. It also flavors baked goods, beverages, and sweets.

Family: Rutaceae

Extraction: Cold pressed from the fresh peel. The scent is distinctively sharp and citrus. All citrus oils degrade quickly due to the high amounts of terpene compounds they contain, so refrigerate quantities that you will not use within a year. The terpene compounds have been removed from "cedro oil," making it more water soluble.

Medicinal action: An antioxidant, preservative, and antiseptic, lemon essential oil helps counter viral and bacterial infections. In one study, it killed all bacteria tested, including *Salmonella* and *Staphylococcus.* In massage oil, it stimulates lymphatic system detoxification. It treats high blood pressure and congested livers, it boosts the immune system, and it improves weight metabolism, although it also stimulates appetite.

Cosmetic/skin use: Lemon is best used on oily hair and complexions and for skin impurities. It treats bruises, boils, insect bites, warts, and skin infections. It can slightly lighten skin pigmentation problems, but only use it if your skin will have no subsequent sun exposure.

Emotional attributes: The scent dissipates feelings of impurity or indecisiveness and can stimulate emotional purging. Like other citruses, it increases one's sense of humor and general well-being, and is an antidepressive.

Considerations: Lemon irritates sensitive skin and may be photosensitizing in some people; it is best applied at night or to skin that will not get sun exposure.

LEMONGRASS

Cymbopogon citratus

Originally from India, lemongrass is an important Southeast Asian medicine that has been well adopted in South America. Grown in Central America, Brazil, and China, it is among the ten best-selling essential oils in the world, at more than fifteen hundred tons a year, for use in soap, cosmetic fragrances, and deodorants. It gives Ivory soap that familiar scent.

Family: Poaceae (Gramineae)

Extraction: Distilled from the partially dried leaves. Lemongrass has a distinctive lemon-herbal, slightly bitter fragrance. The compound citral is extracted from it for a commercial lemonlike fragrance. **Lemongrass Cochin (*C. flexuosus*)** is grown in India for isolation of the compound citral.

Medicinal action: Lemongrass is antiseptic and quite effective in fighting urinary tract infections. In several studies, it inhibited all fungi tested. It eases pain from indigestion, muscle cramps, rheumatism, nerve conditions, and headaches. It is said to help remove lactic acid buildup in tired muscles.

Cosmetic/skin use: Lemongrass counters oily hair, acne, skin infections, scabies, and ringworm. It also has deodorant properties.

Emotional attributes: The fragrance is sedating and soothing, and it helps with stress and nervous exhaustion.

Considerations: Lemongrass can be irritating to skin. It is unlikely that its action as a blood anticoagulant would be problematic when used as a diluted essential oil, but play it safe and don't use lemongrass for a week before having surgery.

Associated Oils

Palmarosa *(C. martini):* Palmarosa's lemon-rose fragrance is reminiscent of the richer, more expensive rose geranium, which it often adulterates. Like lemongrass, it treats stress and nervous exhaustion. A cell regenerator, it balances oil production and can be used on any hair or complexion type, but works especially well for acne, infected skin, or varicose veins. It is a good antifungal, inhibiting all fungi tested in one study. Its rose-scented compound geraniol is extracted for commercial use. The scent varies depending on its quality and age and whether it comes from India, Brazil, the Philippines, or Java.

Citronella *(C. nardus):* It is recorded that while riding an elephant near the Egyptian border in 332 BC, Alexander the Great supposedly became intoxicated when he smelled spikenard being crushed underfoot, which was more likely citronella. Also known as *nard,* it was first exhibited at London's Crystal Palace in 1851 and proceeded to become the primary scent in cleaning products. While many people associate the scent with kitchen cleansers, citronella added to a warm bath was sedative and improved sleep in one study for people who were healthy and those with nervous sleep disorders. Its sedative action proved even stronger when taken with hops extract. It is a physical and emotional purifier, used to treat colds, infections, and oily complexions. In one study, it inhibited all of the fungi that were tested. The inexpensive citronella often adulterates lemon verbena and melissa essential oil, although it is harsher and can irritate skin. In fact, the old preparation *Oleum melissae indicum,* or "oil of Indian melissa," is made with citronella oil. **Java Citronella** *(C. winterianus)* is widely cultivated because is a little sweeter and yields twice the essential oil. It is a source of the compound citronellal.

LEMON VERBENA
Aloysia triphylla; Lippia citriodora

Brought to Europe by the Spanish, lemon verbena was christened *Herb Louisa* after Maria Louisa, wife of King Charles IV of Spain, and later designated *Aloysia* in her honor. It became stylish to scent finger bowls at Victorian banquets with a few lemon verbena leaves.

Family: Lamiaceae (Labiatae)

Extraction: Distilled from the leaves. The sweet scent is lemony, and it is often adulterated with less expensive oils.

Medicinal action: Lemon verbena treats nervous indigestion. It destroys bacterial infections, such as *Staphylococcus,* the intestinal *E. coli,* and even tuberculosis. Historically, like most lemon-scented herbs, it has been used for colds and sinus congestion relief. In South America, the tea is a popular remedy for asthmatics.

Cosmetic/skin use: It is used on oily complexions and to scent body washes and hair rinses. The diluted essential oil treats hard-to-heal wounds, but it can also be irritating to the skin, so caution is advised.

Emotional attributes: The soothing fragrance encourages both sleep and concentration.

Associated Oil

Cape Verbena; Zinziba *(Lippia javanica):* This dark, red-brown essential oil has a pleasant, sweet, almost fruity scent, with a dash of pepper as a top note that is somewhat reminiscent of marigold *(Tagetes)* oil. Medicinally, it is used as a pain reliever, antidepressant, antiseptic, and general restorative, as well as an asthma and malaria treatment. It is emotionally uplifting.

LITSEA

Litsea cubeba

This fruit tree in the laurel family hails from India and Southeast Asia and is known as *May Chang* in China. It is also called tropical verbena (although it is unrelated to lemon verbena except for the lemony scent) and cubeb, but don't confuse it with true cubeb (described under black pepper).

Family: Lauraceae

Extraction: Distilled from the leaves or small, pepperlike fruits.

Medicinal action: This relaxant treats indigestion and reduces excessive perspiration and inflammation. It is an excellent bronchial dilator for asthma, bronchitis, or allergic reactions when diluted into a throat spray or massage oil. It has even been used to help counter anaphylactic shock. In China, where research shows it regulates the heartbeat and can lower high blood pressure, it is also used to relieve pain. The tea treats urinary infections, especially in children.

Cosmetic/skin use: Litsea is an antiseptic so it is used on bacterial and fungal skin infections and sometimes acne.

Emotional attributes: In the East, the flower is made into a tea that is considered both calming and stimulating, characteristics that are also applied to the fragrance. It helps those in emotional turmoil, anxiety, or shock. Traditional Chinese Medicine uses it to open the spleen, kidney, and bladder channels and promote *qi* (chi) flow through these areas.

Considerations: Litsea is a potential skin irritant, so avoid using it on sensitive skin. Don't use litsea with anyone who has glaucoma since it is known to increase eye pressure in animals.

MARJORAM

Origanum majorana; Majorana hortensis

"Sweet" marjoram is native to Asia but is naturalized in Europe, where singers have long preserved their voices with the honeyed tea. A marjoram species was probably the "hyssop" of the bible, used for purification.

Family: Lamiaceae (Labiatae)

Extraction: Distilled from the leaves; oleoresin. The scent is sweet, herby, and a little warm, hinting of camphor. The chemistry can vary depending on the plant's genetic makeup and how it is processed.

Medicinal action: A strong sedative, marjoram eases muscle spasms, muscle tics, menstrual cramps, spasmodic coughs, headaches (especially migraines), and stiff joints. It also helps normalize blood pressure. It counters many viral infections, countering colds, flu, and laryngitis. Studies show it inhibits urinary infection, fungi responsible for some ear infections, and intestinal inflammation. As a potent antioxidant, it preserves the food it flavors.

Cosmetic/skin use: Use marjoram on bruises, burns, insect bites, and inflammation, and to treat fungal and bacterial infections. It also helps repair injured skin.

Emotional attributes: Marjoram helps those who feel emotionally unstable or are prone to hysteria, depression, shock, or irritability, especially due to outside stimulus. The old texts say it works so well that overuse deadens the emotions. Modern aromatherapists use marjoram to ease insomnia, grief, loneliness, rejection, and "broken hearts." Even so, in weddings, it symbolizes honor, happiness, and love.

Associated Oils

Oregano *(O. vulgare):* Closely related botanically, the division between the many species of oregano and marjoram is hazy. Oregano is much more irritating to the skin, but it is a potent antibiotic that effectively acts against respiratory, genital, urinary, and intestinal infections. In one study, it destroyed all the bacteria tested, including *Salmonella* and *Staphylococcus*. Capsules and tablets to destroy digestive infections contain dilute amounts of essential oil so are safe if you follow the package instructions. On the other hand, ingesting a drop of pure essential oil will likely burn the roof of your mouth, and most will be absorbed there, never reaching the digestive tract.

Spanish Marjoram *(T. mastichina):* See Thyme.

Spanish Oregano *(T. capitatus):* See Thyme.

MASTIC

Pistacia lentiscus

Mastic comes from a Mediterranean tree closely related to edible pistachio *(P. vera)*. It has been chewed to sweeten the breath for over two thousand years. The oleoresin once thickened herbal cordials and still finds its way into liqueurs, foods, and expensive perfume.

Family: Anacardiaceae

Extraction: Distilled from the oleoresin. The scent is rich, balsamic, and turpentine.

Medicinal action: The balm was an ancient trade item closely related to the biblical terebinth. A 1719 tincture called Jerusalem Balsam gained fame as a bronchial decongestant and antiseptic, and it was used as a substitute for medicinal turpentine. Mastic is still used extensively in medicine, such as hemorrhoid creams and as a balm that is rubbed on sore muscles, rheumatism, sciatica, and other painful areas. Twelve compounds appear to work synergistically to create an antiseptic and mild analgesic action on whooping cough, colds, sinus infections, and urinary tract disorders, and to prevent tooth decay and decrease infectious *E. coli, Staphylococcus,* and *Bacillus subtilis.* Another use is to relieve lymphatic congestion.

Cosmetic/skin use: Mastic is antiseptic used on wounds and boils, an antifungal for ringworm, and reduces varicose veins and hemorrhoids. It is used to rid the hair of lice and other parasites.

MELISSA OR LEMON BALM

Melissa officinalis

Known to herbalists as "lemon balm," this southern European native flavors many liqueurs, including Chartreuse, Cordial-Médoc, Aromatique, and Alpenkräuter.

Family: Lamiaceae (Labiatae)

Extraction: Distilled from the leaves. The sweet scent is soft, lemony. The ratio of its two main lemonlike components, citral and citronellal, varies considerably depending on where it is grown and the maturity of the plants—citronellal compounds tend to concentrate in older leaves. In addition, both compounds are rapidly lost when the plant is dried and stored. Although the leaves smell pungent, the plant actually contains a relatively low amount of essential oil (0.05 to 0.3 percent). The exception is some Mediterranean cultivars, particularly from Spain, but these still are only 0.4 percent oil. Not easily distilled, the expensive, low-yielding oil is often adulterated with the far less costly lemon, lemongrass, citronella, litsea, lemon catnip, or even lemon eucalyptus.

Medicinal action: Melissa is used to treat lung congestion, high blood pressure, menstrual pain, and sometimes infertility. It counters indigestion, calming digestive tract muscles and providing pain relief. Studies show it decreases inflammation and fights viral and bacterial infections such as *Staphylococcus*.

Cosmetic/skin use: Lemon balm is a very good antiseptic and antioxidant for the complexion, dermatitis, inflammation, allergies, insect bites, and skin infections. In addition, melissa's antiviral properties have been shown in studies to be particularly effective against both herpes virus I and II, as well as the related chicken pox.

Emotional attributes: Melissa was the main ingredient in the medieval Carmelite Water along with lemon peel, nutmeg, coriander, and angelica. It was taken for nervous headaches and neuralgia (and splashed on to improve the complexion). It is still produced as Eau de Mélisse de Carmes and the German Klosterfrau Melissengeist. Melissa's sedative action helps shock, distress, depression, nervousness, anger, fear, forgetfulness, and insomnia. The famous herbal healer Avicenna found that it elevated the mood, and Gerard declared that it "maketh the heart merry, joyful, strengtheneth the vitall spirits."

Associated Oil

Lemon Catnip *(Nepeta cataria):* Grown mainly for essential oil production, lemon catnip has been shown by science to be an excellent cockroach, flea, and mosquito repellent that is less toxic than DEET. Some compounds are similar to melissa, but the scent is harsher.

MYRRH

Commiphora myrrha

This small, scrubby tree from the Middle East and northeast Africa isn't handsome, but the precious gum it exudes makes up for its lackluster look. An important trade item for more than a thousand years, myrrh was a primary ingredient in ancient cosmetics and incense. The Egyptians mummified their dead with it.

Family: Burseraceae

Extraction: Distilled from the gum resin that flows from the incised trunk and hardens into beads.

Medicinal action: Myrrh improves digestion, diarrhea, and immunity. It treats coughs, gum disease, and candida infection, and increases menstruation.

Cosmetic/skin use: Myrrh is effective for chapped, cracked, sensitive, dry, or aged skin, eczema, bruises, infection, varicose veins, and ringworm. It eases inflammation and promotes skin repair, so can be used on wounds, burns, warts, and dermatitis. It is useful for dry hair and dandruff.

Emotional attributes: Myrrh has been used since antiquity to inspire prayer and meditation and to fortify and revitalize the spirit.

Associated Oils

Opopanax *(C. erythraea):* This Somalian and Ethiopian oil is a low-grade myrrh with similar properties that is used to impart a winelike taste to liquor. Don't confuse it with the other plants called *opopanax*; cassie *(Acacia farnesiana),* or the medicinal devil's club *(Oplopanax horridum).*

Guggul *(C. mukul):* See chapter 14.

Copal *(Copaiba officinalis):* This oleoresin (not really balsam) is one of several copals used in their native South and Central America as protective and healing incense. The Catholic Church there uses it in place of myrrh, calling it *Jesuits' Bark oil.* It is collected in bamboo tubes from the heartwood of the rain forest tree. An anti-inflammatory, it treats bronchitis, chronic cystitis, and intestinal infection. It is inexpensive and made into body oil, hair products, and soap.

MYRTLE

Myrtus communis

This attractive North African bush now makes itself at home throughout the Mediterranean. It was a favorite in ancient gardens of Baghdad, Granada, and Damascus. Today it is grown commercially in Morocco, where twigs laid on burning coals flavor grilled foods. In southern Italy, the leaves are pressed into fresh cheese to impart their flavor.

Family: Myrtaceae

Extraction: (distilled from the leaves, twigs, and sometimes flowers) The scent is spicy and slightly camphorous.

Medicinal action: The Corsican liqueur Mirto is flavored with myrtle and sipped as a digestive cordial. Myrtle also treats lung and respiratory infections, spasmodic coughs, muscle spasms, and hemorrhoids.

Cosmetic/skin use: Myrtle was the main ingredient in the sixteenth-century complexion remedy angel's water, and the essential oil is still used in perfumes. It is appropriate for oily and acned complexions and enlarged surface veins.

Emotional attributes: The scent balances energy. The ancient Greeks and Romans honored poets with myrtle to suggest that their fame would never die.

NEROLI

Citrus aurantium var. *amara*

See Orange Blossom.

OAKMOSS

Evernia prunastri

This lichen (a combination of fungus and algae) hangs from trees like Spanish moss. It was found in Egyptian royal tombs. It was popular in sixteenth-century perfumes and remains a fixative in chypre-type perfumes today (named after Cyprus, the home of this moss).

Family: Usneaceae

Extraction: Absolute; concrete; vacuum-distilled from the absolute. It offers an earthy, full, and slightly sweet fragrance. It is collected in Yugoslavia, France, Italy, and Morocco. **Tree Moss** (*E. furfuracea*) produces a sharper scent when it grows on cedar and especially on pine trees.

Emotional attributes: Oakmoss creates a sense of home, attachment, and belonging.

ORANGE

Citrus sinensis

The familiar sweet orange comes from Sicily, Israel, Spain, and the United States, each offering a slightly different characteristic. *Chu-lu,* the first monograph to describe the various citruses, was written in China in 1178. Check the label for the Latin name to assure you get the citrus you want.

Family: Rutaceae

Extraction: Cold pressed from the peel. Inferior oil comes from peel pressed for juice. More water soluble, oil without terpene is used in soft drinks. The scent is typically similar to citrus, perky and lively. All citrus oils degrade quickly due to the high amounts of terpene compounds they contain. Refrigeration is advised if you do not use them within a year.

Medicinal action: Orange treats flu, colds, congested lymph, indigestion, irregular heartbeat, and high blood pressure. It detoxifies and makes a wonderful complement to massage treatments designed to reduce cellulite. In one study, it inhibited all of the fungi that were tested.

Cosmetic/skin use: It is good to use on oily hair and complexions and acne.

Emotional attributes: This sedative fragrance counters depression, anxiety, hysteria, shock, and nervous tension. Researchers have confirmed that orange reduces anxiety and improves one's mood.

Considerations: The oil may be slightly photosensitizing, so it is best to use it when skin will not be exposed to the sun.

Associated Oils

Grapefruit *(C.* x *paradisi):* Oil from this peel encourages weight loss and gallbladder activity, and it is noted for its cleansing action. In one study, the scent of grapefruit stimulated the sympathetic nervous system while at the same time inhibiting nerves in the stomach. It is a favorite of children, and we find it a useful accompaniment for inner-child work.

Lime *(C. aurantifolia):* Native to India and Southeast Asia, this is the most tender citrus tree. Unlike other citruses, the peel can be steam-distilled (nonphotosensitizing) as well as pressed (very photosensitizing). It is easy to detect the scent of cold-pressed lime, which smells like freshly grated limes rather than candy. Lime flavors cola beverages and is used to treat depression.

Tangerine or **Mandarin** *(C. reticulata):* From the peel of the mandarin, this oil aids insomnia, lymph congestion, fat reduction, and indigestion. It is rarely photosensitizing and one of the safest citrus oils for children and pregnant women.

ORANGE BLOSSOM (NEROLI)

Citrus aurantium

One of the many stories about this plant is that neroli was named after the sixteenth-century Italian princess of Nerola, who loved its scent. An Indochina native, it is grown commercially in France, Morocco, Tunisia, and Egypt.

Family: Rutaceae

Extraction: Distilled from the blossoms of the bitter orange tree, not the sweet orange that produces orange oil; concrete; absolute. The fragrance is sweet, spicy, floral, and distinctive. Occasionally, the inferior Neroli Portugal *(C. aurantium* var. *dulcis)* is produced from this sweeter, less-fragrant orange. Little essential oil results from pressing the peel, which oxidizes quickly and degrades and is among the most photosensitizing citrus oils. It is mostly used to flavor digestive aperitifs and the liqueur curaçao.

Medicinal action: Neroli treats muscle pain, circulation disorders such as hemorrhoids and high blood pressure, and indigestion.

Cosmetic/skin use: Neroli is used on all complexion types, especially to regenerate skin cells for dermatitis and mature, sensitive, acne, and couperose skin. It also helps repair scars and varicose veins.

Emotional attributes: One of the best aromatic antidepressants, neroli counters emotional shock, mental confusion, nervous strain, anger, anxiety, fear, and lack of confidence. It redirects one's energy into a more positive direction, countering both fatigue and insomnia. It is used for those who get upset for no apparent reason or those who fear public speaking. It may have hormonal properties and has been used as an aphrodisiac since ancient times.

Associated Oil

Petitgrain *(C. aurantium):* Now distilled from fragrant leaves, unripe fruit, and stems of the bitter orange, this oil originally came from the small, unripe fruit (thus its name, which means "little fruit"). Considered "poor man's neroli," the fragrance is similar, but harsher, sharper, and much less expensive. It is an antidepressant that increases perception and awareness, reestablishing trust and self-confidence. Most oil comes from Paraguay, where the nineteenth-century French botanist Benjamin Balsam first distilled the leaves (petitgrain is produced from the twigs of other citruses—for example, mandarin and lemon petitgrain, although these are not commonly available).

OREGANO

Origanum vulgare

See Marjoram.

PATCHOULI

Pogostemon cablin

Indian women stuff mattresses with patchouli leaves and lay them among clothes to scent them. An effective pest deterrent, patchouli keeps moths and mold out of woolen shawls and rugs. Europeans would not buy imitation rugs because they didn't smell "authentic," of patchouli. Patchouli's heyday was in the 1960s, but the oil still flavors many famous perfumes and some smoking tobacco. Many people have never smelled the high-quality oil used in famous perfumes such as Tabu and Shocking. The oil comes from Indonesia, India, and now, China.

Family: Lamiaceae (Labiatae)

Extraction: Distilled from the fermented leaves; resinoid; CO_2. The fragrance is heavy, earthy, woody, musty, similar to vanilla, and distinctive. Since it is developed through oxidation, the leaves carry little indication of their potential. They are aged before being distilled for up to twenty-four hours. Even then, the translucent yellow oil is harsh, but it turns syrupy brown and more vanilla-scented as it ages. Inferior oil comes from distilling in crude iron vessels rather than stainless steel.

Medicinal action: Patchouli helps reduce appetite, water retention, exhaustion, and inflammation. When taken as an extract, it has been found to improve digestion and prevent nausea by nearly 60 percent. Researchers think the essential oil reduces spasms in digestive tract muscle.

Cosmetic/skin use: As a cell rejuvenator and antiseptic, patchouli is a treatment for acne, eczema, inflamed, cracked, sensitive, or mature skin and skin growths. Use it on dry hair or complexion. An excellent antifungal, it inhibited all fungi tested in one study, including athlete's foot. East Indian women prize it as a scent for their hair and conditioner that prevents dandruff.

Emotional attributes: Patchouli counters nervousness, anxiety, oversensitivity, and depression by putting problems into perspective and releasing pent-up emotions. An aphrodisiac, it helps insomnia while also being mildly stimulating.

PEPPERMINT
Mentha piperita

Peppermint first appeared only in the seventeenth century, when it managed to self-hybridize. It now grows wild throughout Europe, North America, and Australia. After the *British Medical Journal* noted in 1879 that peppermint's menthol compound relieves headaches and neuralgia, menthol cones that evaporated into air and candles scented with it became the rage.

Family: Lamiaceae (Labiatae)

Extraction: Distilled from the leaves. The scent is powerful and minty fresh. Peppermint is one of the few essential oil plants grown and distilled in the United States, where the light cloud cover over central Oregon and Michigan increases oil production, most of which is redistilled to produce a lighter mint flavor for candies, gum, toothpaste, and mouthwash. Several mints are also distilled for perfume.

Medicinal action: Inhaling peppermint steam clears sinus and lung congestion and infection. It alleviates nausea, ulcers, and is a specific remedy for irritable bowel syndrome, for which drugstores sell specially coated, enteric pills that don't dissolve or release the essential oil until they reach the colon. Studies show it enhances digestion by stimulating digestive juices, making digestive tract activity slower and more rhythmical, and destroying viruses, parasites, and bacteria, including salmonella poisoning. In one study, an application of 10 percent peppermint oil on the temples of people suffering from tension headaches provided substantial relief (but take care to keep it out of the eyes). When researchers sponged a combination of peppermint and eucalyptus diluted in alcohol on volunteers' foreheads, their headaches were greatly reduced. Peppermint oil's dual hot and cold action accentuates the warming sensation in liniments and is an excellent remedy for pain.

Cosmetic/skin use: Peppermint stimulates the skin's oil production, so small amounts are appropriate for use on a dry complexion and hair. It also relieves the discomfort of ringworm, herpes simplex, scabies, insect bites, and poison oak, and studies have found it defeats several types of viral and fungal skin infections. When tested against other oils, it proved to be one of the most effective essential oils to kill head lice (one study diluted 2 drops of essential oil in 100 milliliters of equal parts water and vinegar).

Emotional attributes: As a stimulant, the scent counters depression, anxiety, insomnia, shock, mental fogginess, and lack of focus, and unblocks "stuck" emotions. Research volunteers who inhaled a thirty-second puff of peppermint every five minutes found that they were better able to remember and identify complicated patterns on a computer monitor, and brain activity related to seeing and focusing attention was steadier.

Considerations: Watch out—too much oil will burn skin. Do not use more than one or two drops in a bathtub.

Associated Oils

Spearmint *(M. spicata):* Milder in action, spearmint brings back childhood joy and memories. It is the mint of choice for pregnant women and young children, possessing fewer irritating and toxic constituents. The oil's composition varies according to where the plant comes from and how it is grown.

Cornmint *(M. arvensis):* This species is less sweet, but contains much more menthol, making it a good choice for liniments. Cornmint is the source of natural menthol crystals used to produce a stimulating/cooling sensation in liniments, lipstick, hair tonics, and other body-care products. It is cultivated in China and Japan, and in Brazil, by descendants of Japanese immigrants who introduced it there.

Pennyroyal *(M. pulegium):* Pennyroyal occasionally treats fever, itching skin, indigestion, colds, and scant, painful menstruation. The scent relieves dizziness; ancient Romans even wore pennyroyal head garlands to dispel drunkenness. Culpeper dabbed the waters on headaches and the vinegar on bruises and burns. It is used to scent soap and makes a good flea repellent. However, it is potentially toxic and can produce liver toxicity due to its pulegone compounds, so the essential oil should be used with care, if at all. Don't put the oil on your pets since they may lick it and they have very absorbent skin (placing 1 drop of pennyroyal essential oil on your eight-pound cat is the equivalent of using 18 drops of oil on an adult—definitely an overdose). The herbal tea is safer, but pregnant women should avoid even that.

PETITGRAIN

C. aurantium

See Orange Blossom (Neroli).

RAVENSARA

Cinnamomum camphora; "Ravensara aromatica"

Ravensara means "good leaf" in Madagascar, where the seeds are a popular spice. This oil was originally sold as *Ravensara aromatica,* although it is a contrived botanical name. The oil is actually distilled from a chemotype of camphor with a different composition that makes it far less toxic.

Family: Lauraceae

Extraction: Distilled from the leaves and sometimes from the fruit and bark. The scent is similar to a combination of camphor and eucalyptus, but it is softer and more refined.

Medicinal action: Ravensara is a personal favorite of ours for infection. It is an antiseptic treatment for bronchitis, sinus congestion, and other viral infections, such as shingles and viral hepatitis. It makes an excellent massage oil for muscle fatigue and especially for lymphatic problems. It is also thought to boost the immune system.

Cosmetic/skin use: It is useful for acne and infected skin conditions.

Emotional attributes: Like camphor, it counteracts shock and depression and focuses one's attention. Arabs say that camphor reduces sexual desire.

Considerations: This is still an oil to use with some care and not for extended periods of time.

Associated Oils

Camphor *(C. camphora):* Unlike harsh, synthetic mothballs, camphor leaves and bark smell woodsy with a hint of cardamom. In China, statues of Buddha are carved from the wood to inspire devotion; camphor hydrosol is added to wine as a digestive tonic and as flavoring for chicken, which is steamed over the leaves (we've distilled camphor hydrosol for room freshener). Camphor is a heart stimulant and skin irritant, so use it very carefully, if at all. Never use the even more toxic brown or yellow camphor produced from heavier parts of the oil. Ho oil, a sweeter linalol chemotype from Vietnam, is a substitute for endangered rosewood oil. Also use **Borneo (Borneol) Camphor** *(Dryobalanops aromatica)* cautiously. Once used against plague, Marco Polo called it "balsam of disease." Chinese burn the incense during funerals and other important ceremonies and treat wounds, sprains, infectious disease, and nerve pain.

ROSE

Rosa damascena; R. gallica; etc.

The Greek poetess Sappho christened rose the "queen of flowers" in 600 BC. It was one of the favorite medicines of herbalist and visionary Paracelsus, who used it to fight the plague. The Arabs preserved the scent by sealing dried blossoms in clay jars and then sprinkled them with water to freshen them. Rosewater (hydrosol) is a by-product of distillation and a common ingredient in Middle Eastern culinary dishes. One or two tablespoons tastes divine in a variety of sweet dishes such as fruit salad or rice pudding.

Family: Rosaceae

Extraction: Distilled (rose otto) or solvent extracted (rose absolute) from the blossoms. The fragrance is intense, sweet, floral, and easily recognized. It can take up to sixty roses to create 1 drop of this precious oil! Rose oil is costly, not only because the petals have few essential oil glands and so little is produced during distillation, but also because the bushes themselves need so much care and the flowers must be harvested by hand. Also, unlike most essential oils, rose oil is difficult to separate from water because many constituents are very water soluble, so the water is redistilled. The resulting oil congeals at cool temperatures due to its natural waxes. Although originally distilled in Asia Minor, Bulgaria is the world's largest producer, making the most valued rose oil, although China is producing an increased amount. Turkey makes a slightly less expensive oil.

Medicinal action: Honey of Red Rose was once recommended for sore mouths and throats by the official medical references, the *United States* and *British Pharmacopoeia*s. Rose treats asthma, hay fever, nausea, impotency, and it is specific for women's problems, especially menstrual irregularities caused by circulatory congestion. Studies reveal that it may increase sperm count and reduce muscle spasms in the digestive tract. It is even a hangover remedy.

Cosmetic/skin use: A cell rejuvenator, rose is appropriate for all hair and complexion types, including sun-damaged skin. It is useful for most blood vessel problems, including varicose veins and couperose skin. It soothes and heals burns and rashes, and it is a strong antiseptic on bacterial and viral skin infection.

Emotional attributes: The fragrance of rose inspired poets and lovers throughout the ages, and it has been used to "open" the heart and ease grief, heartache, loss, and sadness. During consulting or massage sessions, it helps clients open up and feel more trust about their healing. Employed for relationship conflicts, envy, anger, and intolerance, it is comforting, supportive through crisis, and an aphrodisiac. It also helps alleviate depression, anxiety, fear, insomnia, and lack of confidence.

Considerations: Rose is very nontoxic, but sometimes the essential oil irritates sensitive skin if not well diluted.

Associated Oil

Cabbage Rose *(R. centifolia):* Also called *rose de mai,* this oil is slightly less expensive. Once cultivated extensively in France, cabbage rose now comes mostly from Morocco. This is often the species made into an absolute through solvent extraction, while *R. damascena* is generally distilled.

ROSEMARY

Rosmarinus officinalis

Rosmarinus means "dew of the sea," where this Mediterranean herb loves to grow. Rosemary delights late winter with prolific blooms. The old French name *incensier* came from rosemary's celebrated history as church incense. The stalks, stripped bare of the leaves, make good skewers for barbecue.

Family: Lamiaceae (Labiatae)

Extraction: Distilled from the flowering tops or leaves. The powerful fragrance is herby, sharp, and camphorous. The ratio of compounds in the oil depends on the stage of the plant when it was picked.

Medicinal action: Rosemary is very antiseptic. Until the twentieth century, the fragrant leaves were burned to purify French hospitals. With more antioxidant proper-

ties than most fruits and vegetables, rosemary has been developed into a food preservative through technology that isolates a fraction of the plant to produce a water-soluble extract. Rosemary is one of the best stimulants for the nervous system, adrenal glands, digestion, and poor circulation. It treats lung congestion, sore throats, and canker sores. In penetrating liniments, it eases muscle and rheumatism pain.

Cosmetic/skin use: Rosemary was the main ingredient in the fourteenth-century Hungary water, used for complexion care and as a cologne. Rosemary helps sluggish, underactive skin and is used on dry, mature, and couperose complexion types and varicose veins. It is a potent antibacterial, antiviral, and antifungal for skin. Researchers found that rosemary is a beneficial antioxidant in creams or lotions to minimize free radical damage and protect the skin from cellular damage. They speculated that it even plays a role in helping genes improve skin cells' stress tolerance to oxidation. It also helps reduce cellulite, dermatitis, scars, inflammation, and skin parasites. An age-old dandruff and hair loss remedy for all hair types, rosemary branches were even used as hairbrushes.

Emotional attributes: Rosemary is known as the "herb of remembrance," made famous when Shakespeare's Ophelia said, "There's rosemary, that's for remembrance . . ." The smoke was inhaled for brain weakness. Rosemary's reputation for improving memory is borne out in modern scientific studies showing that its antioxidant actions slow the breakdown of acetylcholine in the brain (many Alzheimer's patients have low levels of this neurotransmitter). The fragrance improves memory, confidence, perception, and creativity, and helps balance mind and body. It also prevents dizziness, grief, dark thoughts, and nightmares, and helps you remember good dreams. Commoners burned rosemary instead of frankincense when they prayed. Everyone carried it to symbolize both love and death at funerals.

Considerations: Rosemary can be overstimulating and may increase blood pressure, although this common warning has probably been exaggerated. It has been shown to accelerate estrogen's action, but only in mice receiving very large doses. Although it does not induce miscarriage, it is often recommended that pregnant women stick to using it as a culinary spice.

Associated Oils

Rosmarinus officinalis has several chemotypes:

Borneol Type: This oil helps overcome fatigue and infections and is a heart tonic.

Camphor Type: This camphorlike scented oil is a vein decongestant, mucolytic, cardiac tonic, and diuretic. This and borneol oil are the stronger and harshest chemotypes due to the camphor compound.

Cineol Type: This oil is especially effective for lung congestion, cystitis, and chronic fatigue.

Verbenone Type: For sinus infections and as a mucolytic and antispasmodic, this helps balance the endocrine and nervous systems. It is suitable for oily or regenerative skin care, but contains some potentially harsh ketones.

Rosmarinus pyramidalis: This oil has respiratory applications, but it is specific for ear and sinus problems.

ROSEWOOD

Aniba roseodora

The French call this South American rain forest tree *bois de rose,* or "wood of rose." Rosewood was first distilled in 1875 in French Guiana, but it became so popular that all the trees were cut. It reminds us that the rain forest is a valuable resource needing protection. We recommend using rose geranium, palmarosa, coriander, or ho wood mixed with rose as substitutes. See our concerns in the section on sustainability on page 151.

Family: Lauraceae

Extraction: Distilled from wood chips. The pleasant fragrance is sweet, woodsy, and rosy.

Medicinal action: Rosewood eases headaches and fights colds, fevers, nausea, and many types of infections, including vaginitis.

Cosmetic/skin use: Rosewood rejuvenates cells and is suitable for use on all complexion types.

Emotional attributes: An antidepressant, rosewood encourages tranquility and constructive emotional work.

SAGE

Salvia officinalis

Familiar as a culinary herb, sage comes from Spain and Asia Minor. Only a few of the many species are distilled. We've made wonderful hydrosols from pineapple sage *(S. elegans).*

Family: Lamiaceae (Labiatae)

Extraction: Distilled from the leaves. The scent is spicy, sharp, and very herby. An oleoresin is produced from the exhausted material that has been distilled.

Medicinal action: During the Renaissance, it was asked, "How can a man die who has sage in his garden?" pointing to sage's usefulness in treating so many ailments. In ancient Crete, the burning leaves were inhaled to relieve asthma. A decongestant with antiseptic properties, the diluted oil or herbal tea makes an excellent sore throat gargle. Sage's antioxidant properties are on par with rosemary, and the herb was used to preserve food, as well as to digest it. It also has hormonal estrogenic action, decreasing excessive menstruation, lactation, and alleviating menopause symptoms, especially hot flashes.

Cosmetic/skin use: Sage reduces perspiration, oily skin and hair, and acne, and is said to encourage hair growth. It also treats insect bites, boils, and bacterial skin infections. Its drying action makes it good in a deodorant, but read "Considerations" first.

Emotional attributes: The sixteenth-century herbalist John Gerard said of sage, "It is singularly good for the head, brain . . . it quickeneth the senses, memory." It looks like the herb does slow loss of short-term memory by preventing breakdown of the chemical messenger acetylcholine in the brain and blocking an enzyme called AChE (acetylcholinesterase) that is associated with memory loss and that seems to play a role in Alzheimer's and possibly other degenerative brain diseases. It does so without disrupting other brain activity or damaging the liver. Sage's anti-inflammatory and antioxidant properties may be useful in treating other problems associated with Alzheimer's. Sage also helps those suffering from excessive sexual desire, grief, physical overexertion, and insomnia and it encourages inward focus.

Considerations: Sage was a medieval tonic to reduce nervous tics, but since the essential oil contains high quantities of the compound thujone, a neurotoxic ketone, it can be toxic to the nervous system and kidneys. That means anyone prone to seizures or nervous system problems should avoid using it as an essential oil and stick to the culinary herb. Even then, it is recommended to drink sage tea no more than few times a week. Sage is also irritating to skin and mucous membranes, so use it topically in low dilutions.

Associated Oil
See Clary Sage.

Spanish Sage *(S. lavandulaefolia):* Less toxic and irritating than common sage, this oil is useful for acne, eczema, and dermatitis, and it helps relieve arthritis, poor circulation, and the flu. The distinctive lavender fragrance is so strong, it can be mistaken for lavender.

SANDALWOOD
Santalum album

One of the oldest perfume materials, sandalwood has been in use for at least two thousand years.

Family: Santalaceae

Extraction: Distilled; CO_2. The scent is balsamic, soft, warm, and woodsy. The tree begins producing oil after thirty years, and only from the heartwood and some roots. Mysore, India, has high quality oil, which the government tries to regulate, but wild trees have been endangered for some time. We recommend cultivated Australian or Indonesian sandalwood. In India, the oil is often distilled with another plant at the same time to create an attar, although this term is not always used correctly.

Medicinal action: Once a gonorrhea treatment, sandalwood is still used for genital and urinary infections. It also counters inflammation, hemorrhoids, persistent coughs, nausea, throat problems, and some types of nerve pain and fungal infections.

Cosmetic/skin use: Suitable for all hair and complexion types, sandalwood is especially useful on rashes, inflammation, and mature, dry, acne-prone, or chapped skin, and dry hair. It hastens the repair of damaged skin and reduces scarring. The essential oil inhibits herpes simplex virus from replicating in the laboratory, working on the virus before it is absorbed and in a different manner than the drug acyclovir. Rather than directly killing the infection, it seems to help cells protect themselves by reinforcing their protective envelopes and modulating liver processes.

Emotional attributes: Sandalwood improves depression, anxiety, stess, and insomnia. It helps promote spiritual practices, peaceful relaxation, openness, and "grounding," and it comforts mourners during funeral ceremonies.

Associated Oils

Australian Sandalwood *(S. spicatum)*. Australian is very similar to Indian sandalwood. Two newer oils from Australia are *S. yasi* and *S. austracalidonicum.*

Amyris *(Amyris balsamifera):* This small Haitian tree called *West Indian rosewood* often scents "sandalwood" soap.

SPEARMINT

M. spicata

See Peppermint.

SPIKENARD

Nardostachys jatamansi

Ancient Egyptians and Romans made this expensive essential oil into the very popular *nardinum* ointment, which Mary Magdalene lavishly poured over Christ's feet and is mentioned in the bible's Song of Solomon.

Family: Valerianaceae

Extraction: Distilled from the rhizome; CO_2. The scent is earthy and strong, reminiscent of both valerian and patchouli. Properly produced oil is greenish, while *N. grassilis* is pale yellow. It grows in Pakistan and the Himalayan mountains (see our concerns in the section on sustainability on page 151).

Medicinal action: Considered a nerve and liver tonic, spikenard treats nervous indigestion, insomnia, headaches, and heart palpitations.

Cosmetic/skin use: Spikenard has a long history of use for hair loss, scalp irritation, skin inflammation, rashes, and psoriasis. It is beneficial for all skin and hair types, but especially on a dry or mature complexion.

Emotional attributes: Spikenard relieves emotional tension and insomnia. It is traditionally applied to the feet for "grounding." Studies indicate that it increases growth of

nerve endings and that its sedative action blocks nerve cells called ganglions without depressing the parasympathetic nervous system that controls many of the body's automatic responses.

Associated Oils

Valerian *(Valeriana officinalis):* Isovaleric acid is the compound responsible for a strong and pungent scent that has been compared to dirty socks, so valerian is not often used in aromatherapy, although carefully blending small amounts with softer-smelling oils is very effective. Studies show that the oil decreases mental stress and relaxes the brain, muscles, and nervous system. The herb has been shown to decrease theta waves and increase beta waves, in a manner very similar to the sedative drug diazepam, but without the drug's intensity or side effects. A CO_2 extract is available. Ayurvedic medicine uses Indian valerian *(V. wallichii).*

TEA TREE

Melaleuca alternifolia

European explorers made tea out of the leaves of this large Australian tree, so they named it *tea* tree (which is sometimes spelled *ti*). It was once given to soldiers for their first aid kits.

Family: Myrtaceae

Extraction: Distilled from the leaves. The scent is similar to its relative eucalyptus, but softer. Poor-quality oil smells more like melted rubber.

Medicinal action: Tea tree's main use is to counter bacterial, fungal (including candida and thrush), and viral infections, with numerous studies backing it. It became popular after researchers found that it reduced mouth infection, and marketers introduced tea tree toothpaste, mouthwash, and even toothpicks. It also treats the flu and lung, genital and urinary, vaginal, sinus, mouth, and respiratory infections. Contact with blood and pus actually increases its antiseptic properties, and it boosts production of the immune system's interleukin, while reducing tumors. In other studies, it decreased prostaglandins, which are responsible for causing inflammation, by as much as one-third.

Cosmetic/skin use: Tea tree is ideal for oily skin and hair and to eliminate dandruff and scalp dermatitis. It is especially useful in healing wounds, acne, dermatitis, diaper rash, warts, scabies, and various bacterial and fungal infections. It is one of the most nonirritating antiseptic oils, although this varies with the particular species. A 3 percent concentration has been shown to be effective on herpes simplex virus. Also use it on the related shingles and chicken pox viruses. Researchers found that it protects skin from radiation burns during cancer therapy and, in one study, suppressed inflammatory skin disorders associated with immune system problems and skin cancer. It also relieves the inflammation and discomfort of sunburn and insect bites. Researchers found that tea tree kills mites and ticks and is one of the best essential oils to destroy head lice.

Emotional attributes: The scent builds strength, especially before an operation and during postoperative shock.

Associated Oils

The numerous species and subspecies all have an interesting, paperlike bark that curls off the trunk.

Cajeput *(M. cajuputi):* The name *cajeput* comes from the Malaysian *caju-puti,* meaning "white bark." It is a vein decongestant and is harsher than tea tree oil.

MQV *(M. quinquenervia):* This sweeter-smelling "tea tree" works for respiratory problems and is considered a good immune system tonic. It is wonderful in an aromatherapy diffuser.

Niaouli *(M. viridiflora):* Called *Gomen oil* because it was once shipped from that West Indies port, niaouli is now harvested in Australia. It is considered especially effective in fighting viruses such as herpes. It also has a sweeter, more pleasant fragrance.

Manuka *(Leptospermum scoparium):* Also known as New Zealand tea tree, manuka is very antiseptic and antifungal, especially on lung and urinary tract infections and skin infections such as *Staphylococcus* and ringworm. It is antiviral against the herpes simplex virus. Studies have shown that the oil is an antioxidant, antihistamine, lung expectorant, and anti-inflammatory. The scent is used to counter fear and low libido. In Maori, *maukanuka* means "anxiety," reflecting its traditional use as a nervine and sedative. It may act on the same receptors as benzodiazepine drugs to relax the mind. The lemon-scented **Lemon Manuka** *(L. citratum)* has similar properties.

Lemon Tea Tree *(L. petersonii):* Despite its name, this is another manuka, with a refreshing citrus scent. It is antiseptic and well suited for treating acne, oily skin, insect bites, and respiratory problems.

Kanuka *(Kunzea ericoides,* formerly *Leptospermum ericoides):* In New Zealand, kanuka leaves are traditionally used in vapor baths to relieve colds, inflammation, and fever. The sap has long been considered a blood purifier, and the oil treats urinary tract infections. Kanuka is similar to manuka, but it contains monoterpene compounds instead of manuka's larger and heavier sesquiterpenes.

THUJA

Thuja occidentalis

See Cedarwood.

THYME

Thymus vulgaris

Ancient Greeks complimented each other as "smelling like *thymbra,*" their word *thymian* meant "to burn as incense," and *thymiatechny* described the "art of using perfumes as medicine." Rudyard Kipling wrote of the "wind-bit thyme that smells like the perfume of the dawn in paradise."

Family: Lamiaceae (Labiatae)

Extraction: Distilled from the leaves; absolute. The scent is strong, herbaceous, sweet, and medicinal. Thyme can contain a considerable quantity of essential oil, with up to 6 percent in summer-harvested French thyme. When first distilled, thyme oil is red, quite hot, and a harsh skin irritant, although a stronger antiseptic than white thyme, but it is usually redistilled, yielding clear *white* thyme. Several species are available as *red* thyme, such as *Thymus vulgaris* and *T. satureioides.*

Medicinal action: Thyme is a potent antioxidant, antibacterial, antifungal, and a favored treatment for mouth infection, including thrush. Find its compound thymol in cough drops, warming vapor rubs such as Vicks, and gargles such as Listerine, which comparison studies rated as very effective in destroying mouth bacteria. Thyme relieves lung congestion and was once a specific whooping cough remedy. Researchers tell us that it helps destroy the *Helicobacter pylori* bacteria responsible for stomach ulcers and the common vaginal infections candida and *Trichomonas,* even in low concentrations. Thyme kills intestinal worms, and it works against drug-resistant *Campylocbacter jejuni,* the most common bacterial cause of diarrhea. The twelfth-century herbalist and abbess Saint Hildegard of Bingen recorded a vapor balm recipe using thyme and sage to ease pain and kill lice.

Emotional attributes: Thyme relieves mental instability, fear, melancholy, and nightmares and prevents memory loss and inefficiency. It is considered to be fortifying to the spirit.

Considerations: Be careful! Thyme oil burns delicate membranes and irritates skin unless you use a gentle chemotype (see below) or dilute well.

Associated Oils

Thymus vulgaris has many chemotypes and at least a hundred varieties (double that if you count the cultivars):

Geraniol Type: This gentler antiseptic treats vaginitis, cystitis, acne, eczema, and earaches. It is a uterine and cardiac tonic with a mildness (comparable to the linalol type) from the abundance of the compound geraniol.

Linalol Type: This nontoxic antiseptic treats bronchitis, acne, nervous fatigue, psoriasis, prostate problems, candida, and urinary tract infections. Its compound linalol is nonirritating, making it gentle enough for children and skin care.

Thymol Type: Stimulating and very antibacterial, this chemotype is common, although the thymol compound makes it potentially irritating to skin and mucous membranes and gives it a harsh aroma.

Thujanol Type: This type is high in thujanol and terpenes, but low in the more-irritating and somewhat-toxic phenols such as thymol. It treats viral infections, with French research showing it to be effective against sexually transmitted disorders, such as chlamydia and the condyloma virus that causes venereal warts.

Thyme Species

Moroccan; Sweet Thyme *(T. satureioides):* This species contains 70 to 80 percent borneol, an immune-supporting alcohol. It is a digestive stimulant that also settles nerves and is used to treat chronic fatigue syndrome. In one study, the red version of this oil killed all bacteria tested, including *Salmonella* and *Staphylococcus.*

Spanish; Wild Marjoram *(Thymus mastichina):* Several species of thyme, including this North African one, are sold as "marjoram." It is an antiseptic for upper-respiratory infections, but not a sedative or muscle relaxant like sweet marjoram. It is also much harsher and less expensive.

Spanish Oregano *(Thymus capitatus):* Called *origan* in the perfume trade, this is really thyme with a scent similar to oregano. It can irritate the skin and should be used very cautiously, if at all.

TUBEROSE

Polianthes tuberosa

One of the most expensive flower oils, the intensely fragrant tuberose from Mexico is also grown in India and the Tropics. The Aztecs prized it as medicine, and Hawaiian leis are often made with it. It is used mostly for fragrance, in which it has found international fame in perfumes such as White Shoulders and Chloé. The name comes from its tuberous root.

Family: Agavaceae

Extraction: Produced through enfleurage at one time; now is available as concrete; absolute. This solvent-extracted oil has a slightly "green" fragrance. The scent is floral, very sweet, and similar to honey, with a slight hint of camphor. Sometimes the oil is made from the slightly less odorous double-petaled garden flower.

Emotional attributes: The fragrance is sensual and an aphrodisiac. Its East Indian name *rat ki rani* means "mistress of the night."

VANILLA

Vanilla planifolia

This tropical native Mexican orchid is now grown in Tahiti, Java, and Madagascar. Orchids are considered the most highly evolved flowers, and this is the only one with an edible fruit. When first transplanted on the island of Réunion, vanilla didn't produce pods because the hummingbirds and bees that pollinate it don't live there. A hand pollination method developed in 1841 is still used today. In the Tonga Islands, vanilla beans are extracted in coconut oil for body lotion.

Family: Orchidaceae

Extraction: (resinoid; absolute; oleoresin; CO_2) These extracts are quite thick, making it difficult to work with them unless they have been thinned, usually with a solvent. Many aromatherapy products are made instead with the vanilla extract used in cooking. The scent is sweet, balsamic, creamy, and typically vanilla.

Emotional attributes: Vanilla's fragrance is consoling and soothing, and it improves one's confidence and helps dissolve pent-up anger and frustration. An aphrodisiac, it can unleash hidden sensuality. It is usually considered a stimulant, exciting the brain and even preventing sleep in some people, although it also used to subdue hysteria. Studies show that children like this aroma, possibly because chemists found it is the closest natural scent to mother's milk.

VETIVER; VETIVERT

Vetiveria zizanioides

Vetiver is not a picturesque plant with its grasslike leaves, but the aromatic roots are its treasure. In India, the roots are woven into door and window screens called *tatties* or *khustaties* and fans. The British occupation of India made vetiver water and cologne popular in nineteenth-century England and North America. The perfume Mousseline des Indes took its name from Indian muslin scented with vetiver to protect it from insects. Two Victorian perfumes, Maréchale and Bouquet de Roi, were also based on vetiver. Modern perfume uses it to add a deep note and it fixes (stabilizes) the scent. Vast areas of India are covered with the wild plants, which reduce soil erosion.

Family: Poaceae (Gramineae)

Extraction: Distilled from the root; CO_2. Vetiver has an earthy, heavy scent. The essential oil is quite different depending on which country produces it. The main sources are Réunion, Haiti (with a highly regarded roseate note in its oil), and India (with wild roots that are often preferred for their balsamic, woody scent). Inferior oil is made from old vetiver screens. Brazil is also cultivating vetiver.

Medicinal action: Vetiver eases muscular pain, sprains, and liver congestion, and is a circulatory stimulant. It has a cooling action on fevers and other "hot" disorders such as inflammation.

Cosmetic/skin use: Vetiver treats acne, wounds, and dry skin.

Emotional attributes: The scent is uplifting, relaxing, and comforting, releasing deep fear and tension. It cools the body and mind of excessive heat and grounds, centers, and gives individuals who tend to feel nervous, anxious, or overly sensitive a sense of security.

WINTERGREEN

Gaultheria procumbens

See Birch.

YLANG-YLANG

Cananga odorata

Ylang-ylang, meaning "flower of flowers," is a Philippine native. The flowers are grown for the perfume trade.

Family: Annonaceae

Extraction: Distilled from the flowers; absolute; concrete. The intensely sweet scent is heady (described by some as similar to bananas) and floral. It is very cloying and long lasting. The oil varies greatly because of climatic and botanical differences, with some of the best originating in Réunion. The commercial grades are *Extra* (the finest, first distillation), followed by *One, Two,* and *Three. Complete* mixes all the grades together. An inexpensive cananga oil (type macrophylla) is inferior because it is rich in terpene and low in ester compounds.

Medicinal action: A strong sedative, ylang-ylang is antispasmodic and helps lower blood pressure.

Cosmetic/skin use: Ylang-ylang is a tonic that balances oil production for all skin and hair types, although it is most often recommended to correct dry conditions. A Victorian-era hair tonic called Macassar oil contained ylang-ylang, and it was so oily that doilies were placed on high-backed chairs to protect the fabric from stains.

Emotional attributes: The fragrance is very relaxing, but can also reverse fatigue. It makes the senses more acute and tempers depression, fear, jealousy, anger, and frustration. It is an aphrodisiac in low dilutions.

Considerations: High concentrations can produce headaches or nausea.

Materia Medica Essential Oils at a Glance

This list will help you easily locate all of the essential oils covered in this chapter or in chapter 14. This chapter includes a descriptive paragraph for each primary oil. Secondary oils, which are related botanically or chemically to primary oils but used less often, are described as subheadings under primary oils. In the list below, all of the oils are in alphabetical order. Primary oils are in bold and secondary oils are indented. Botanical names tend to change over the years, so some oils have two Latin names.

Agarwood (*Aquilaria agallocha*): See chapter 14.
Ajowan (*Trachyspermum ammi; Carum copticum*): See chapter 14.
Allspice (*Pimento doica; P. officinalis*): See Bay.
Ambrette (*Hibiscus abelmoschus; Abelmoschus moschatus*): See chapter 14.

Amyris (*Amyris balsamifera*): See Sandalwood.

Angelica (*Angelica archangelica*)

Angelica, Indian (*Angelica glauca*): See chapter 14.

Anise (*Pimpinella anisum*)

Anise, Star (*Illicium verum*): See Anise.

Anise, Turkish (*Pimpinella anisetum*): See Anise.

Balsam, Canadian (*Abies balsamea*): See Fir.

Balsam of Peru (*Myroxylon balsamum* var. *pereirae*): See Benzoin.

Balsam of Tolu (*Myroxylon balsamum*): See Benzoin.

Basil (*Ocimum basilicum*)

Basil, Hairy or Hoary (*Ocimum canum; O. americanum*): See Basil.

Basil, Holy (*Ocimum tenuiflorum; O. sanctum*): See Basil and chapter 14.

Basil, Réunion (*Ocimum basilicum*): See Basil.

Bay (*Laurus nobilis*)

Bay Rum (*Pimenta racemosa*): See Bay.

Benzoin (*Styrax benzoin*)

Bergamot (*Citrus bergamia*)

Birch (*Betula lenta*)

Black Pepper (*Piper nigrum*): See Black Pepper and chapter 14.

Cade (*Juniperus communis*): See Juniper.

Cajeput (*Melaleuca cajuputi*): See Tea Tree.

Calamus, Indian (*Acorus odorata*): See chapter 14.

Camphor (*Cinnamomum camphora*): See chapter 14.

Camphor, Borneo (*Dryobalanops aromatica*): See Ravensara.

Cananga (*Cananga odorata* type *macrophylla*): See Ylang-Ylang.

Cape Snowbush (*Eriocephalus africanus*): See Chamomile.

Cape Verbena; Zinziba (*Lippia javanica*): See Lemon Verbena.

Caraway (*Carum carvi*)

Cardamom (*Eletteria cardamomum*): See Cardamom and chapter 14.

Carrot Seed (*Daucus carota*)

Cassia (*Cinnamomum cassia; C. aromaticum*): See Cinnamon.

Cassie (*Acacia farnesiana*): See Cinnamon.

Catnip, Lemon (*Nepeta cataria*): See Melissa.

Cedarwood (*Cedrus* species)

Cedarwood, Moroccan (*Cedrus libani*): See Cedarwood.

Cedarwood, Tibetan (*Cedrus deodara*): See Cedarwood and chapter 14.

Cedarwood, Virginia (*Juniperus virginiana*): See Juniper.

Cedro Oil (*Citrus limon*): See Lemon.

Celery Seed (*Apium graveolens*): See chapter 14.

Chamomile, Cape (*Eriocephalus punctulatus*): See Chamomile.

Chamomile, German (*Matricaria recutita: M. chamomilla*)

Chamomile, Moroccan or Ormenis (*Chamaemelum mixtum; Anthemis mixta; Ormenis mixta*): See Chamomile.

Chamomile, Roman (*Chamaemelum nobilis; Anthemis nobilis*): See Chamomile.

Cilantro (*Coriandrum sativum*): See Coriander.

Cinnamon (*Cinnamomum verum; C. zeylanicum*)

Cistus; Labdanum (*Cistus ladaniferus*)

Citronella (*Cymbopogon nardus*): See Lemongrass.

Clary Sage (*Salvia sclarea*)

Clove Bud (*Syzygium aromaticum*, formerly *Eugenia caryophyllata*)

Copal (*Copaiba officinalis*): See Myrrh.

Coriander (*Coriandrum sativum*)

Cornmint (*Mentha arvensis*): See Peppermint.

Costus (*Saussurea lappa*): See chapter 14.

Cubeb (*Piper cubeba; P. officinalis*): See Black Pepper.

Cumin (*Cuminum cyminum*): See chapter 14.

Cumin, Black (*Nigella sativa*): See Carrier Oils.

Cyperus (*Cyperus scariosus*): See chapter 14.

Cypress (*Cupressus sempervirens*)

Davana (*Artemesia pallens*): See chapter 14.

Dill (*Anethum graveolens*): See Fennel.

Elemi (*Canarium luzonicum*): See Frankincense.

Eucalyptus (*Eucalyptus globulus*)

    Eucalyptus, Australian (*Eucalyptus australiana*): See Eucalyptus.

    Eucalyptus, Blue Mallee (*Eucalyptus polybractea*): See Eucalyptus.

    Eucalyptus, Grey (*Eucalyptus radiata*): See Eucalyptus.

    Eucalyptus, Gully Gum (*Eucalyptus smithii*): See Eucalyptus.

    Eucalyptus, Lemon (*Eucalyptus citriodora*): See Eucalyptus.

    Eucalyptus, Peppermint; Dives (*Eucalyptus piperita; E. dives*): See Eucalyptus.

Fennel (*Foeniculum vulgare*): See Fennel and chapter 14.

Fenugreek (*Trigonella foenum-graecum*): See chapter 14.

Fir (*Abies alba* and other species)

    Fir, Siberian (*Abies siberica*): See Fir.

Frankincense (*Boswellia carterii*)

    Frankincense, Indian; Boswellia (*Boswellia serrata*): See Frankincense and chapter 14.

Galanga; Galangal (*Alpina officinalis; A. galanga*): See Ginger and chapter 14.

Galbanum (*Ferula galbaniflua*): See chapter 14.

Geranium (*Pelargonium graveolens*)

    Geranium, Cape Rose (*Pelargonium capitatum* x *radens*): See Geranium.

    Geranium, Lemon (*P. odoratissimum*): See Geranium.

Ginger (*Zingiber officinale*): See Ginger and chapter 14.

Grapefruit (*Citrus* x *paradisi*): See Orange.

Guggul (*Commiphora mukul*): See chapter 14.

Hedychium; Ginger Lily (*Hedychium spicatum*): See chapter 14.

Helichrysum (*Helichrysum angustifolium; H. italicum*)

Hemlock (*Tsuga canadensis*): See Fir.

Ho Oil (*Cinnamomum camphora*): See Ravensara.

Hyssop (*Hyssopus officinalis*)

Inula, Sweet (*Inula graveolens; I. odorata*)

Jasmine (*Jasminium officinale* and *J. grandiflorum*): See Jasmine and chapter 14.

    Jasmine, Sambac (*Jasminium sambac*): See Jasmine.

Juniper (*Juniperus communis*)

Kanuka (*Kunzea ericoides; Leptospermum ericoides*): See Tea Tree.

Keawa; Screw Pine (*Pandanus tectoriu; P. odoratissimus*): See chapter 14.

Lavandin (*Lavandula* x *intermedia: L.* x *hybrida*): See Lavender.

Lavender (*Lavandula angustifolia; L. vera; L. officinale*)

    Lavender, Spike (*Lavandula latifolia; L spica*): See Lavender.

    Lavender, Stoechas (*Lavandula stoechas*): See Lavender.

Lemon (*Citrus limon*)

Lemon Balm (*Melissa officinalis*): See Melissa.

Lemon Verbena (*Aloysia triphylla; Lippia citriodora*)

Lemongrass (*Cymbopogon citratus*)

    Lemongrass, Cochin (*Cymbopogon flexuosus*): See Lemongrass.

Lime (*Citrus aurantifolia*): See Orange.

Litsea (*Litsea cubeba*)

Lotus (*Nelumbo nucifera*): See chapter 14.

Lovage (*Levisticum officinale*): See Angelica.

Manuka (*Leptospermum scoparium*): See Tea Tree.

Manuka, Lemon (*Leptospermum citratum*): See Tea Tree.

Marigold, French (*Tagetes minuta; T. erecta; T. patula*): See Carrot Seed.

Marjoram (*Origanum majorana; Majorana hortensis*)

    Marjoram, Spanish (*Thymus mastichina*): See Thyme.

    Marjoram, Spanish (*Thymus mastichina*): See Marjoram.

Mastic (*Pistacia lentiscus*)

Melissa or Lemon Balm (*Melissa officinalis*)

Mugwort, Greater (*Artemisia arborescens*): See Chamomile.

Myrrh (*Commiphora myrrha*)

Myrtle (*Myrtus communis*)

Neroli (Orange Blossom) *(Citrus aurantium)*:
  See Orange Blossom.

Nutmeg *(Myristica fragrans)*: See chapter 14.

Oakmoss *(Evernia prunastri)*

Olibanum *(Boswellia papyrifera)*: See Frankincense.

Opopanax *(Commiphora erythraea)*: See Myrrh.

Orange *(Citrus sinensis)*

Orange Blossom (Neroli) *(Citrus aurantium)*

Orange, Bitter *(Citrus aurantium)*: See Orange Blossom.

Oregano *(Origanum vulgare)*: See Marjoram.

Oregano, Spanish *(Thymus capitatus)*: See Marjoram.

Oregano, Spanish *(Thymus capitatus)*: See Thyme.

Palmarosa *(Citrus martini)*: See Lemongrass.

Patchouli *(Pogostemon cablin)*

Pennyroyal *(Mentha pulegium)*: See Peppermint.

Pepper Tree, Peruvian *(Schinus molle)*: See Black Pepper.

Peppermint *(Mentha piperita)*

Petitgrain *(Citrus aurantium)*: See Orange Blossom.

Pine *(Pinus species)*: See Fir.

Pine, Ocean *(Pinus palustris)*: See Fir.

Pine, Scotch; White *(Pinus sylvestris)*: See Fir.

Plai *(Zingiber cassumunar)*: See Ginger.

Ravensara *(Cinnamomum camphora; "Ravensara aromatica")*

Rose *(Rose damascena)*
  Rose, Cabbage *(Rosa centifolia)*: See Rose.

Rosemary *(Rosmarinus officinalis)*

Rosewood *(Aniba roseodora)*

Sage *(Salvia officinalis)*
  Sage, Spanish *(Salvia lavandulaefolia)*: See Sage and chapter 14.

Sandalwood *(Santalum album)*
  Sandalwood, Australian *(Santalum spicatum)*:
    See Sandalwood.

Spearmint *(Mentha spicata)*: See Peppermint.

Spikenard *(Nardostachys jatamansi)*

Spruce, Black *(Picea mariana)*: See Fir.

Storax; Styrax *(Liquidambar orientalis)*: See Benzoin.

Tangerine or Mandarin *(Citrus reticulata)*: See Orange.

Tansy, Blue *(Tanacetum annuum)*: See Chamomile.

Tea Tree *(Melaleuca alternifolia)*

Terebinth *(Pinus palustris and others)*: See Fir.

Thuja *(Thuja occidentalis)*: See Cedarwood.

Thyme *(Thymus vulgaris)*
  Thyme, Moroccan *(Thymus satureioides)*: See Thyme.

Tuberose *(Polianthes tuberosa)*

Turmeric *(Curcuma longa)*: See chapter 14.

Valerian *(Valeriana officinalis)*: See Spikenard.

Vanilla *(Vanilla planifolia)*

Vetiver; Vetivert *(Andropogon zizanioides; Vetiveria zizanioides)*: See Vetiver; Vetivert and chapter 14.

Wintergreen *(Gaultheria procumbens)*: See Birch.

Ylang-Ylang *(Cananga odorata)*

Charts

THE FOLLOWING CHARTS distill the information presented in this book into an easy-to-use format. They will help you choose at a glance the best essential oils for your project. We think that the creative—and most fun—part of aromatherapy is designing your own formulas. These custom-made blends are also the most effective because you add your intention to them.

To use the charts, choose a condition you would like to treat and read down that column to see what oils are suggested. In most cases there are more oils listed than you need for one formula, so look up each one in chapter 15, "Materia Medica." Reading about all of the attributes of each oil will make it obvious which one is best suited for your blend. You can also base your selection on the availability of the oils, perhaps choosing ones that you already have, that are easily available, or that fit your price range. Once your essential oil blend is completed, information in chapter 5, "Guidelines for Using Essential

Oils and Herbs," will help you decide which base is the most appropriate to dilute the blend and the best way to use it.

You can also use these charts to learn more about a particular essential oil by reading across the column to see the conditions that it treats. This will help you choose which essential oils to purchase. Use these charts to help you put together an aromatherapy collection for a particular purpose, say for a first-aid kit or a complexion-care kit for a specific skin type. You may be surprised how many things you can do with just four or five essential oils.

For the charts, we selected essential oils that are used most often. After you have some expertise in formulating, you will probably want to expand your selection to other essential oils and may even find yourself making your own charts. We find that charts are not only an excellent learning tool, but prove very handy even after you have years of aromatherapy experience.

FRAGRANCES FOR EMOTIONS

See chapter 4 for more information.

	ANGER	ANXIETY	FATIGUE	DEPRESSION	FEAR	FORGETFULNESS	GRIEF	HYPERSENSITIVITY	INSOMNIA	NERVOUSNESS	PANIC/SHOCK	STRESS/OVERWORK	IRRITABILITY	key word
angelica			X	X								X		perception
anise						X			X			X		thoughtfulness
basil	X		X									X		confidence
bay						X					X			purpose
benzoin		X								X		X		protection
bergamot		X		X					X			X		noncompulsiveness
cardamom		X	X			X						X		warmth
cedarwood		X	X					X				X	X	stamina
chamomile	X	X		X	X			X	X			X		resistance
cinnamon		X										X	X	invigoration
clary sage				X				X			X	X	X	exhilaration
clove			X			X						X		direction
cypress		X	X	X			X		X				X	purpose
eucalyptus			X								X	X		energy
fennel		X				X			X			X		clarity
frankincense		X	X				X		X	X		X		faith
geranium	X	X		X				X	X					balance
helichrysum			X	X								X		fortitude
hyssop	X				X		X							strength
jasmine	X	X	X	X					X			X		fantasy
juniper		X					X					X		renewal
lavender	X	X	X	X		X		X	X	X	X	X		tranquility

FRAGRANCES FOR EMOTIONS

	ANGER	ANXIETY	FATIGUE	DEPRESSION	FEAR	FORGETFULNESS	GRIEF	HYPERSENSITIVITY	INSOMNIA	NERVOUSNESS	PANIC/SHOCK	STRESS/OVERWORK	IRRITABILITY	key word
lemon			X	X		X						X		purity
lemon verbena				X		X			X	X		X		purity
litsea		X				X					X			regrouping
marjoram		X	X	X			X	X	X	X		X		comfort
melissa	X	X			X	X			X	X		X	X	stability
myrrh		X		X				X				X		devotion
neroli	X	X	X	X	X			X	X	X		X	X	confidence
nutmeg		X								X		X		mindlessness
orange/lime		X		X							X	X	X	happiness
patchouli		X	X	X									X	compromise
peppermint		X	X	X		X				X	X	X		energy
petitgrain		X		X					X		X			expansion
pine		X		X										direction
rose	X	X		X	X		X	X		X	X	X		comfort
rosemary		X				X	X			X				perception
sage							X		X			X		focus
sandalwood			X	X					X	X		X		centering
spikenard		X		X					X					peacefulness
thyme					X	X				X		X		awareness
vanilla	X	X								X		X		constructiveness
vetiver				X							X			grounding
ylang-ylang	X		X	X					X		X	X	X	acceptance

ESSENTIAL OILS FOR PHYSICAL PROBLEMS

See chapter 6 for more information. Double checks indicate especially potent oils.

	Circulation / Blood Pressure Problems	Headaches	Hormonal Imbalances	Indigestion	Infections: Bacterial	Infections: Fungal	Infections: Viral	Inflammation	Lung / Sinus Congestion	Menstrual Problems	Pain / Muscle Cramps
angelica			X	X					X	X	
anise			X	X	X						
basil	X	X	X	X	X	XX	X		X	X	
bay	X	X			XX		XX		X		X
benzoin					X			X	X		
bergamot					X	XX	XX				
black pepper	X			X	X	X	X		X		X
caraway				X	X	X	X		X	X	X
cedarwood					X				X		
chamomile		X		X	X	X	X	XX		X	X
cinnamon		X		X	X	XX	X				X
clary sage		X	X		X			X		X	
clove	X	X		X	XX	XX	X		X		X
coriander		X		X		X	X				
cypress					X				X		
eucalyptus		X			XX	XX	XX		X		X
fennel			X	X	X			X	X		
frankincense					X	X		X			X
geranium		X			XX	XX	XX	XX			
ginger	X	X		X	X				X	X	X
helichrysum					XX	X		XX			X
hyssop					X		XX		X		

ESSENTIAL OILS FOR PHYSICAL PROBLEMS

	CIRCULATION / BLOOD PRESSURE PROBLEMS	HEADACHES	HORMONAL IMBALANCES	INDIGESTION	INFECTIONS: BACTERIAL	INFECTIONS: FUNGAL	INFECTIONS: VIRAL	INFLAMMATION	LUNG / SINUS CONGESTION	MENSTRUAL PROBLEMS	PAIN / MUSCLE CRAMPS
juniper				X	X		XX	X	X		X
lavender	X	X		X	XX	X	XX	XX		X	
lemon					XX	X	X				
lemon grass		X		X	XX	XX	XX				X
lemon verbena				X	X				X		X
marjoram	X	X		X	XX	X	X	XX	X		X
melissa	X	X		X	X	XX	XX	X			
myrrh				X	XX	X	X	X			
myrtle					XX			X	X		X
neroli	X		X			X	X	X			
orange	X			X	XX		X				
patchouli					X	X					X
peppermint		X		X	XX	XX	X		X		
ravensara					XX		X		X		X
rose				X	X	X	X	XX		X	
rosemary				X	X		XX		X	X	X
sage			X		XX		XX			X	
sandalwood				X	X	X	X	X			X
thyme		X		X	XX	XX	XX		X		
tea tree					XX	XX	XX	XX			
ylang-ylang	X	X			X	X					

ESSENTIAL OILS FOR SKIN PROBLEMS

See chapter 6 for more information.

	ALLERGIES	BITES	BOILS	BURNS	DERMATITIS	CELL DAMAGE	RASHES/ITCHING	SCARS/STRETCH MARKS	SKIN GROWTHS	VEINS, ENLARGED	WARTS	WOUNDS
basil			X									
carrot seed					X		X	X	X			
cedar		X			X		X					
chamomile	X	X	X	X	X	X	X	X	X	X		
cistus			X		X	X		X				X
clary sage						X						
cypress										X		
eucalyptus		X	X			X		X				
frankincense		X						X	X	X		X
geranium				X		X		X				
helichrysum	X	X		X	X	X		X	X			
lavender	X	X		X	X	X	X	X		X	X	X
litsea	X											
mastic			X							X		X
myrrh										X		X
neroli					X	X						
orange								X				
patchouli								X				
peppermint		X					X					
rose				X	X	X	X					X
rosemary		X				X	X					
sandalwood						X	X	X	X			
tea tree		X		X	X		X				X	X
thuja											X	
thyme		X			X						X	

ESSENTIAL OILS FOR HAIR CARE

See chapter 8 for more information.

	NORMAL HAIR	DRY HAIR	OILY HAIR	DANDRUFF	HAIR GROWTH	HIGHLIGHTS	SCALP DERMATITIS
basil			X		X		
cedar	X	X	X		X		X
chamomile	X	X	X			X	X
clary sage	X	X	X		X		
cypress			X				X
geranium	X	X	X	X			
juniper			X	X			
lavender	X	X	X	X			X
lemon			X			X	
lemongrass			X			X	
patchouli	X	X	X	X			
peppermint		X			X		
rose	X	X	X				
rosemary	X	X		X	X		X
sage			X	X	X		
sandalwood	X	X					X
spikenard	X	X	X		X		
tea tree			X	X			X
ylang-ylang		X		X	X		

ESSENTIAL OILS FOR COMPLEXION TYPES

See chapter 9 for more information.

	Normal Skin	Dry Skin	Oily Skin	Combination Skin	Acne	Couperose Skin	Mature Skin / Wrinkles	Sun-Damaged Skin	Sensitive Skin
basil			X		X				
bergamot			X						
carrot		X				X	X	X	X
cedar	X	X	X	X					
chamomile	X	X	X	X	X	X		X	X
cistus		X			X		X	X	
clary sage	X	X	X	X	X		X		
cypress			X						
eucalyptus			X		X				
fennel							X		
frankincense		X				X	X	X	X
geranium	X	X	X	X	X		X		
helichrysum						X	X	X	X
jasmine	X	X	X	X			X		X
juniper			X		X				
lavender	X	X	X	X	X		X	X	X
lemon			X		X				
lemongrass			X		X				
lemon verbena		X							
myrrh							X		X
myrtle			X	X	X	X			
neroli	X	X		X	X	X	X		X
orange			X						
palmarosa	X	X	X	X	X				
patchouli	X	X	X	X	X		X		X
peppermint		X			X				
ravensara			X		X				
rose	X	X	X	X		X	X		X
rosemary	X	X	X	X	X		X		
sage			X		X				
sandalwood		X			X		X	X	
spikenard	X	X	X	X	X		X		
tea tree			X		X				
vetiver		X							
ylang-ylang		X			X				

Appendix:
Botanical Names of Herbs

This list gives the botanical names for the herbs that are mentioned throughout the book. The botanical names of the essential oils are given in chapter 15.

Alkanet .... *Alkanna tinctoria*
Aloe vera .... *Aloe barbadensis*
Arnica .... *Arnica montana*
Astragalus .... *Astragalus membranicus*

Barberry .... *Berberis vulgaris*
Blackberry .... *Rubus* species
Black cohosh .... *Cimicifuga racemosa*
Black currant .... *Ribes nigrum*
Black haw .... *Viburnum prunifolium*
Black walnut .... *Juglans nigra*
Bladderwrack .... *Fucus vesiculosus*
Blue cohosh .... *Actuea racemosa*
Borage .... *Borago officinalis*
Burdock .... *Arctium lappa*

Calendula .... *Calendula officinalis*
California poppy .... *Eschscholzia californica*
Cascara .... *Frangula purshiana*
Catnip .... *Nepeta cataria*
Celery .... *Apium graveolens*
Chaste berry .... *Vitex agnus-castus*
Chickweed .... *Stellaria media*
Cleavers .... *Galium aparine*
Comfrey .... *Symphytum officinale*

Corn silk .... *Zea mays*
Cramp bark .... *Viburnum opulus*

Dandelion .... *Taraxacum officinalis*
Devil's claw .... *Harpagophytum procumbens*
Dong quai .... *Angelica sinensis*

Echinacea .... *Echinacea purpurea*
                                       or *E. angustifolia*
Elder .... *Sambucus nigra*
Elecampane .... *Inula helenium*

False unicorn .... *Chamaelirium luteum*
Fenugreek .... *Trigonella foenum-graecum*
Flax seed .... *Linum usitatissimum*

Garlic .... *Allium sativum*
Gentian .... *Gentiana lutea*
Ginkgo .... *Ginkgo biloba*
Ginseng .... *Panax ginseng*
Goldenrod .... *Solidago* species
Goldenseal .... *Hydrastis canadensis*
Gotu kola .... *Centella asiatica*
Green tea .... *Camellia sinensis*
Grindelia .... *Grindelia* species

Hawthorn .... *Crataegus laevigata*
Henna .... *Lawsonia* species
Hops .... *Humulus lupulus*

Horehound	*Marrubium vulgare*	Raspberry	*Rubus idaeus*
Horseradish	*Armoracia rusticana*	Red clover	*Trifolium pratense*
Horsetail	*Equisetum arvense*	Reishi mushroom	*Ganoderma lucidum*
Jewelweed	*Impatiens capensis*	Safflower	*Carthamus tinctorius*
		Sarsaparilla	*Smilax officinalis*
Kava	*Piper methysticum*	Sassafras	*Sassafras albidum*
		Saw palmetto	*Serenoa serrulata*
Lady's mantle	*Alchemilla vulgaris*	Schizandra	*Schisandra chinensis*
Licorice	*Glycyrrhiza glabra*	Shepherd's purse	*Capsella bursa-pastoris*
Linden	*Tilia* species	Shiitake mushroom	*Lentinula edodes*
		Siberian ginseng	*Eleutherococcus senticosus*
Marshmallow	*Althea officinalis*	Slippery elm	*Ulmus fulva*
Meadowsweet	*Filipendula ulmaria*	St. John's wort	*Hypericum perforatum*
Milk thistle	*Silybum marianus*	Strawberry	*Fragaria vesca*
Motherwort	*Leonurus cardiaca*		
Mugwort	*Artemisia vulgaris*	Usnea	*Usnea barbata*
Mullein	*Verbascum thapsus*	Uva-ursi	*Arctostaphylos uva ursi*
Mustard	*Brassica nigra*		
		Valerian	*Valeriana officinalis*
Neem	*Azadirachta indica*	Vervain	*Verbena officinalis*
Nettle	*Urtica dioica*		
		Wild cherry bark	*Prunus serotina*
Oregon grape root	*Mahonia aquifolium*	Wild indigo	*Baptisia tinctoria*
		Wild oat	*Lactuca virosa*
Parsley	*Petroselinum crispum*	Wild yam	*Dioscorea villosa*
Partridge berry	*Mitchella repens*	Willow	*Salix alba*
Passionflower	*Passiflora incarnata*	Witch hazel	*Hamaemelis virginiana*
Pau d'Arco	*Tabebuia* species		
Plantain	*Plantago major* or *P. lanceolata*	Yarrow	*Achillea millifolium*
		Yellow dock	*Rumex crispus*

Bibliography

GENERAL BIBLIOGRAPHY

Aftel, Mandy. *Essence and Alchemy.* New York: North Point Press, 2001.

Al-Samarqandi. *The Medical Formulary.* (thirteenth century) Reprint. Edited by Levey, Martin, and Noury al-Khaledy. Oxford: Oxford University Press, 1967.

Alpers, William C. *The Era Formulary.* New York: D. O. Hayes & Co., 1914.

Arctander, Steffen. *Perfume and Flavor Materials of Natural Origins.* Montclair, NJ: Self-published, 1960.

Atal, C. K., and B. M. Kapur, eds. *Cultivation and Utilization of Aromatic Plants.* Jammu-Tawi, India: Regional Research Lab, Council of Scientific & Industrial Research, India, 1982.

Bauer, Kurt, Dorothea Garbe, and Horst Surburg. *Common Fragrance and Flavor Materials.* Weinheim, Germany: VCH, 1990.

Calkin, Robert, and J. Stephan Jellnek. *Perfumery: Practice and Principles.* New York: John Wiley & Sons, 1994.

Chase, Deborah. *The Medically Based No-Nonsense Beauty Book.* New York: Alfred A. Knopf, 1974.

Cooke, Jean, Ann Kramer, and Theodore Rowland-Entwistle. *History's Timeline.* New York: Crescent Books, 1981.

Cooley, Arnold J. *The Toilet and Cosmetic Arts in Ancient and Modern Times.* New York: Burt Franklin, 1970. (Originally published 1866.)

Craker, Lyle E., and James E. Simon, eds. *Herbs, Spices and Medicinal Plants: Recent Advances in Botany, Horticulture, and Pharmacy* 1, Phoenix, AZ: Oryx Press, 1986.

D'Andrea, Jeanne. *Ancient Herbs in the J. Paul Getty Museum Gardens.* Malibu, CA: J. Paul Getty Museum, 1982.

Donato, Giuseppe, and Monique Seefried. *The Fragrant Past: Perfumes of Cleopatra and Julius Caesar.* Rome, Italy: Istituto Poligrafico e Zecca dello Stato, 1989.

Dorland, Gabrielle. *Scents Appeal.* Medham, NJ: Wayne Dorland, 1993.

Dorland, Wayne E. *The Flavors and Fragrance Industry.* Mendham, NJ: W. E. Dorland, 1977.

Duraffourd, Paul. *The Best of Health, Thanks to Essential Oils.* Perigny: La Vie Claire, 1984.

Engen, Trygg. *The Perception of Odors.* New York: Academic Press, 1982.

Gattefossé, René-Maurice. *Gattefossé's Aromatherapy.* Essex, Eng.: C. W. Daniel, 1993.

Genders, Roy. *Perfume Through the Ages.* New York: Putnam, 1972.

Gerard, John. *The Herball, or Generall Historie of Plantes.* (1597) Enlarged by Thomas Johnson. London: Adam Islip, Joice Norton, and Richard Whitakers, 1633.

Gibbons, Boyd. "The Intimate Sense of Smell." *National Geographic,* Sept. 1986.

Gilbert, PhD, Avery N., and Charles J. Wysocki. "The Smell Survey Results." *National Geographic,* 1987.

Gloess, Verlagsgesellschaft, et al. *The H&R Book of Perfume; Fragrance Guide Feminine Notes; Fragrance Guide Masculine Notes; Guide to Fragrance Ingredients* Hamburg: Johnson Pub., 1984.

Greer, Mary. *The Essence of Magic: Tarot, Ritual, and Aromatherapy.* North Hollywood, CA: Newcastle Pub., 1993.

Grieve, Maude. *A Modern Herbal,* vols. I–II. New York: Dover Pub., 1971.

Guenther, Ernest. *The Essential Oils,* vols. I–IV. Malabar, Florida: Robert E. Krieger Pub., 1948 (reprinted 1972).

Gumbel, Dietrich. *Principles of Holistic Skin Therapy with Herbal Essences.* Heidelberg: Karl F. Haug Pubs., 1986.

Hildegard. *Manuscript.* (twelfth century) Reprint. Edited by Strehlow, Wighard and Gottfried Herzka. Santa Fe, NM: Bear & Co., 1987.

Hirsch, Alan. *Scentsational Sex.* Boston, MA: Element, 1998.

Howes, David. New Guinea: An Olfactory Ethnography. In *Dragoco Report,* 2, 1992: 71–81.

Kapoor, L. D. *Handbook of Ayurvedic Medicinal Plants.* Boca Raton, FL: CRC Press, 1990.

Kaufman, William. *Perfume.* New York: E. P. Dutton, 1974.

Keville, Kathi, ed. *The American Herb Association Quarterly*, vols. 7:1–22:1. Nevada City, CA: American Herb Association, 1988–2007.

———. *Herbs: An Illustrated Encyclopedia*. New York: Friedman-Fairfax, 1997.

Landing, James E. *American Essence: History of the Peppermint and Spearmint Industry in the U.S.* Kalamazoo, MI: Kalamazoo Public Museum, 1969.

Langenheim, Jean. *Plant Resins*. Timber Press. Portland, OR, 2003.

Lautié, Raymond, and André Passebecq. *Aromatherapy: The Use of Plant Essences in Healing*. Wellingborough, Eng.: Thorsons, 1979.

Lavabre, Marcel. *Aromatherapy Workbook*. New York: Inner Traditions, 1989.

Lawless, Julia. *The Encyclopedia of Essential Oils*. Rockport, MA: Element Books, 1992.

Le Guérer, Annick. *Scent: The Mysterious and Essential Powers of Smell*. New York: Turtle Bay Books, 1992.

Leung, Albert Y., and Steven Foster. *Encyclopedia of Common Natural Ingredients Used in Food, Drugs and Cosmetics*. New York: Wiley-Interscience, 1996.

Manniche, Lise. *Sacred Luxuries*. Ithaca, NY: Cornell University, 1999.

Maury, Marguerite. *Marguerite Maury's Guide to Aromatherapy: The Secret of Life & Youth*. London: C. W. Daniel, 1989.

Morris, Edwin T. *Fragrance: The Story of Perfume from Cleopatra to Chanel*. New York: Charles Scribner's, 1984.

Parry, Ernest. *The Chemistry of Essential Oils and Artificial Perfumes*, vols. I–II. London: Scott, Greenwood and Son, 1918.

———. *Parry's Cyclopedia of Perfumery*, vols. I–II. Philadelphia: P. Blakiston's Son & Co., 1925.

Piesse, G. W. Septimus. *The Art of Perfumery: Odors of Plants*. Philadelphia: Presley Blakiston, 1880.

Pool, Lawrence J. *Nature's Masterpiece: The Brain and How It Works*. New York: Walker, 1987.

Poucher, William. *Perfumes, Cosmetics and Soaps*. Princeton, NJ: Van Nostrand, 1926.

Richtman, W. O. *Aromatic Waters: 1809–1900*. Milwaukee, WI: Pharmaceutical Review Publishing, 1902.

Rimmel, Eugene. *The Book of Perfume*. London: Chapman & Hall, 1865.

Sacks, Oliver. *The Man Who Mistook His Wife for a Hat*. New York: Summit Books, 1985.

Schnaubelt, Kurt. *The Aromatherapy Course*. San Rafael, California. Self-published, 1985.

School of Salernum. *Regimen Sanitatis Salernitanum*. (Illuminated fourteenth-century text). Translated by John Ordronaux. Reprint. Philadelphia: J. B. Lippincott, 1870.

Teranishi, Roy, Ron G. Buttery, and Hiroshi Sugisawa, eds. *Bioactive Volatile Compounds from Plants*. Washington, D.C.: American Chemical Society, 1993.

Theophrastus. *Enquiry into Plants*. 2 vols. ("Concerning Odors," fourth century BC.) Reprint. Edited by Sir Arthur Hort. London: W. Heinemann, 1916.

Throop, Priscilla. *Hildegard von Bingen's Physica*. Rochester, VT: Healing Arts Press, 1998.

Tisserand, Robert, and Tony Balacs. *Essential Oil Safety: A Guide for Health Care Professionals*. London: Churchill Livingstone, 1995.

Valnet, Jean. *The Practice of Aromatherapy*. Rochester, VT: Healing Arts Press, 1990.

Van Toller, Steve, and George H. Dodd, eds. *Perfumery: The Psychology and Biology of Fragrance*. London: Chapman & Hall, 1988.

Vogel, Vergil J. *American Indian Medicine*. Norman, OK: University of Oklahoma Press, 1970.

Whitfield, Dr. Philip, and D. M. Stoddart. *Hearing, Taste and Smell: Pathways to Perception*. New York: Torstar Books, 1984.

Williams, David. *Perfumes of Yesterday and Today*. Port Washington, NY: Micelle Press, 2004.

Windholtz, Martha, et al., eds. *The Merck Index: An Encyclopedia of Chemicals and Drugs*. 16th ed. Whitehouse Station, NJ: Merck, 2002.

Winter, Ruth. *The Smell Book: Scents, Sex and Society*. Philadelphia: J. B. Lippincott, 1976.

———. *A Consumer's Dictionary of Cosmetic Ingredients*. 3rd rev. ed. New York: Crown Pub., 1989.

Woolley, S. W., and G. P. Forrester. *Pharmaceutical Formulas*. 2 vols. 10th ed. London: Chemist and Druggist, 1929.

Wren, R. C. *Potter's New Cyclopedia of Botanical Drugs and Preparations*. Saffron Waldon, Eng.: C. W. Daniel, 1985.

BIBLIOGRAPHY BY CHAPTER

Chapter 2: The Sense of Smell

Almagor, U. "Odors and Private Language: Observations on the Phenomenology of Scent." *Human Studies* 13 (1990): 106–121.

Engen, T., and D. McBurney. "Magnitude and Category Scales of the Pleasantness of Odors." *Journal of Experimental Psychology* 68 (1964), 435–440.

Gibbons, B. "The Intimate Sense of Smell." *National Geographic* (Sept. 1986), 324–360.

Green, T. "Marketing Scents." *Smithsonian* (June 1991), 53–61.

Hines, D. "Olfaction and the Right Cerebral Hemisphere." *Journal of Altered States Consciousness* 3, no. 1 (1997), 47–59.

Howes, D. "New Guinea: An Olfactory Ethnography." *Dragoco Report* 2 (1992), 71–81.

Jesse, J. "The Sense of Smell Awakens Nostalgia." *Dragoco Report* 3 (1982), 76.

Kirk-Smith, M. D., C. Van Toller, and G. H. Dodd. "Unconscious Odor Conditioning in Human Subjects." *Biological Psychology* 100 (1983), 221–223.

Lawless, H. T. "A Sequential Contrast Effect in Odor Perception." *Bulletin of the Psychonomic Society* 29, no. 4 (1991), 317–319.

Max, B. "This and That: The Essential Pharmacology of Herbs and Spices." *Trends in Pharmacological Sciences* 13 (1992), 15–20.

McClintock, M. N. "Menstrual Synchrony and Suppression." *Nature* 299 (1971), 244–245.

Solvason, H. B., et al. "A Behavioral Augmentation of Natural Immunity: Odor Supports a Pavlovian Conditioning Model." *International Journal of Neuroscience* 61, nos. 3–4 (Dec. 1991): 277–88.

Synnot, A. "A Sociology of Smell." *Canadian Review of Sociology and Anthropology* 28, no. 4 (1991), 437–459.

Weintraub, P. "Sentimental Journeys." *Omni* 8, no. 7 (1986), 48–52.

Ziporyn, T. "Taste and Smell: The Neglected Senses." *Journal of the American Medical Association* 247, no. 3 (1982), 277–285.

Chapter 4: Scent and Psyche

Atanasova-Shopova, S., and K. Roussinov. "Central Neurotropic Effects of Lavender Essence." *Izv. Inst. Fiziol. Bulg. Akademia Nauk.* 13 (1970), 69–77.

Atanasova-Shopova, A., and K. Roussinov. "Effects of *Salvia sclarea* Essential Oil on the Central Nervous System." *Izv. Inst. Fiziol. Bulg. Akademia Nauk.* 13 (1970), 89–95.

Buchbauer, G., et al. "Aromatherapy: Evidence for Sedative Effects of the Essential Oil of Lavender after Inhalation." *Journal of Biosciences* 46, nos. 11–12 (1991), 1067–1072.

———, et al. "Fragrance Compounds and Essential Oils with Sedative Effects upon Inhalation." *Journal of Pharmaceutical Sciences* 82, no. 6 (1993), 660–664.

Crowther, D. "Complementary Therapy in Practice." *Nursing Standard* 5, no. 23 (1991), 25–27.

Daly, C. D., and R. S. White. "Psychic Reactions to Olfactory Stimuli." *British Journal of Medical Psychology* 10 (1930), 70–87.

Dodd, G. H., and Steven Van Toller. "The Biology and Psychology of Perfume." *Perfumer and Flavorist* 8 (1983), 1–14.

Duncan, L. "Observations on Eldercare in the USSR." *Geriatric Nursing,* vols. 7–8 (1982), 257–259.

Engen, T., et al. "Long-Term Memory of Odors with and without Verbal Descriptions." *Journal of Experimental Psychology* 100 (1973), 288.

Harder, U. "Physiological/Psychological Background to the Reactions to Fragrance." *Contact* 32 (1984), 14–22.

King, J. R. "Have Scents to Relax!" *World Medicine* 19 (1983), 29–31.

Lorig, T. A., and M. Roberts. "CNV Brain Wave Patterns." *Chemical Senses* 15, no. 5 (1990), 537–545.

Lyman, M., and M. A. McDaniel. "Effects of Encoding Strategy on Long-Term Memory for Odours." *Quarterly Journal of Experimental Psychology* 38 (1986), 753–765.

Macht, D., and Giu Ching Ting. "Experimental Inquiry into the Sedative Properties of Some Aromatic Drugs and Fumes." *Journal of Experimental Therapeutics* 18, no. 5 (1921), 361–372.

Marshall, M. "Stress Management in Dermatology Patients." *Nursing Standard* 5, no. 24 (1991), 29–31.

Pratt, J. "Notes on the Unconscious Significance of Perfume." *International Journal of Psychoanalysis* 23 (1942), 80–83.

Roberts, A., and J. M. Williams. "The Effect of Olfactory Stimulation on Fluency, Vividness of Imagery and Associated Mood." *British Journal of Medical Psychology* 65, no. 2 (1992), 197–199.

Rovesti, P. P. "Aromatherapy and Aerosols." *Soap, Perfumery, and Cosmetics* 46 (1973), 47–57.

Sanderson, H., and J. Ruddle. "Aromatherapy and Occupational Therapy." *British Journal of Occupational Therapy* 55(8) (1992), 310–314.

Tasev, T., et al. "Neurophysical Effect of Bulgarian Essential Oils from Rose, Lavender, and Geranium." *Folia Medica* 11, no. 5 (1969), 307–317.

Warm, J. S., et al. "Effects of Olfactory Stimulation on Performance and Stress in a Visual Sustained Attention Task." *Journal of the Society of Cosmetic Chemists* 42 (1991), 199–210.

Chapter 5: Guidelines for Using Essential Oils and Herbs

Abuharfeil, N. M., et al. "Augmentation of natural killer cell activity in vitro against tumor cells by wild plants from Jordan." *Journal of Ethnopharmacology* 71, nos. 1–2 (2000), 55–63.

Chen, Y., et al. "Study of effects of oil from Hippophae rhamnoides in hematopoiesis." *Zhong Yao Cai* 26, no. 8 (2003), 572–75.

El Tahir, K. E., et al. "Respiratory effects of volatile oil of Nigella." *General Pharmacology* 24, no. 5 (1993), 1115–1122.

Hanafy, M. S., and J. Hatem. "Studies on antimicrobial activity of Nigella seed." *Ethnopharmacology* 34, nos. 2–3 (1991), 275–78.

Kenny, S., et al. "GLA with tamoxifen as primary therapy in breast cancer." *International Journal of Cancer* 85, no. 5 (2000), 643–48.

Yang, B., et al. "Effects of dietary supplementation with sea buckthorn seed and pulp oils on atopic dermatitis." *Journal of Nutritional Biochemistry* 10, no. 11 (1999), 622–30.

Chapter 6: Therapeutics

Aggag, M. E., and R. T. Yousef. "Antimicrobial Activity of Chamomile Oil." *Planta Medica* 22 (1972), 104–144.

Bassett, I. B., et al. "The Antiseptic Properties of Tea Tree Oil on Acne." *Medical Journal of Australia* 153 (1990), 455–458.

Belaiche, P. "Germicidal Properties of the Essential Oil of *Melaleuca alternifolia*." *Phytothérapie* 15 (1985), 9–11.

Buchbauer, G. "Aromatherapy: Do Essential Oils Have Therapeutic Properties?" *Perfumer and Flavorist* 15 (1990), 47–50.

Gobel, H., et al. "Effect of Peppermint and Eucalpytus Oil on Headache." *Cephalalgia* 14, no. 13 (1994), 228–234.

Harries, N., et al. "Carminative Actions of Volatile Oils." *Journal of Clinical Pharmacy* 2 (1978), 171–177.

Holtmann, S., et al. "The Anti-Motion Sickness Mechanism of Ginger." *Acta Oto-Laryngologica* 108, nos. 3–4 (1989), 168–174.

Kabara, J. "Aroma Preservative: Essential Oils and Fragrances as Anti-Microbial Agents." *Cosmetic Sciences* 1 (1984), 237–273.

Kar, A., and S. R. Jain. "Antibacterial Evaluation of Some Indigenous Medicinal Volatile Oils." *Qualitas Plantarum Materia Vegetable* 20, no. 3 (1971), 231–237.

Kishore, N., et al. "Fungitoxicity of Essential Oils Against Dermatophytes." *Mycoses* 36, nos. 5–6 (1993), 211–215.

Lima, E. O., et al. "The *in vitro* Antibacterial Activity of Essential Oils." *Mycoses* 36, nos. 9–10 (1993), 333–336.

Morliere, P. "*In vitro* . . . Photosensitizing Properties of Bergamot Oil." *Journal of Photochemistry and Photobiology* 7, nos. 2–4 (1990), 199–208.

Ogunlana, E. O., et al. "Effect of Lemongrass on *E. coli* Cells." *Microbios* 50, no. 202 (1987), 43–59.

Ong, S. G. "Treating of Influenza with Volatile Oils Extracted from Chinese Plants." *Science Record* 2, no. 7 (1958), 233–238, and 3, no. 3 (1959), 120–127.

Prospero, G. "UV Sunscreen Properties in *Helichrysum*." *Cosmet. Toil.* 91, no. 3 (1976), 42.

Raharivelomanana, P. J., et al. "Study of the Antimicrobial Action of Various Essential Oils." *Archives de l'Institut Pasteur de Madagascar* 56, no. 1 (1989), 261–271.

Shwaireb, M. H. "Caraway Oil Inhibits Skin Tumors." *Nutrition and Cancer* 19, no. 3 (1992), 321–325.

Chapter 9: Facial Care

von Woedtke, T., et al. "Aspects of the antimicrobial efficacy of grapefruit seed extract and its relation to preservative substances contained." *Pharmazie* 54, no. 6 (1999), 452–56.

Chapter 15: Materia Medica

Beddows, C. G., et al. "Preservation of alpha-tocopherol in sunflower oil by herbs and spices." *International Journal of Food Sciences and Nutrition* 51, no. 5 (2000), 327–39.

Beiswanger, B. B., et al. "Comparative efficacy of stabilized stannous fluoride dentifrice peroxide/baking soda, and essential oil mouthrinse for prevention of gingivitis." *Journal of Clinical Dentistry* 8, no. 2 (1997), 54–61 and 46–53.

Benecia, F., and M. C. Courreges. "Antiviral activity of sandalwood oil against Herpes simplex viruses." *Phytomedicine* 6 (1999), 119–23.

Billing, J., and P. W. Sherman. "Antimicrobial functions of spices." *Quarterly Review of Biology* 73, no. 1 (1998), 3–49.

Buck, D. S., et al. "Comparison of two topical preparations for treatment of onychomycosis." *Journal of Family Practice* 38 (1994), 601–5.

Caelli, M., et al. "Tea tree oil as an alternative topical decolonization agent for methicillin-resistant *Staphylococcus aureus*." *Journal of Hospital Infection* 46, no. 3 (2000), 236–37.

Calabrese, V., et al. "Biochemical studies of a natural antioxidant isolated from rosemary and its application in cosmetic dermatology." *International Journal of Tissue Reactions* 22, no. 1 (2000), 5–13.

Caldefie-Chézet, F. "Potential antiinflammatory effects of *Melaleuca alternifolia* on human peripheral blood leukocytes." *Phytotherapy Research* 20, no. 5 (2006), 364–70.

Cox, S. D., et al. "Tea tree oil." *Journal of Applied Microbiology* 88, no. 1 (2000), 170–5.

Dias, P. C., et al. "Antiulcerogenic activity of crude hydroalcoholic extract of Rosmarinus officinalis." *Journal of Ethnopharmacology* 69, no. 1 (2000), 57–62.

Dorman, H. J., et al. "Antimicrobial agents from plants: F.v. and C.m. essential oils." *Planta Medica* 88, no. 2 (2000), 308–16.

Dryden, M. S., et al. "Randomized, controlled trial of tea tree topical preparations vs. standard topical regimen for clearance of MRSA." *Journal of Hospital Infection* 56, no. 4 (2005), 283–6.

Goel, N., et al. "An olfactory stimulus modifies nighttime sleep in young men and women." *Chronobiology International* 22, no. 5 (2005), 889–904

Hart, P. H., et al. "Terpinen-4-ol, the main component of the essential oil of *Melaleuca alternifolia* (tea tree oil), suppresses inflammatory mediator production by activated human monocytes." *Inflammation Research* 49, no. 11 (2000), 619–26.

Hay, I. C. et al. "Randomized trial of aromatherapy: Successful treatment for alopecia areata." *Archives of Dermatology* 134 (1998), 1349–1352.

Inouye, S., et al. "Antibacterial activity of essential oils and their major constituents against respiratory tract pathogens by gaseous contact." *Journal of Antimicrobial Chemotherapy* 47, no. 5 (2007), 565–73.

Jandourek, A., et al. "Efficacy of melaleuca oral solution for the treatment of fluconazole refractory oral candidiasis in AIDS patients." *AIDS* 12 (1998), 1033–37.

Kim, M. J., et al. "Effects of aromatherapy on pain, depression, and life satisfaction of arthritis patients/massage for relief of constipation in the elderly." *Taehan Kanho Hakhoe Chi* 35, no. 1 (2005), 186–94 and 56–64.

Kulevanova, S., et al. "Investigation of antimicrobial activity of essential oils of several Macedonian Thymus species." *Bollettino chimico farmaceutico* 139, no. 6 (2000), 276–80.

Kulik, E., et al. "Antimicrobial effects of tea tree oil on oral microorganisms." *Schweiz Monatsschr Zahnmed* 110, no. 11 (2000), 124–30.

Kuriyama, H., et al. "Immunological and Psychological Benefits of Aromatherapy Massage." *Evidence-based Complementary and Alternative Medicine* 2, no. 2 (2005), 179–184.

Law, M. R., and A. K. Hackshaw. "Environmental tobacco smoke." *British Medical Bulletin* 52 (1996), 22–34.

Lee, I. S., and G. J. Lee. "Effects of lavender aromatherapy on insomnia and depression in women college students." *Taehan Kanho Hakhoe Chi* 36, no. 1 (2006), 136–43.

Lee, K. G., and T. Shibamoto. "Determination of antioxidant potential of volatile extracts isolated from various herbs and spices." *Journal of Agricultural and Food Chemistry* 50, no. 17 (2002), 4947–52.

Mantle D., et al. "Adverse and beneficial effects of plant extracts on skin and skin disorders." *Adverse Drug Reactions and Toxicological Reviews* 20, no. 2 (2001), 89–103.

Schnitzler, P., et al. "Antiviral activity of Australian tea tree oil and eucalyptus oil against herpes simplex virus in cell culture." *Pharmazie* 56, no. 4 (2001), 343–47.

Tabak, M., et al. "In vitro inhibition of Hp by extracts of thyme." *Journal of Applied Microbiology* 80, no. 6 (1996), 667–72.

Veal, L. "The potential effectiveness of essential oils as treatment for headlice, *Pediculus humanus capitis*." *Complementary Therapies in Nursing and Midwifery* 2 (1996), 97–101.

Yang, K. K., et al. "Antiemetic principles of *Po.c.*" *Phytomedicine* 6, no. 2 (1999), 89–93.

Yip, Y. B., and S. H. Tse. "Effectiveness of acupressure with aromatic lavender essential oil for sub-acute, non-specific neck pain." *Complementary Therapies in Clinical Practice* 12, no. 1 (2006), 18–26.

Resources

Aromatherapy Associations and Journals

Aromatherapy Times
Suite 7B, Walpole Court,
Ealing Green, London,
England W5 5ED
www.ifaroma.org

Aromatherapy Today
Jennifer Jefferies and Toni Esser
PO Box 4298
Elanora, Qld, Australia 4221
www.aromatherapytoday.com

Canadian Federation of
Aromatherapists
www.cfacanada.com

International Federation of
Aromatherapists
www.ifaroma.org

International Journal of Aromatherapy
www.elsevier.com/wps/find/journal_
browse.cws_home

*International Journal of Clinical
Aromatherapy*
www.ijca.net

*International Journal of Essential Oil
Therapeutics*
www.ijeot.com

Making Scents
Jeffrey Schiller
3541 W. Acapulco Lane
Phoenix, AZ 85053
602-938-4439
www.aromaherbshow.com/index_056
.htm

National Association for Holistic
Aromatherapy
www.naha.org

Perfumer and Flavorist Journal
Allured Publishing Corp.
336 Gundersen Drive, Suite A
Carol Stream, IL 60188 USA
630-653-2155 (phone),
630-653-2192 (fax)
www.allured.com
www.perfumerflavorist.com

Aromatherapy Education and Essential Oils/Products

Alexandra Avery
4717 S.E. Belmont St.
Portland, OR 97215
800-669-1863
www.alexandraavery.com

Alliance of International
Aromatherapists
www.alliance-aromatherapists.org

American Herb Association
PO Box 1673
Nevada City, CA 95959
530-265-9552
www.ahaherb.com
*Current list of herb and aromatherapy
courses/products:*
AHA Directory of Mail Order Herb &
Aromatherapy Products $4
AHA Directory of Herb & Aromather-
apy Education $3.50
AHA List of Recommended Books $2

Aromatherapy International
Bill Georgaqui
West End Place
150 Staniford St. #632
Boston, MA 02114
800-722-4377
www.aromausa.com

Atlantic Institute of Aromatherapy
Sylla Sheppard-Hanger
16018 Saddlestring Drive
Tampa, FL 33618
813-265-2222
www.atlanticinstitute.com

Aura Cacia
Frontier Natural Products Co-op
PO Box 299
Norway, IA 52318
800-669-3275
www.auracacia.com

Australasian College of Health Sciences
Dorene Peterson
5940 SW Hood Ave.
Portland, OR 97239
800-487-8839
www.achs.edu

A Woman of Uncommon Scents, Inc.
PO Box 103
14613 Timmons Road
Roxbury, PA 17251
800-377-3685
www.awomanofuncommonscents.com

College of the Botanical Healing Arts &
Elizabeth Jones Essential Oils
PO Box 7542
Santa Cruz, CA 95061
800-710-7759
www.elizabethvanburen.com
www.cobha.org

EIM Laboratories
Christian Duraffourd and Jean-Claude
Lapraz
357 W. Center, Ste. 204
Pocatello, ID 83204
www.eimcenter.com

EO/Small World Trading Company
15A Koch Rd.
Corte Madera, CA 94925
800-570-3775
www.eoproducts.com

e3
145 Hummingbird Ln.
Talent, OR 97540
888-482-7662
www.essentialthree.com

Jeanne Rose
219 Carl St.
San Francisco, CA 94117
415-564-6785
www.jeannerose.net

Kathi Keville
Oak Valley Herb Farm
PO Box 2482
Nevada City, CA 95959
530-265-9552

also herb seminars
www.ahaherb.com

Living Libations
Nadine Artemis
610 Heron St.
Toronto, Ontario, Canada M5R 2R7
www.livinglibations.com

Laboratory of Flowers & Aromatherapy
Seminars
Michael Scholes
310-827-7737
www.labofflowers.com

Pacific Institute of Aromatherapy
Kurt Schnaubelt, Monika Haas
PO Box 6723
San Rafael, CA 94903
415-479-9120
www.pacificinstituteofaromatherapy
.com

Precious Aromatherapy
Paula Dzykowski
800-877-6889
www.aromatherapy.com

Santa Fe Fragrances
Christine Malcolm
PO Box 282
Santa Fe, NM 87504
505-474-0302
www.santafefragrance.com

Simplers' Botanical Co.
PO Box 2534
Sebastopol, CA 95473
800-652-7646
www.simplers.com

White Lotus Aromatics
Christopher McMahon
602 S. Alder Street
Port Angeles, WA 98362 USA
www.whitelotusaromatics.com

Natural Perfumes and Custom Blending

Aftelier Perfumes
Mandy Aftel
1442A Walnut Street #369
Berkeley, CA 94709
www.aftelier.com

John Steele
3949 Longridge Ave.
Sherman Oaks, CA 91423
818-986-0594

Essential Oil Distillers

Essential Oil Company
Robert Siedel
8225 SE 7th Ave.
Portland, OR 97202
800-729-5912
www.essentialoil.com

FloraGenics Distillation Systems
PO Box 538
Pescadero, CA 94060
877-446-3567
www.floragenics.com

Gary Stadler
PO Box 675561
Rancho Santa Fe, CA 92067
www.heartmagic.com

Pope Scientific, Inc.
351 N. Dekora Woods Blvd.
PO Box 80019
Saukville, WI 53080
414-251-0900
www.popeinc.com

Aromatherapy Websites

Alternative Medicine Foundation
www.amfoundation.org/herbinfo.htm

Aromatherapy Internet Resources
www.holisticmed.com/www/
aromatherapy.html

Aromatherapy Registration Council
www.aromatherapycouncil.org

Aromatherapy Trade Council (UK)
www.a-t-c.org.uk

Essential oil research
www.aromatherapydatabase.com

International Federation of
Aromatherapists
www.ifaroma.org

Tony Burfield's Aroma Pages
www.tonyburfield.co.uk www.users
.globalnet.co.uk/~nodice/
www.cropwatch.org

Fragrance/Cosmetic Resources

Association for Chemoreception Sciences
www.achems.org

Cosmetic Toiletry and Fragrance
Association
www.ctfa-online.org

EO resource index
www.bojensen.net/EssentialOilsEng/
EssentialOils.htm

Fragrance Foundation
www.fragrance.org

Fragrance Materials Association
of the US
www.fmafragrance.org

International Fragrance Association
www.ifraorg.org

Leffingwell & Associates
www.leffingwell.com

Monell Institute
www.monell.org

Perfumers World
(Perfumery course)
www.perfumersworld.com

PubMed Scientific Research (National
Institutes of Health)
www.ncbi.nlm.nih.gov

Research Institute for Fragrance Materials
www.rifm.org

Sense of Smell Institute
www.senseofsmell.org

Regulatory Agents

Aromatherapy Trade Council
www.a-t-c.org.uk

Business for Social Responsibility
www.bsr.org

Cosmetic Ingredient Review
www.cir-safety.org

Food and Drug Administration
www.fda.gov

Organic Trade Association
www.ota.com/index.html

REACH (Registration, Evaluation and
Authorization of CHemicals) legislation
www.reachlegislation.com

United Plant Savers
www.unitedplantsavers.org

U.S. Cosmetics Regulations
www.cfsan.fda.gov/~dms/cos-toc.html

Herbal Sources

American Botanical Council and
magazine
www.herbalgram.org

American Herb Association
www.ahaherb.com

American Herbalists Guild
www.americanherbalistsguild.com

American Herbal Products Association
www.ahpa.org

Herb Research Foundation
www.herbs.org

Medical Herbalism magazine
www.medherb.com

Herbal Correspondence Courses

California School of Herbal Studies
www.cshs.com

Foundations of Herbalism
Christopher Hobbs
www.foundationsofherbalism.com

The Science and Art of Herbalism by
Rosemary Gladstar
www.sagemountain.com

Index

teas, 50, 81, 82

tinctures, 50–51

vinegars, 51

whole vs. essential oils, 175–76

Herpes, 66

High performance liquid chromatography (HPLC), 151

Hildegard of Bingen, Saint, 8

Hippocrates, 5

Hirsch, Alan R., 16, 19, 22

Hoary basil *(Ocimum canum; O. americanum)*, 178

Hobbs, Christopher, 62

Hoffmann, David, 60

Holy basil *(Ocimum tenuiflorum; O. sanctum)*, 164, 178

Honeys, aromatic, 121

Hormonal imbalances, 222–23

Horseradish *(Cochlearia armoracia; Armoracia rusticana)*, 41

Hot rock therapy, 74

Human papillomavirus (HPV), 66

Hung Chu, 6

Hydrodiffusion, 144

Hydrolats, 101–2, 142

Hydrosols
in the kitchen, 121–22

production of, 141

in skin care, 101–2

storing, 121

Hypersensitivity, 220–21

Hyposmia, 15

Hyssop *(Hyssopus officinalis)*, 193–94, 220, 222

I

IBAMA *(Brazilian Institute of Environment and Renewable Natural Resources)*, 153

Ice Cream, Strawberry-Rose, 123

Immortelle. *See* Helichrysum

Immune system, 69

Incas, 9

India, 9

Indian angelica *(Angelica glauca)*, 164

Indian calamus *(Acorus calamus)*, 154, 165

Indian frankincense *(Boswellia serrata)*, 167, 191

Indian myrrh *(Commiphora mukul)*, 168

Indian valerian *(Valeriana wallichii)*, 210

Indigestion, 222–23

Infections, 222–23

Inflammation, 68, 222–23

Inhalants, 44, 57

Insects
bites of, 68, 224

repellants for, 68–69

Insomnia, 29–30, 220–21

International Flavors and Fragrance (IFF), 21, 23, 24, 27

International Union for Conservation of Nature (IUCN), 152

Inula, sweet *(Inula graveolens; I. odorata)*, 40, 194

Irritability, 220–21

Itching, 224

J

Jaborandi *(Pilocarpus jaborandi)*, 41

Japan, 6–7, 30–31

Jasmine *(Jasminium officinale; J. grandiflorum)*, 194
as aphrodisiac, 20

in Ayurvedic medicine, 168

chakras and, 172

for cosmetic/skin use, 194, 226

for emotions, 194, 220

extraction of, 194

therapeutic activity of, 194

Jatamansi. *See* Spikenard

Java citronella *(Cymbopogon winterianus)*, 198

Jellinek, Paul, 29

Jesus Christ, 6

Jitterbug Perfume Spritzer, 122

Jojoba, 45

Juniper *(Juniperus communis)*, 195
in Ayurvedic medicine, 168

chakras and, 172, 174

considerations for, 195

for cosmetic/skin use, 195, 225, 226

for emotions, 195, 220

extraction of, 195

therapeutic activity of, 195, 223

K

Kajima, 30–31

Kanuka (Kunzea ericoides), 211

Kapha, 163, 170

Kava *(Piper methysticum)*, 82

Keawa *(Pandanus tectoriu; P. odoratissimus)*, 169

Kenyan juniper *(Juniperus procera)*, 154

Keratinization, 84

Ketones, 159, 160

Keville, Kathi, 48, 62

Khella *(Ammi visnaga)*, 40

Kidney stones, 61–62

King, John J., 27

Knasko, Susan, 11

Korean angelica *(Angelica gigus)*, 176

Krasnow, V., 31

Kripke, Margaret, 110

Kukui nut oil, 45

Kyphi, 4, 27

L

Labdanum. *See* Cistus

Labows, John N., 14

Lactation, 65

Lanolin, 115

Lapraz, Jean-Claude, 53

Larsen, Jan-Helge, 77

Laudanum, 185

Lavandin *(Lavandula x. intermedia; L. x hybrida)*, 196

Lavender *(Lavandula angustifolia; L. vera; L. officinale)*, 195–96
chakras and, 173, 174

components of, 157

for cosmetic/skin use, 102, 196, 224, 225, 226

doshas and, 167

for emotions, 29, 196, 220

extraction of, 195–96

Lavender Lemonade, 122

Lavender Sunrise Body Powder, 90

therapeutic activity of, 53, 63, 196, 223

Lecithin, 115

LeGuerer, Annick, 12

Lemon *(Citrus limon)*, 197
chakras and, 173

considerations for, 197

for cosmetic/skin use, 197, 225, 226

doshas and, 167

for emotions, 197, 221

extraction of, 197

Lavender Lemonade, 122

Lemon-Geranium Sponge Cake, 124

therapeutic activity of, 197, 223

Lemon balm. *See* Melissa

Lemon catnip *(Nepeta cataria)*, 201

Odors. *See also* Fragrances
    classifying, 129
    cultural differences and, 11
    gender preferences for, 18, 19
    health and, 14–15
    impact of, 12
    intensity of, 132
    personal, 17
    processing of, by the brain, 12–13
    reactions to, 11
Olive oil, 45, 46
Opopanax *(Commiphora erythraea),* 201
Orange *(Citrus sinensis),* 202
    considerations for, 202
    for cosmetic/skin use, 202, 224, 226
    doshas and, 167
    for emotions, 202, 221
    extraction of, 202
    Orange-Rosemary Sorbet, 122
    therapeutic activity of, 202, 223
Orange blossom. *See* Neroli
Oregano *(Origanum vulgare),* 199–200
Origan, 213
Origins, 24
Ormenis *(Chamaemelum mixtum; Anthemis mixta; Ormenis mixta; O. multicaulis),* 184
Overwork, 220–21
Oxides, 159, 160
Oxygen bars, 31

P

Pain, 60, 222–23
Palmarosa *(Cymbopogon martini),* 167, 198, 226
Panic, 220–21
Parosmia, 15
Parsley *(Petroselinum sativum; Carum sativum),* 41, 82
Passionflower *(Passiflora incarnata),* 82
Patchouli *(Pogostemon cablin),* 203–4
    as aphrodisiac, 20
    chakras and, 172
    for cosmetic/skin use, 204, 224, 225, 226
    for emotions, 204, 221
    extraction of, 204
    therapeutic activity of, 204, 223
Peach Blush, 122
Peanut oil, 46

Pecan oil, 45
Pelvic inflammatory disease (PID), 64
Pennyroyal *(Mentha pulegium),* 40, 205
Penoel, Daniel, 155
Pepper, black *(Piper nigrum),* 165, 180–81, 222
Peppermint *(Mentha piperita),* 204–5
    chakras and, 172
    considerations for, 205
    for cosmetic/skin use, 205, 224, 225, 226
    doshas and, 167
    for emotions, 205, 221
    extraction of, 204
    Peppermint Tapioca, 123
    Refreshing Mint Julep, 122
    therapeutic activity of, 53, 204, 223
Peppermint eucalyptus *(Eucalyptus dives),* 189
Perfumes. *See also* Blending
    alcohol concentrations of, 137
    carriers for, 136
    categories of, 129–30
    colognes vs., 136
    fixatives for, 131–32
    history of, 2–10, 136, 138–39
    natural ingredients in commercial, 140
    odor classification and, 129
    producers of natural, 235
    representational vs. abstract, 129
    top, middle, and base notes in, 130–31
    wearing, 137
Peruvian pepper tree *(Schinus molle),* 181
Petitgrain *(Citrus aurantium),* 167, 172, 203, 221
Pets, 39
Phenols, 158, 160
Pheromones, 17–18, 19
Phlebitis, 54
Photosensitivity, 37–38, 40
Piesse, Charles, 129
Pillows, dilly, 70
Pine *(Pinus* sp.), 167, 190, 221
Pitta, 163, 170
Plai *(Zingiber cassumunar),* 193
PMS (premenstrual syndrome), 62
Poison oak, ivy, or sumac, 67
Polo, Marco, 8
Pomegranate oil, 47
Poucher, William A., 133
Poultices, 58, 68
Powders, 90

Pregnancy
    essential oils for, 38, 65
    massage during, 76
    safety and, 38
Preservatives, 118, 119
Prokofiev, Sergei, 22
Prostatitis, 65
Proust, Marcel, 31–32

R

Rashes, 67, 224
Raspberry oil, 47
Ravensara *(Cinnamomum camphora),* 205–6, 223, 226
Rectifying, 144
Redken, 24
Regulatory agents, 236
Reproductive system, 62–66
Resinoids, 146
Respiratory system, 56–58
Rheumatism, 59
Rice bran oil, 45, 46
Roman chamomile *(Chamaemelum nobile),* 173, 184
Rome, ancient, 3, 5–6
Room sprays, 44, 58
Root chakra, 171–72
Rose *(Rosa damascena; R. gallica),* 206–7
    as aphrodisiac, 20
    chakras and, 172, 173
    components of, 157
    considerations for, 207
    for cosmetic/skin use, 102, 206, 224, 225, 226
    for emotions, 207, 221
    Exotic Rose Cream, 117
    extraction of, 206
    Midnight at the Oasis Balls, 123
    reconstructed, 149
    Strawberry-Rose Ice Cream, 123
    therapeutic activity of, 63, 206, 223
Rose de mai, 207
Rose hip seed *(Rosa rubiginosa),* 47
Rosemary *(Rosmarinus officinalis),* 207–8
    chakras and, 174
    chemotypes of, 208
    considerations for, 208
    for cosmetic/skin use, 102, 207, 224, 225, 226
    doshas and, 167

About the Authors

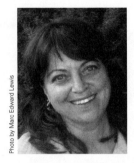

Photo by Marc Edward Lewis

KATHI KEVILLE has studied herbs and aromatherapy since 1968. Her early fascination with the fragrant plants in her herb garden led to her involvement in aromatherapy. She now cultivates 150 herbs—many mentioned in this book—in her fragrance gardens in Nevada City, California. She teaches aromatherapy and herbal seminars there and throughout North America and operates Oak Valley Herb Farm, a mail-order herb business specializing in aromatherapy products. Kathi was trained as a masseuse and she consults and formulates for the aromatherapy massage and body-care industry. She is director of the American Herb Association, an honorary life member of the American Aromatherapy Association, the National Association of Holistic Aromatherapists, and the former National Institute of Holistic Aromatherapy, a founding member of United Plant Savers, and was a founding member of the American Herbalists Guild. She has written over 150 magazine articles. Kathi also appears in her aromatherapy garden on the aromatherapy TV series *Everybody Nose* on the Veria satellite channel. She is the author or coauthor of *American Country Living: Ultimate Lifestyle Compendium; Aromatherapy for Dummies; Aromatherapy: For Healing the Body & Mind; Complete Book of Herbs: Herbs to Enrich Your Garden, Home & Health; Ginseng; Herbs: A Guide to Growing, Cooking and Decorating; Herbs: American Country Living; Herbs: An Illustrated Encyclopedia; Herbs for Chronic Fatigue; Herbs for Health & Healing; Pocket Guide to Aromatherapy;* and *Women's Herbs, Women's Health,* with Christopher Hobbs.

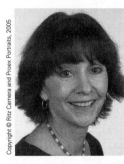

Copyright © Ritz Camera and Proex Portraits, 2005

MINDY GREEN has worked in the natural products and complementary health care industry since the early 1970s. She has owned an herb store and natural foods restaurant in Victoria, BC, was co-owner of the California School of Herbal studies, served as education and research director at the Herb Research Foundation's non-profit medical library in Boulder, Colorado, and as program specialist at the University of Colorado Hospital Anschutz Cancer Center. She is a nationally certified Registered Aromatherapist, a founding member of the American Herbalists Guild, and associate editor of the American Herb Association Newsletter. A licensed esthetician and massage therapist, she has founded and owned several herb and essential oil businesses. She has served on the education committees of the Aromatherapy Registration Council and the National Association of Holistic Aromatherapists, and is on the advisory board of the Australasian College of Health Sciences, and the Board of Directors of United Plant Savers. Mindy is the Clinical Aromatherapist for the Aveda Corporation in Minneapolis, Minnesota. As an herbalist and environmental activist, she loves learning and teaching on the subject of all things botanical, and contributing to the awareness of global health. Mindy is the author of two other books, *Calendula* and *Natural Perfumes.*